E-Co-Affectivity

SUNY series in Ancient Greek Philosophy

Anthony Preus, editor

E-Co-Affectivity
Exploring *Pathos* at Life's Material Interfaces

MARJOLEIN OELE

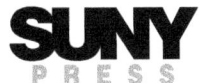

Cover art: iStock by Getty Images.

Published by State University of New York Press, Albany

© 2020 State University of New York

All rights reserved

No part of this book may be used or reproduced in any manner whatsoever without written permission. No part of this book may be stored in a retrieval system or transmitted in any form or by any means including electronic, electrostatic, magnetic tape, mechanical, photocopying, recording, or otherwise without the prior permission in writing of the publisher.

For information, contact State University of New York Press, Albany, NY
www.sunypress.edu

Library of Congress Cataloging-in-Publication Data

Names: Oele, Marjolein, author.
Title: E-co-affectivity : exploring *pathos* at life's material interfaces / Marjolein Oele.
Description: Albany : State University of New York Press, 2020. | Series: SUNY series in ancient Greek philosophy | Includes bibliographical references and index.
Identifiers: LCCN 2019028129 | ISBN 9781438478616 (hardcover) | ISBN 9781438478609 (pbk. : alk. paper) | ISBN 9781438478623 (ebook)
Subjects: LCSH: Emotions (Philosophy) | Senses and sensation.
Classification: LCC B105.E46 O35 2020 | DDC 113/.8—dc23
LC record available at https://lccn.loc.gov/2019028129

10 9 8 7 6 5 4 3 2 1

For my parents,
Jacoba Oele-Ruissen (1929–2012), and Laurens Oele (1923–2017)
And my brother,
Bastiaan Laurens Oele
For fueling my desire to know and care amid
a world in need of compassion

Contents

List of Illustrations		ix
Acknowledgments		xi
Introduction		1
Chapter 1	Plants and Affectivity: The Middle-Voiced Lives of Plants	17
Chapter 2	Animals and Affectivity: *Aisthēsis*, Touch, Trauma, and Bird Feathers	49
Chapter 3	Generative Human Affectivity: The Placenta as Place-and-Time-Making In-Between	79
Chapter 4	Skin and Human Sapient Affectivity: Skin, Webbed Existence, Temporal Depth, and Trust	107
Chapter 5	E-Co-Affectivity beyond the Anthropocene: On Soil and Soil Pores	139
Notes		165
Works Cited		231
Index		247

Illustrations

Figure 1.1	Arugula plants in the stage of seedling, when the roots develop and spread and rapid growth occurs. Pixabay Creative Commons.	34
Figure 1.2	Half-alive oak tree. Flickr Creative Commons. Photo by Odd Wellies.	41
Figure 1.3	Nitrogen-fixing nodule: A root nodule that lives in symbiosis with nitogren-fixing bacteria. Flickr Creative Commons. Photo by London Permaculture.	44
Figure 2.1	Different types of bird feathers. Illustration by Andrew Leach; property of Cornell Lab of Ornithology.	65
Figure 2.2	Faultbars in the feathers of a Grey Heron (*Ardea cinerea*) and White Cockatoo (*Cacatua alba*). Photo by Jørgen Mortensen.	69
Figure 2.3	Faultbars in the feather of a European Blackbird (*Turdus merula*). Photo by Jørgen Mortensen.	69
Figure 2.4	Two horned owls allopreening: the owl on the left is assisting the other owl with preening. CC Creative Commons. Photo by Terry Llovet.	73
Figure 3.1	Placenta Post-Partum in Clinical Hospital Setting. Photo by Gerard Kuperus.	83
Figure 4.1	"Expanded Self," 2015. Artwork by Sonja Bäumel. Being in the world as an individual really means being a multibeing community in a vital process of permanent exchange.	128

Figure 5.1	Soil. Pixabay Creative Commons.	151
Figure 5.2	Soil pores allow water and gas to move through soil. Flickr Creative Commons. Photo by John A. Kelley, USDA Natural Resources Conservation Service.	152
Figure 5.3	*Soil quasi bricks*, 2003. Artwork by Ólafur Elíasson. ARoS Aarhus Kunstmuseum, Denmark, 2004. Photo by Poul Pedersen.	163

Acknowledgments

With a book title such as *E-Co-Affectivity*, it would be insensitive, if not outright wrong, *not* to acknowledge the soil and the various milieus that have informed, shaped, and inspired this project. If there was ever a place and time to address the factor of togetherness (the "co" of co-affectivity) that goes beyond simple addition to truly constitute a community, and if there was ever a place and time to address the home and milieu (the "eco" of eco-affectivity) that has made this very project possible, then here and now is the place and time to acknowledge this.

Addressing the academic home and milieu within which I have come into my own, I have to thank the University of San Francisco and its various institutional support mechanisms for promoting my academic research. First, being awarded NEH Chair at USF in 2016–17 allowed me time to finalize the draft and draw the main lines of this book manuscript together, as well as the opportunity to share my work with a broad public at USF, including colleagues, students, and staff. Second, over several years, USF's Faculty Development Fund provided generous funding for research support, including financial support for travel to conferences and compensation for my research assistants. Third, at USF I have found an inspiring group of scholars who have provided encouragement over the past few years as I conceptualized and executed *E-Co-Affectivity*. I have spent many hours with each of my colleagues in weekly writing teams, weekend retreats, and summer writing programs, brainstorming ideas and providing mutual support. I owe deep gratitude to each and every one of my writing partners. Also, a special thank you is due to my colleagues in the philosophy department for their willingness to listen, discuss, critique, and encourage my efforts in each step of the process.

The other academic context instrumental in fostering this research is the Pacific Association for the Continental Tradition (PACT). Often, at PACT's annual meetings my ideas were tested and consequently reshaped, and I had many thoughtful conversations that pushed this project further. At PACT, I owe special thanks to Geoffrey Ashton, Kim Carfore, Michael Eng, Tim Freeman, Josh Hayes, Chris Lauer, Danielle Meijer, Sam Mickey, Bob Mugerauer, Dorothea Olkowski, Emily Parker, Amanda Parris, Elizabeth Sikes, Peter Steeves, Sam Talcott, Brian Treanor, and Jason Wirth.

Outside of USF and PACT, acknowledgment is due to the Ancient Philosophy Society (APS), for offering a forum for continental interpretations of ancient philosophy and for inspiring me to carve my own path in reading ancient texts. More recently, as I increasingly found my work intersecting with topics in environmental philosophy, I have found a new vital home in the International Association for Environmental Philosophy (IAEP), and I owe thanks to IAEP for allowing me the space and time to present and discuss ideas that became part of this book.

I would also like to express my gratitude to the following journals for their kind permission to reproduce earlier versions of chapters 3 and 5. An earlier version of chapter 3 was published as "Openness and Protection: A Philosophical Analysis of the Placenta's Mediatory Role in Co-Constituting Emergent Intertwined Identities" in *Configurations* 25, no. 3 (July 2017): 347–71. And an earlier, shorter version of chapter 5 was published as "E-Co-Affectivity beyond the Anthropocene: Rethinking the Role of Soil to Imagine a New 'Us'" in *Environmental Philosophy* 16, no. 2 (Fall 2019): 291–317.

A special word of thanks is due to two research assistants who became my closest interlocutors, editors, and collaborators during this project: Darcy Allred and Daniel O'Connell. In the final stages, Darcy offered astute, thorough, and careful proofing and editing, keeping me on task and focused. Dan's research support extended from the book's conception through its completion. Enabled by virtual networks spanning the globe, his insights stimulated innovation, and his suggestions allowed me to keep the arc of the argumentation in view while pointing to crucial areas where my analysis needed to gain further traction. It would not be an exaggeration to say that this book would not be what it is without Dan's loyal and generous research support.

During the publication process, the support from my editor at SUNY Press, Andrew Kenyon, has been remarkable. His enduring trust in me and enthusiasm for this project kept me grounded and hopeful. I also want to acknowledge the three anonymous peer reviewers who provided astute and thoughtful comments on earlier drafts of this manuscript. I am thankful for their comments, which allowed the ultimate version to be sharper in focus and argument, and more closely embedded in the philosophical literature.

Finally, as I think about the familial home that allowed me the time and energy to reinvent myself as a writer and scholar, I owe deep thanks to my lifelong companion and comrade-in-all-things-life-and-philosophy, Gerard, our children, Lars and Imma, and my feline desk-and-lap partner, Harry. I also want to acknowledge the extended Oele and Kuperus family, and the family of friends I acquired over the years, who encouraged me in my passion for this book project: Mylène Berlijn, Karen Einbinder, Carole Heath, Rachaelle Hilhorst, Nathan Hobbs, Shay Kim, Christian Lotz, Ad and Angela Peperzak, Corinne Painter, Jackie Scott, and Ronald Sundstrom.

The first home, or *oikos*, that undergirded my existence and enveloped me with love and trust needs special mention: my parents and my brother Bas. To them this book is dedicated.

Introduction

Inasmuch as the essence of community is affectivity, the community is not limited to humans alone. It includes everything that is defined in itself by the primal suffering of life and thus by the possibility of suffering. We can suffer with everything that suffers. This pathos-with is the broadest form of every conceivable community.

—Michel Henry, *Material Phenomenology* (2008, 134)

The student of nature is concerned with all the works (*erga*) and affections (*pathē*) of a certain sort of body and a certain sort of material.

—Aristotle, *De anima* (II.1, 403b12)

Hence, the philosopher should be intrigued by this concretization of a depth that does not fear to place itself at the very limit, where the self joins together with (its) other [. . .], where the self also positions itself facing a universe that permeates it, and about which it is informed, thanks to sensorial (or transitional) mediation.

—François Dagognet, *La Peau Découverte* (1993,13)

The thick, heavy soil in which we bury our loved ones carries with it deep, affective resonance. As a regenerative body, the soil provides a sense of consolation related to, yet far different from, a memorial service. Where memorial services speak individual words and invoke distinct memories and affects as related to the unique person who is now dead, the soil touches us in a very different affective register, and draws us, even in or precisely by its concreteness, toward a wider living community of which we are all part.

The soil's distinct concreteness is what Aristotle might call—with a demonstrative—"some this" (*tode ti*): its particular density, its distinct feeling in one's hands and under one's feet, its smell, its weight, its texture.[1] For this reason, no burial is phenomenologically the same: even when occurring in the same place, even when involving the same burial ground or the same family grave, the soil's density, smell, weight, and texture vary in each case.

The figure of soil is an example of an interface that I investigate in this book, and its specific investigation occurs in the very last chapter. Like the other interfaces that I examine, soil offers me the opportunity to investigate the medium, the material in-between, the concrete interface where the main topic of this book—affectivity—lives and breathes. Soil, similar to the other interfaces I investigate, thus seeks to offer a localized, material place to engage affectivity, and simultaneously shows how every interface is not simply an existing place or surface, but a place of ontogenesis: always emerging, creative, porous, and fluid.

The benefit of focusing on the concrete interface is that the account of affectivity can be more flexible and faithful to the uniqueness of each concrete form of affectivity and can concretely show *how and where* ontogenesis takes place through affective responses. To exemplify: the material interface of a human living being (its skin) is not just the meeting place of exteriority and interiority, but a constantly emerging in-between where exteriority and interiority emerge and intersect. Every interface is material, but is also "more" than its current materiality in *co-creating* place, time, and being. For instance, the material genetic traces of previous generations (e.g., the cells of one's mother's mother) left behind by the placenta as organ of the in-between map collective time onto individual time and project beings accordingly into the future.

Contrasting soil, if only briefly, with the concept of "earth" may serve to explain what my account of interfaces and affectivity is trying to do in general and what it seeks to avoid. I seek to draw attention in this book to the concrete tangible interface that mediates and co-creates affective responses and emerging existences in ever new ways. In this, I seek to resist the tendency for certain forms of phenomenology to be overly anthropocentric or to overlook the concrete materiality—and related science—of the phenomena discussed. To illustrate: while my general phenomenological insights are indebted to Heidegger, what I am resisting in choosing soil over earth is Heidegger's focus on earth and his tendency to grasp earth along the lines of a native ground ("urgrund") or "home"[2] specific to human culture, or to grasp it in quasi-mystical terms as the obscure ground of our abode: "the spontaneous forthcoming of that which is continually self-secluding and to that extent sheltering and concealing."[3] Such renditions of earth are to me both too provincial (in the political and also in the anthropocentric sense), and simultaneously too ecstatic and transcendent.[4] It is for this reason that I focus on soil and its concrete, material, "messy" aspects: in being both local and global, in connecting the living and the nonliving, and in giving rise to a community of corelated beings rather than simply individuated beings, the focus on soil rather than earth allows for a different kind of philosophy of affectivity. It is an account of affectivity that stands at the interface, seeking to investigate how time and place and beings emerge as they are, concretely, being affected together.

As my initial account of the interface of soil here perhaps shows, my approach to affectivity through the figure of the material interface includes not only philosophy, but also science. This approach is in large part due to the three different, but ultimately converging, pathways that have inspired my intellectual career and this book. The first path—that of my interest in the topic "affectivity"—has the longest bearing in that it has been with me for nearly my entire adult life. It led as it were to my first academic "love"— the study of medicine—and my consequent training as an MD. Ranging from the most mundane and treatable diseases to the most unsettling ones, those pathologies shifted my life's perspective and drove me inward toward reflection, seeking answers that the discipline of medicine could not offer, even if it provided sound treatments. Enter the second pathway: that of my formative years in graduate school in philosophy and a direct encounter with Aristotle, whose thoughts on *pathos* took me in and surprised me in terms of depth and breadth. His categorical distinctions, his phenomenal observations of particulars, and his endoxic approach enveloped me and became my world for many years. This second path could not have been as productive and rich in meaning had it not been for the third: my sustained immersion in Continental Thought, and especially the encounter with Heidegger's early lecture courses and his ability to make Aristotle speak to so many actual phenomena and topics in continental philosophy today.

Eventually, these pathways cross-fertilized themselves, also sparked by a new attempt to find my own voice and immersion in recent publications on new materialism.[5] I sought to make my continentally inspired reading of Aristotle relevant to contemporary scientific studies of plants, animals, pregnancy, and humans. Inspired by new materialism's turn to the intricacies of bodies, I recovered my passion for reading scientific studies in my attempt to uncover the various tiers and kinds of affectivity in living beings. Along the way, Aristotle's categories remained in sight, but a distinct need made itself pressing: to acquire distance from them, to read them more playfully and more deconstructively, and to use them with care and sensitivity. Thus was born a book whose title would no longer find its center of gravity in Aristotle (as envisioned in the work's original title, *Rethinking Affectivity with Aristotle*), but centrally turned to the matter, that is, *E-Co-Affectivity*, itself.

As I was pulled more and more to the phenomena themselves, I felt the distinct desire to address this topic not only on the level of conceptual analysis, but also on the level of personal affect, if only briefly, at the beginning of each chapter. The affective charge of such autobiography has many purposes: it announces the topic in a formulaic fashion, it reaches out to connect to the reader on a personal level, and it simultaneously emphasizes in its affective charge the very content of the book's topic: that affectivity can never be understood without this *felt* dimension, and that each interface and topic as I address it is also lived and made known in multiple ways.

The *title* of this book, *E-Co-Affectivity*, while fitting, still sits somewhat uneasily with me. The reason is that the term "affectivity" is too much associated with philosophical idiom, and does not have direct resonance and coinage in colloquial language: we may use associated nouns such as "liking" (or "affection") or verbs such as "to affect," but the broader cohesion and immediate, intuitive appeal that I seek in the term "affectivity" is absent.[6] This is unfortunate, especially as this monograph draws on an immediately recognizable, central phenomenon of all lives: the fact that all living beings—including human beings—become who they are through interaction and reciprocity with that which affects them as mediated by the interface.

I use the term "affectivity" within a wide spectrum of meanings, similar to the Greek term *pathos*. In terms of etymology, our term *pathos* originates in the ancient Greek root πάθος (suffering, feeling, passion, illness, qualitative change) and παθ- is the stem of πάσχειν, to suffer (which is of unknown origin).[7] I have often wondered: if we could only reinstate and reemploy the Ancient Greek term *pathos*[8] and its verbal cognate *paschein*, then that would really capture the broad range within which I seek to grasp the fundamental *affectivity* operating in all forms of life. Reaching in meaning from incidental change and emotion to illness and excruciating suffering, the term *pathos* covers an amazing array true to the dynamics of life's emergences and transformations. Unfortunately, however, *pathos* has lost its broad scope in our current use of the term, since as used now, *pathos* refers mostly to the (rhetorical) appeal to emotions such as pity and sadness.[9] Still, *pathos* found its way into the subtitle of this book as a nod to the historical background and conceptual riches it provides to the concept of affectivity.

Thus, focusing on its definition, "affectivity" covers a broad terrain, similar to its Greek root *pathos*, and can include such things as illness, suffering, qualitative change, and emotion. Central to the concept of affectivity is a complex kind of causal relationship. *Instead of seeing affectivity merely in terms of the passive effect of a cause, the kind of affectivity I propose puts at its center stage the receptive, responsive power of living beings to react to what happens to them, which may include their ability to participate in, and shape, how they are affected.* Thus, this conception of affectivity can be understood as a kind of responsiveness or reactivity to the world. My account of affectivity speaks both to the ability to be affected and the ability to affect, and the complex relationship between the two.[10] It recognizes that, on an organic level, living beings become who they are through mutual interaction with, and strategic affective responses to, that which affects them.[11]

With the term "e-co-affectivity," I seek to emphasize that affectivity neither occurs in a vacuum nor pertains to singular, discrete entities: it implies a certain place or milieu (hence "eco," as in the Greek "oikos") and connection to others (hence "co"), whose mediation may have either destructive, or constructive, or ambiguous effects. The hyphenation I use speaks to the fact that the influence of place and community cannot be tightly distinguished from the happenings of affectivity as such: they are rather aspects of *one* phenomenon in which they participate: e-co-affectivity. And while in many chapters I provide a descriptive account of the effects of the milieu and community within which affectivity takes place, the fifth chapter adds to this a prescriptive, ethical lens in that it seeks to formulate a new epoch beyond the anthropocene that is sensitive to the larger ecological, communal concerns at stake.

In terms of *significance*, the turn to affectivity is important because it speaks to the fact that all living beings become who they are through reciprocity with that which affects and moves them. We need only to think about processes of generation, of being born, of being fed, addressed, and cared for,[12] to instantly recognize this affective dimension of our lives.[13] By turning to affectivity we acquire a fuller and deeper insight into the underpinnings of *how living beings are always in motion*, that is, how they come to be, grow, interact, react, suffer, and die. This focus is much needed to complement, if not strategically undermine, modern philosophy's focus on static and insular activity, autonomy, and disembodied freedom. And twentieth-century continental philosophers such as Heidegger, Levinas, and Butler have provided important conceptual tools—through concepts such as *Befindlichkeit*, thrownness, the face of the Other, radical passivity, and precarity—to break through modern philosophy's shortcomings in this respect.

Still, those conceptual tools can be sharpened and adjusted, and *E-Co-Affectivity* in that regard both builds on certain ideas of above-mentioned theorists and refines and adjusts others. For instance, while Heidegger prioritizes within his account of affectivity the question of being and the question this poses to individual Dasein, my account of affectivity emphasizes becoming over being, and points toward communal rather than individual becoming for its central focus of action. These shifts—from being to becoming, and from individual to community—hold ethical implications as well, in that they focus our attention on the emergent co-relationships between beings and ask for considerations of an e-co-political climate in which the various forms of affective lives and their interdependence are given a chance for transformation. This is in line with what Barad has called an *ethics of responsivity*, which concerns "responsibility and accountability for the lively relationalities of becoming of which we are a part."[14] And, as Michel Henry conveys, the essence of community lies in a constitutive *pathos-with*:

> Inasmuch as the essence of community is affectivity, the community is not limited to humans alone. It includes everything that is defined in itself by the primal suffering of life and thus by the possibility of suffering. We can suffer with everything that suffers. This pathos-with is the broadest form of every conceivable community.[15]

Following Barad's and Henry's insights, in this book I will try to show how community, which I define very broadly as "life in association with human and non-human others,"[16] is best to be grasped along the lines of co-affective-emergence as mediated by a material interface, and that our ethics should be responsive to the co-affectivity at the heart of this community.

While the articulation of the need to address the meaning of affectivity is all but new and has been integral to twentieth- and twenty-first-century continental thought and its so-called "affective turn," what is innovative about this book is *thinking through the concrete, living places where affectivity happens*. In this, the book does not so much engage with the thoughts on affectivity by thinkers such as Butler, Heidegger, Irigaray, and Sloterdijk in their own right, but rather focuses on *the meaning and productive results of this engagement in the context of specific living beings*. Additionally, by drawing on a broader and deeper spectrum of affectivity in line with Aristotle's usage and as applied to multiple forms of life, I move explicitly beyond a narrow, psychological interpretation of affect as passion, mood, feeling, and emotion. This allows me to seek intersections among various forms of affectivity and to place them within the larger context of ecological concerns, thereby allowing for a productive place to rethink and reconstitute the meaning of specific forms of affectivity within the larger context of e-co-affectivity.

Hence, the contribution of this book is to articulate and unlock the meaning, depth, and complexity of affectivity in living beings, ultimately focusing on the very materiality of the interfaces that co-generate and co-constitute those living beings. Interfaces separate, mix, and generate two universes as they meet "within."[17] Interfaces provide material conditions that generate certain forms of being; simultaneously, they are never static but prone to change, creativity, and (individual, species, and communal) engineering.[18] For instance, in my account of human skin, I show that the sapience and sentience attributed to humans has been informed, from the earliest beginning, by the interaction of internally emergent and externally emergent factors in the changing interface that became human skin.

The benefits of such a *situated* focus on affective ontologies are many. For one, instead of a generic discourse on affectivity, the ontology I provide through mapping affective responses can be more flexible and faithful to the uniqueness of each concrete form of affectivity. Second, such a situated discourse can concretely show *how and where* form, abstraction, and choice emerge out of affective materiality (e.g., on the level of the individual, the species, the community, etc.). Third, this focus brings to the fore aspects of local ontogenesis and spatiotemporal synthesis that crucially inform the work of affective interfaces. Fourth, this book seeks to think through different categories of affective change and tries to show how they may interact and contaminate each other on the local level. For instance: to what degree can incidental, qualitative change be distinguished from change on the level of the underlying substance, and to what degree can change on the level of *aisthēsis* be distinguished from qualitative change exactly?[19] Thus, this book demonstrates both the need for using such categorical inventions and the need to "break them down." This deconstruction is aimed so that, as Haraway puts it, "richer and more responsive invention, speculation and proposing—worlding—can go on."[20] In short, I seek to use categorical distinctions that are not fixed but open to revision, aiming for a more refined grasp of phenomena productive not only on the level of theory, but also with regard to our ongoing practical interactions with human and nonhuman others.

The *structure* of the book follows the need for a situated focus on affective ontologies. Accordingly, it is divided in chapters, each of which analyzes different forms of affectivity in different life forms. The book begins by focusing on plants, moves on to discuss touch in bird feathers, considers next the ontogenetic boundary that is the human placenta, and uncovers the meaning of the skin as sapient and sentient interface crucial to human affectivity. While this movement from plants to nonhuman animals to human animals might suggest a *scala naturae*, this book seeks to disrupt such an ontological or ethical hierarchy. In each chapter, my goal is for my analysis to acquire complexity in its own terms, and to do justice to each form of life examined, with possible moments of intertwinement and cross-pollination with other analyses. And, by ending this book with the figure of soil as a messy, porous, un-grounding ground, I foreclose any avenues that could suggest a prioritization of human sapient affectivity; instead, soil serves the purpose of pointing to a broader material interface that emphasizes relationality and mediation among various forms of life as well as relationships to the inorganic, without prioritizing any.

In fact, precisely by *appearing* to be dedicated to hierarchized groupings as found in the Aristotelian tradition, while actually analyzing each form of life at the level of the concrete, material interface, this book is uniquely qualified to undermine the power of hierarchy and point at the equalizing power of matter, without giving up on agency,[21] or on nuance and distinctions[22] among strata and falling back into pure *adequatio* among the various forms of life.[23] While we can distinguish certain similarities and differences in the affectivity of living interfaces, such as those of feather and human skin, the difference or complexity in strata can themselves not be evaluated in terms of better or worse.[24]

The fifth, and final, chapter of this book is different from the previous four. It does not focus on one particular form of life, although it does highlight one particular material interface: soil. It seeks to sketch the outlines of a new and robust sense of *e-co-affectivity* that is both deep and broad in ethical and political appeal. If we take threats such as climate change seriously within our living, singular eco-sphere,[25] then a politics of e-co-affectivity needs to warn against the reduction of and threat to its symbiotic communities. Ultimately, I focus on the material interface of soil as a place to produce and engineer a new epoch beyond the anthropocene. The soil's ontogenetic powers and its complex inner workings provide the locale for us to engage with emergent potentialities and to create more porous and enduring ways to form new communities.

The *research questions* that drive the investigation of affectivity in this book focus on examining the kinds and modalities of affectivity, how they relate to each other, and whether—by interacting—there might be risks of (productive) contamination, conflation, and deconstruction. This means, for example, that the chapter devoted to plants (chapter 1) examines both the positive, affective force of growth, as well as the potentially negative affective force of illness and trauma. For the chapter on birds (chapter 2), this involves an investigation of sensitivity in the form of touch, and thinking through the ways in which touch is a unique form of affectivity yet also indicative of other forms of affectivity.

However, given that forms of affectivity can be modified, communicated, and shared, my analysis also seeks to move beyond an assessment of affectivity simply in terms of binary values, such as positive or negative, and incidental versus substantial. My analysis, rather, seeks to provide evidence for *categorical contamination* between kinds and modalities of affectivity, thereby uncovering not only further semantic complexity to the present but also providing alternative pathways for becoming anew.

Another research question turns on the need to capture affectivity beyond the passive-active bifurcation. In his *Categories*, Aristotle casts motion in terms of the correlated categories *poiein* ("to act") and *paschein* ("to be affected," "to be acted upon").[26] What would an alternative ontology of motion, one that is no longer subject- or action-oriented, and one that allows for dynamic and flexible ontogenesis, look like? Might the middle voice be an attractive alternative, and, if so, why and how might it be particularly productive for plants (chapter 1)? Would it allow us to move away from the centralized singular and allow us to cast affectivity in terms of polyphonic communal places that generate meaning? And what might be the weaknesses of the middle voice: might the "zone of indistinction" it suggests not all too easily lead to a flat ontology and ethics, contrary to the ethical and political e-co-affectivity that may be needed for a future beyond the anthropocene (chapter 5)?

When thinking through the *locality* of affectivity, the issue of the meaning of the boundary and the concrete place of the in-between come to the fore. This raises the following questions: What can interfaces such as the interstitial space between feathers (chapter 2), the placenta (chapter 3), and skin (chapter 4) tell us about affectivity and place- and time-making? How can living interfaces allow for the emergence of form and transcendence? And more generally: How does an account of affectivity articulate *the immanent unfolding of form and meaning through matter*?

When we further explore such interfaces, the following questions emerge: How can animal identity be born out of difference in mediation with this interstitial space? How can pain, trauma, and social, evolutionary, and intimate practices leave their traces in this space (chapter 2)? What can the placenta—if articulated correctly as the exemplary generative organ of the in-between—teach us about ontogenetic affectivity? And can we discern further material traces of its constitutional work, perhaps in our living physiology, pathology, and social relationships (chapter 3)? And what happens to our understanding of human affectivity if we zoom in on the uniquely human material interface of bare skin? In what way does this affective, sapient inter(sur)face (re)create our time, place, and being? How does it foreclose or open up future possibilities (chapter 4)?

Finally, given all these different forms of affectivity, how can we think of affectivity on a larger, ethical, and political level, one that aims beyond the here and now and that we may call (synthetically and provocatively) that of *e-co-affectivity beyond the anthropocene*? How may we think through the web of affective relationships without denying the uniquely human task to shift in affective response and act and feel differently in light of our current environmental predicaments (chapter 5)?[27]

In terms of its *methodology*, *E-Co-Affectivity* makes use of concepts in twentieth- and twenty-first-century Continental Thought in conjunction with insights from Aristotle, but does not engage with those concepts on their own terms. Rather, borrowing categories and schematic abstractions from both Continental Thought and Aristotle, I seek to draw close to and clarify life's affective phenomena. Accordingly, each chapter needs to vary and experiment with such abstractions to speak to the specifics of the subject matter. By providing different analytic tools in each chapter, I seek to employ a flexible, conceptual apparatus that can do justice to what the *logos* of the phenomena demands.[28] Exemplifying, the chapter on the placenta will benefit most from conceptual accounts and critiques of mimesis and place-making, while the chapter on birds will benefit most from a deconstructive reading of Aristotle's account of *pathos* and *aisthēsis*. Thus, while weaving a story about affectivity in various life forms, this book seeks to prevent each chapter from being too quickly assimilated into a *general* story about affectivity as such, and seeks to outline the uniqueness of each account as far as possible toward what I call *provisional* ontologies—provisional insofar as the ontologies I describe are based on our access to the phenomena, and are changeable given the flux of reality and constant ontogenesis.

Given the need for each chapter to vary and experiment with abstractions as prompted by the subject matter, my engagement with sources in the phenomenological tradition will offer an eclectic selection, based in part on what each chapter, and each interface, appears to demand. This means, for instance, that for the chapter devoted to skin I incorporate less frequently cited thinkers such as Dagognet and Serres, over against more well-known accounts of "flesh" by Merleau-Ponty, to acquire depth and precision in analyzing skin. And for the chapter on soil, which seeks to engage the notion of compassion within a broader, material, ecological context, I pull from thinkers such as Haraway, Stengers, and Stiegler, rather than appealing to the more conventional phenomenological account of Heideggerian "earth."[29]

In relation to the field of "affect studies" or "affect theory," my work on affectivity shows affinity with some of its approaches, especially where it turns to the body, such as Clough's emphasis on the body and emotion as part of what she dubbed the "affective turn,"[30] as well as her focus on "affectivity as a substrate of potential bodily responses, often autonomic responses, in excess of consciousness."[31] Similarly, I am sympathetic to Brian Massumi's work *Parables for the Virtual*, which, in drawing on Deleuze's reading of Spinoza, offers a theory of affect that is explicitly embodied: he defines affects as "virtual synesthetic perspectives anchored in (functionally limited by) the actually existing, particular things that embody them."[32] Since my work draws toward the embodied concrete affectivity of various forms of life, my approach has less affinity with that strain of affect theory that turns to affect in the more narrow sense of emotion or feeling,[33] and specifically as felt by humans,[34] even as such theory speaks with nuance of the complex and "sticky" nature of affect, as Ahmed for instance does in defining affect as "what sticks, or what sustains or preserves the connection between ideas, values, and objects."[35]

Since this book investigates affective responses, and specifically as emerging in different kinds of living beings, it also invites comparison with theorists that draw on affect as embodiment and extend this thought to the broader ecological community. For their historical lineage, such theorists often follow "the line of thought from Gilles Deleuze and Félix Guattari back through Baruch Spinoza and Henri Bergon."[36] One recent instance of work that examines affect in Spinoza and connects it to the wider ecological community is Hasana Sharp's *Spinoza and the Politics of Renaturalization*. This book traces Spinoza's thought on affect and the community of affects, and understands human vulnerability along the lines of vulnerability in beasts, rocks, and vegetables, aiming to facilitate "social harmony and political emancipation."[37] In Sharp's view, what follows from Spinoza's account of action as affect is that "human action is not an individual exercise but the consequence of an enabling affective milieu, comprising infinitely many human and nonhuman forces."[38]

While my approach to the question of affectivity in different forms of life thus converges with aspects in affect theory that focus on the body and that trace its historical lineage through Spinoza scholarship, and aligns strategically with projects such as Sharp's that analyze affects as part of a wider account of both human and nonhuman forces, my trajectory is distinct in that it takes its origin in Aristotle. Using Aristotle to conceptualize affectivity in various life forms is refreshing given the more prevalent usage of the Deleuze/Spinoza trajectory, and has various advantages, which I outline here.

First, in the figure of Aristotle we find a thinker who has always embraced the concrete phenomena of life. This is especially the case if we read Aristotle through the lens of Heidegger, who interprets Aristotle as a thinker of life-in-motion.[39] For instance, in his 1924 summer lecture course *Basic Concepts of Aristotelian Philosophy*, Heidegger encourages us to trace the meaning of Aristotelian concepts back to their "indigenous ground" (their *Bodenständigkeit*) rather than through their formal definitions. This original ground is primarily not theoretical, but experiential, according to Heidegger, and lies "in the commerce of life with its world."[40] This has made it possible to make Aristotle's categories more conversant with phenomenological interests in the changeable nature of living beings, which allows us to move Aristotle's philosophy in the direction of a more fluid ontogenetic metaphysics.[41] Additionally, with Aristotle's interest in concrete observations and science, we find good transition points to integrating science and concrete phenomena discussing all forms of life.

Second, my reading of Aristotle will seek to think with Aristotle against Aristotle (similarly to how Habermas has urged to "think with Heidegger against Heidegger"), so as to think along routes that have been inspired by Aristotle, but are not necessarily Aristotle's. A return to Aristotle may help us in rethinking both some of the problematics at the root of the concept of affectivity as well as what, in its current reformulation, may have been forgotten and what may bring us forward. By reading Aristotle carefully and with nuance, through the method of "affirmative deconstruction,"[42] as Bianchi proposes, we may reclaim some of Aristotle's insights that are relevant and helpful for our current day (for instance, his account of the constitutive nature of touch, and his account of direct and indirect co-suffering), while problematizing others (such as his account of the active-passive distinction and the various hierarchical stratifications of affective change).

Notably, the conceptual turn I make in this work to Aristotle (and, to a lesser extent, Plato) not only functions to structure my engagement with contemporary questions, but also serves to *add* to the study of Aristotle and Plato, namely by showing their relevance and how contemporary questions can uncover forgotten or new aspects to their accounts. For instance, my discussion of the phenomenon of *aisthēsis* in chapter 2 relies on some of Aristotle's pertinent ideas regarding the centrality of touch, but contemporary questions I ask also show problems in Aristotle's analysis and the need for Aristotle scholarship to rethink categorical distinction along the lines of what I call *categorical contamination*.

Third, my account of affectivity addresses issues related to community, and I am using the term "community" here in the broad sense of "life in association with human and non-human others," very much in the sense of how ecology defines community: "a group of organisms growing or living together in natural conditions or occupying a specified area."[43] To give fuller depth to this concept, Plato's and Aristotle's concepts of community (*koinōneia*) and the formation of a city-state (*polis*) are helpful, in particular because they access community not as an occurrence *after* the fact that individuals are constituted, but rather as a *constitutive relational* element of individuals' lives. As Aristotle writes, the *polis* holds logical and ontological priority over the family and the individual (*Politics* 1253a18). While I seek to highlight a broader sense of community than merely Aristotle's focus on the human community, and while I want to address the co-emergence of community and individuals rather than seeing the community as taking sole logical and ontological priority, I would like to hold on to Plato's and Aristotle's sense that individual life is dependent on communal life, and that we would do well to understand individual life as being informed by a broader communal form of life. In my view, Simondon's account of collectivity as it forms the individual (in the form of a preindividuated reality) helpfully complements my reading of community in Aristotle and Plato.[44]

Fourth, both Plato and Aristotle address issues of place, and since any discourse on community and affectivity will have to address place, their discourses on community and place-making are important. As Sallis writes in relation to the building of the city (*polis*) in *logos* in the *Republic* (369e): "the city involves not just an assembly of men, not just a community of associates (*koinōnoi*), but their assembly at a common dwelling place. The city is precisely this place where they live together."[45] Place here is not simply an external element to the community, but a constitutive element. As we see articulated in Plato's *Republic*, where the first two people to build the city engage the soil by cultivating and tilling it, "the constitution (*politeia*) of the city both determines and is determined by this location."[46] Especially in chapter 3, I will address this issue of place-making and community and will invoke Plato to make my point. And, ultimately, in chapter 5, I will articulate that conceptualizing community and affectivity as emerging from a communal, mediating interface holds ethical and political implications, since it entails not only the ethical imperative of being attentive to the suffering of others, but the need to reconstitute the meaning and structure of ethics and politics.

As for its *methodology with regard to science*, when this book incorporates scientific discoveries into its train of thought, it does so by finding inspiration in Elizabeth Grosz's work, which seeks to integrate and connect ideas from fields such as biology and physics with postmodern thinkers such as Deleuze and Irigaray. For instance, Grosz's *Becoming Undone: Darwinian Reflections on Life, Politics, and Art*[47] offers a new account of life as openness, by carefully engaging with Darwin's evolution theory, and bringing that in conversation with ideas on determinism and freedom in Deleuze, Bergson, and Irigaray.

Similar to Grosz, I see science not just as a way of offering examples for my theory while also making the concepts immanent to the everyday, but I am using its explanations to *redefine* concepts. For instance, in the chapter on pregnancy and the placenta, recent discoveries speak to the fact that cells of the embryo do not reside only in the uterus, but can be found in the bloodstream, heart, brain, and lungs of the pregnant mother. Vice versa, cells of the mother become part of the fetus' body as well. Such microchimerism, as it is called, may both be involved in destruction of maternal tissue or rebuilding it after trauma. Thus, microchimerism urges us to reconsider the concept and meaning of hospitality, and how life is not lived individually, or even in community with others, but emerges and becomes with and through one another.

As this discussion of microchimerism shows, I seek to let my writing emerge from an *interdisciplinary space*, with horizontal, nonhierarchical relationships between the disciplines. The result, I hope, is an argument where concepts are not just hovering "above" everyday life, but where they are in fact immanently embodied in and emerging from the matter itself.

Chapter 1

Plants and Affectivity

The Middle-Voiced Lives of Plants

I wished to speak to you of the feeling I sometimes have of being Plant myself, a Plant that thinks but that does not distinguish its diverse potencies, nor its form from its force, nor its port from its place. Forces, forms, size, and volume, and duration are but a single river of existence, a tide whose liquid expires in hard solidity, whilst the dim will of growth rises and bursts and would again become will—in the light and innumerable form of seeds.

—Paul Valéry, "Dialogue with a Tree" (1971, 172)

One of the most compelling reasons for wishing to be in the place of the seed is, it seems to me, that germination commences in the middle, in the space of the in-between. That is to say: it begins without originating and turns the root and the flower alike into variegated extensions of the middle . . .

—Michael Marder, *Plant-Thinking: A Philosophy of Vegetal Life* (2013, 63)

[The middle voice] is one that in its recall unsettles the dominance of active and passive voices, one that obstructs the kind of clarity that we expect.

—Charles Scott, "The Middle Voice in *Being and Time*" (1988, 160)

Introduction

Only after the garden was landscaped and its plants took root did our house really become a home. Place and time became visible as the fountain grasses found humid footing in the former riverbed, and the blueberry bushes appeared to resonate with the seasons. The nectarine tree and the plum tree pull me into a spatial and temporal vortex. Planted in the years that our children were born, they point at a shared beginning, a shared life, a shared place and time before being and understanding.

From here, life unfurls, but unevenly, joltingly, sometimes painfully. The later planted plum tree now towers over the nectarine tree, its leaves curled in illness. The plum tree nearly became a victim of its own success, a heavy scar remaining after a heavily overloaded branch almost broke off and dangled from its ripped open stem.

Growing, touching, rooting, connecting. Much is at stake in this time and place that may allow for the creation of a new "us."

It is hard to notice them—*really*. But it is equally hard *not* to notice them. The plants we live among and that form the continuous backdrop and nutritive support to our lives are also very much hidden from us, even if they compose 99.7 of the Earth's biomass[1] and have increasingly become the site of capital investment and technological and genetic manipulation.[2] Literally, they remain invisible in terms of their hidden root systems, their abilities to hibernate, and their hardly visible buds that are full of potentialities; figuratively, they escape our notice as much still remains to be discovered about the fascinating dynamic being that is a plant. In addition to the paradox of presence and absence, the plant presents us with a host of other contradictions: seemingly silent, its leaves rustle distinctively; while sessile it quietly grows and moves; suffering terrible losses, it endures and blooms with ever greater power.

What is arguably the most fascinating paradox that plant life exhibits is the tension it presents between its emphatically open, passive existence and its hardly visible, active, tenacious life that expresses itself in processes such as photosynthesis and absorption of nutriments, but also in actively enduring, responding, resisting, and adapting to changes in its environment, and in growth. As the "indeterminate, undefined, or open growth" of plants shows, plants are constantly becoming, and without enduring growth—and constant ontogenesis—could not even *be*.[3] With respect to its passive and open existence, the life of a plant is lived in full exposure to exteriority. It lives in full dependence on external factors such as the sun, the wind, insects, and nutriments in soil and atmosphere.

The (unknown) author of *De plantis*[4] already argued this much, and emphasizes that the plant, unlike the animal, is, even for its own generation, dependent on "outside action" (*pragmatos tinos eksoterikou*), and "needs this at certain seasons of the year" (*De plantis* 817a19–21). Similarly, Theophrastus addressed the dissemination of seeds by rain and floods, as well as the effects of weather and soil on plants in his *Enquiry into Plants*.[5] If not only nutrition but also generation requires "the outside," then the plant cannot be characterized other than fundamentally dependent and receptive. It is in its openness and dependence on the other that the plant is seen to be extremely vulnerable. If external circumstances such as temperature, soil, air quality, or insect population change, a plant is easily affected and damaged, and might consequently suffer demise.

Despite its dependence on the "outside," however, recent research reveals that plants are far more active and responsive than their "mere dependence" on so-called outside factors seems to suggest. Plants are not only very active in processes such as photosynthesis[6] and absorption of water and minerals, but they also actively endure, respond, communicate,[7] and resist changes in their environment. For instance, in response to damaging insects or viruses or bacteria, plants can produce odors such as methyl jasmonate or methyl salicylate[8] to communicate potential harm to other yet untainted parts,[9] or to other plants.[10]

Further, plants can deter herbivores from feeding on them through structural defense, for instance by producing thorns and prickles, by growing surface hairs, by hardening their leaves (sclerophylly), and by depositing minerals in their tissues.[11] Plants such as the *Nicotiana attenuata* "attract predators that control herbivores" through emitting odors and having the predators eat the eggs left on their leaves by herbivores.[12] Finally, while previous research simply denied that plants may feel pain and suffer, due to complete immersion "in their immediate modes of life"[13] and the absence of a nerve system with noci-receptors and a lacking sense of awareness,[14] current research's unlocking of the ways in which plants defend and respond to parasites or to predators in their own, vegetative ways offers a more nuanced perspective on affectivity in plants, grasping a plant's responsiveness to harm and suffering based on its own materiality and organizational structure, without relying necessarily on interpretations of pain (e.g., noci-receptors) and suffering (e.g., consciousness of pain) that are based on category mistakes.

Thus, if we follow along their adaptive and responsive strategies with more detail, we find evidence to prove that plants are masters of adaptability and can successfully rewrite their present and future in light of both positive, and negative, (traumatic) events.[15] Plants are masterful in enduring, responding to, and resisting changes. In this, as Hallé writes, "Plants have a long history of countering difficulty. Unlike animals, they do not flee, turning challenges to their advantage through a combination of internal genetic variability and longevity."[16] While firmly located in one spot, their place of engagement constantly changes yet has traces of permanence, too, tapping into various registers of (epi-)genetics, symbiosis (with elements, other plants, and other living beings), individuation, and community.

In this chapter I argue that the concept of the *middle voice* offers a way out of the conceptual pressure to understand plants as either mostly *passive* beings (e.g., in terms of their dependence on the "outside") or as overly *active* beings (e.g., in terms of their active photosynthetic processes and their ability to feed themselves);[17] additionally, the middle voice offers a helpful conceptual ground to grasp vegetative affectivity as including "choice." In my reading, the middle voice is not only a useful conceptual tool, but I propose that the middle voice is *materialized* in the ambiguous inner-outer positionality of the plant. While, from a human perspective, the distinction between active, passive, and middle voice might be a theoretical issue,[18] I seek to articulate that plants *live and embody* the open, futural, participatory existence of the middle voice. If we define, following Benveniste and Eberhard's intuitions, a middle-voiced existence as participating in a process that encompasses oneself, then the plant instantiates such middle voice existence in most (if not all) of its affective processes.

Beyond and before activity and passivity, the middle voice allows us to focus on "the processual level"[19] of movements and stresses the quality and nature of the process rather than unduly pondering *who* is doing *what* to *whom*. In particular, since the middle voice replaces the traditional discourse of agency with one that is focused on *locality*, the middle voice offers a nuanced yet broad conception of plants that sees them neither as impassive things nor simply as "subjects of their world"[20] (nor, lyrically, as "wily protagonists in the drama of their own lives—and ours.")[21] Instead, the middle voice allows us to grasp plant life from the perspective of a dynamic happening or an affective continuous unfolding process, in which a plant is neither the agent nor simply the patient, but an internally immersed, decentralized, yet coherent and continuous part of a process. The additional benefit of the middle voice is that it allows us to conceptually *interconnect* otherwise far-different affective processes in plants, such as nutrition, growth and withering, and disease and suffering.

Since, as Mancuso and Viola formulate it, "in the plant world, all faculties are present almost everywhere and no part is truly indispensable,"[22] and since a plant has not one, but "multiple command centers,"[23] the middle voice also provides an opportunity to grasp the plant's affective processes in terms of a stretched out, dispersed, yet coherent and communal self, ruled by "swarm intelligence"[24] rather than that of a singular, identical subject. Moreover, the middle voice may also explain the plant's relationship to its community, in terms of, for instance, its openness toward sharing resources, protecting its community, and willingness toward grafting and hybridization. Thus, while the middle voice, as such, offers a helpful conceptual framework for thinking about the affective ontology of plants by focusing on locality rather than subjectivity, the middle voice also clears room to mark and signal movements and moments of vegetative "choice," where vegetative existence marks its constancy through differentiation from, resistance to, and receptivity of that which happens to it.

In the following, I will first address the essential characteristics of the middle voice, to subsequently analyze how the middle voice offers a new perspective on plants in terms of nutrition and growth.

The Middle Voice

> An anonymous world formed by "someones" also leads to the passivity of each one in relation to affects coming from the outside, and does not allow the experience expressed by the middle voice, which requires us to pass from the outside to the inside of the self.
>
> —Luce Irigaray, *In the Beginning, She Was* (2013, 160)

The concept of the *middle voice* is originally a linguistic category, immanent to older languages such as Ancient Greek and Sanskrit, but extinct as a distinct verbal form in modern Western languages.[25] The middle voice has acquired some philosophical renown in the twentieth and twenty-first centuries in figures such as Heidegger, Gadamer, Derrida, Agamben, and Irigaray.[26] What has attracted philosophers to the middle voice is its ability to think beyond the division between active and passive that seems so deeply rooted in Western thinking. Linguists have argued that the passive voice is a later development of the middle voice.[27] This would imply that *before* or *beyond* the separation between the active and the passive, there is the possibility of another verbal category that offers an alternative way to grasping the relationship between subject and process.[28] Benveniste's linguistic examination of the middle voice has proven influential in that it tries to imagine what this verbal category means, although he also makes clear how difficult it is to sidestep the "traditional terminology" that is steeped in the opposition active-passive.[29]

Benveniste's account traces the middle voice in Ancient Greek and Sanskrit, remarks on its morphological absence in modern languages (such as English),[30] and demarcates its meaning in conjunction with its antonym, the active voice. He proposes to substitute the terms "active" and "middle" with the notions of an *external* and an *internal* voice or diathesis. For the relation between subject and process, this is the difference between the active and the middle voice:

> In the active, the verbs denote a process that is accomplished outside the subject. In the middle, which is the diathesis to be defined by the opposition, the verb indicates a process centering in the subject, the subject being inside the process.[31]

The key difference between the two voices is whether the subject is outside the process, or interior to it. Benveniste cites verbs in both Sanskrit and Ancient Greek that are only expressed in the active voice (e.g., be, live, flow, give) and that "do not require participation of the subject." By contrast, some verbs in Sanskrit and Ancient Greek, such as be born, lie, sit, and suffer, are found only in the middle voice and situate the subject as the "seat of the process":

> [T]he subject is the center as well as the agent of the process; he achieves something which is being achieved in him—being born, sleeping, lying [helpless or dead], imagining, growing, etc. He is indeed inside of the process of which he is the agent.[32]

While Benveniste's explanation might unduly put emphasis on the subject as *agent*—this is, in fact, what we are trying to bypass in our analysis of plants, at least in the more conventional sense of the word "agent"—what is extremely worthwhile in his analysis is his effort to change the *form* and approach of the discourse on processes. Instead of asking who is the agent or patient, the shift is toward *where* the subject is in relation to the process of the verb. Thus, as Eberhard writes, Benveniste's account of the middle voice allows for a shift "away from subjectivity toward locality."[33] This does not mean that the subject acquires less emphasis. Rather, as Eberhard clarifies, the internal diathesis "puts the subject in the sphere of the verb: he or she is inside his or her action, and he or she is subject of the process happening to him or her. What changes is the question that puts itself to the subject, and the key is the medial balance between subject and event."[34]

Charles Scott's account of the middle voice is in particular very helpful to transition thinking about the middle voice in regards to plants. Modern languages often render middle verbs in terms of reflexive statements, and Scott argues that the middle voice is actually to be located beyond reflexivity,[35] and alludes to enactments that are immediate. In his view, the middle voice "is able to articulate nonreflexive enactments that are not "for" themselves or "for" something else. As a formation it does not need to suggest intention outside of its movement or a movement toward an other . . . It is the voice of something's taking place through its own enactment."[36] As examples for such nonreflexive, transitive uses of the middle voice, linguists often appeal to bodily actions such as washing, since the process of washing involves the whole entity acting and being acted upon, rather than being easily distinguished in an acting (initiating) and affected part, which is the case for the reflexive, intransitive use of the middle voice.[37]

These words are promising for an account of plant affectivity. For, if it is true that a *centralized, nuclear* subject cannot be easily discerned in plants (and, thus, neither reflexivity), while simultaneously activity and responsivity cannot be denied to them, then the middle voice offers us a helpful conceptual tool to grasp plant affectivity. Plants prove themselves masters of sensitivity, responsiveness, adaptability, and transformation. It is especially their responsiveness and dependence on their surrounding that brackets emphasis on the autonomous reflexive character of self-affection. Surely, identity is applicable, but also alterity. What is at stake is the plant, but not simply a return to itself. Thus, Scott's otherwise cryptic words about the middle voice acquire lucidity when applied to plants: for Scott, the middle voice "can indicate a whole occurrence's occurring as a whole without self-positing or reflexive movement."[38]

Because plants are so immensely participating and immersed in their activities, their activities remain mostly "hidden," and need to be brought out. The middle voice explains in part this apparent withdrawal, and Scott's words with their focus on "whole occurrence" emphasize the subject's participation in the activities without standing *over* against them. Still, Scott's formulation of the middle voice also points at a problem, according to some critics, shortchanging the subject and making its voice "mute."[39] In applying the middle voice to plants without recognition of this problem, we might be prone to similar criticism, resulting in a vision of plant life that is similarly without a voice, and without a corresponding "choice."

If anything, this "muteness" has to be prevented without compromising the power of the middle voice. What the middle voice should allow us to do in our analysis of plant affectivity is an initial consideration of vegetative affective ontogenesis as necessarily dynamic and processual, but simultaneously opening up to a place where plants may articulate affective depth and constancy, and thus articulate their voice through creativity and choice in their responsivity. Perhaps the place of becoming that is plant life illustrates with remarkable clarity the fact that ontogenesis is always *relational*, dependent on a milieu and what Simondon would call a "pre-individuated" place[40] whose ongoing influence produces ever new, transformative, creative ways of being. And where the middle voice may point very well toward this relational process of becoming in plants, we would do well to emphasize that this process also includes room for creativity and invention, "a process of 'form-taking' of the new in action."[41]

The next section will investigate nutrition in plants, and seek to prove that the middle voice is not only well suited to explain this central and pivotal aspect of a plant's life, but is also able to complicate the biological discourse that sees plants as self-feeders. Through a deconstructive reading of Aristotle, I will argue that vegetative nutritional processes depend on a zone of temporal and spatial mediation, which results in a "deposed" subject whose existence is decentralized, plural, and composed of a network of individuations.

Plants, Nutrition, and the Middle Voice

If we define, following Benveniste's initial explorations and Eberhard and Scott's refinements, a middle-voiced existence as *participating in a process that encompasses the subject*, then many of the processes plants engage in appear to fit this paradigm. One such example is nutrition. As I will articulate here, the middle voice is not only well suited to explain vegetative nutrition, but, in combination with a deconstructive reading of Aristotle, offers important complications to and corrections of the standard scientific language and understanding of plants as self-feeders. In my reading, the discourse of self-feeding is complicated by the inclusion of zones of temporal and spatial indeterminacy. In these zones, what is active and what is passive seek to meet, but find themselves suspended in an undecidable space where affective processes endlessly overlap and withdraw. This is exactly the indeterminacy that the middle voice seeks to capture, allowing us to envision the processual nature of nutrition (i.e., that nutrition happens as a process) far more clearly without unnecessarily focusing on *who* is doing *what* to *whom*. Simultaneously, this focus on process over agency should not obfuscate the important and unique voice that each plant has in this process, for instance in determining the "logic" of its production and distribution of sugars and its absorption and retaining of water. This "logic" must take into account how much water has been absorbed by its roots and how much is transpired through its leaves, and needs to continuously move the sugars produced by photosynthesis.[42]

In current biological terminology, the relationship that plants have to nourishment is classified as based on "autotrophy" (self-feeding)[43] as opposed to animals, which are called "heterotrophs" (feeding on others). Most plants convert solar energy into chemical energy through photosynthesis;[44] it is thus assumed that plants feed themselves (and others) through their own self-sufficient activities, transforming energy and producing carbohydrates and oxygen. While animals depend on plants and/or other animals for their food,[45] plants, by contrast, "asking nothing from anyone, collecting and concentrating a form of energy available to all . . . produce living material without respite."[46]

In other words, plants have a remarkable capacity that other living beings lack, namely, the ability to rely for their own nutrition upon "radical other" inanimate sources such as the sun, water, minerals, and carbon dioxide, and to make their own organic food suitable to their own matter. From inorganic to organic, the plant stands at the literal "root" of life, and the plant not only seeks out and eats its food, but also produces its own food. When we would prioritize this ability to be independent of others in producing one's food,[47] and thus zoom in on the fact that plants are auto-trophs, plants could easily move to the *top* of the food chain rather than hovering at the bottom.[48]

Philosophical underpinnings for this current biological conception of plants as self-feeders can be found in Aristotle's texts. The additional benefit of looking into Aristotle's theory is that his theory also offers sophisticated complications to the idea of self-feeding; the complications he offers, I will argue, provide a more nuanced and complex notion of the affective nutritive ontology of plants.

First of all, Aristotle casts the process of nutrition in terms of the interaction between activity (*poiein*) and passivity (*paschein*) and argues that food (*trophē*) is the third factor by way of which activity and passivity are connected:

> Now there are three [aspects]: the thing fed (*to trephomenon*), that by which it is fed (*hōi trephetai*), and that which feeds (*to trephon*). That which feeds is soul in the primary sense; the thing fed is the body which has that [i.e., the soul], and that by which it is fed is the food. (*DA* II.4, 416b20–24)[49]

It is the "usefully ambiguous"[50] term *trophē*[51] in combination with ancient Greek's verbal flexibility that allows for identity and differentiation between the three factors involved in nutrition. These three key elements are all connected to the same verbal root *troph-*, but show differentiation in their respective endings: the active (*to trephon*), the middle/passive (*to trephomenon*), and dative (*hōi trephetai*).[52] Thus, the process of nutrition finds itself in a zone of identity and difference, with identity constituted by contribution to the same process, and difference determined by whether one instigates the process (the so-called active voice or "subject"), whether one is subjected to the process (the so-called passive voice or "object"), or whether one *materially enables* the active and the passive voice to connect (the so-called instrumental "dative").

Scrutinizing this nutritive process more thoroughly by looking at the de facto contributors in this process, Aristotle actually offers us an account of nutrition in which the main focus of the process is on the organism itself and the fact that it feeds and is fed by itself. In his vision, nutrition's active and passive voices are fundamentally collaborating and enacted by the *same* living, ensouled embodied being. Aristotle's account of nutrition thus allows us to explore the internal cultivation of nutritive affectivity: while holistically one process involving the same being, nutrition is *hetero-affective* in being divided in two.

In his view, nutrition finds its principal organizational *archē* in the soul,[53] its embodied *archē* in the body,[54] and its enabling, interconnecting medium and substrate in food.[55] Thus, the process of nutrition seems self-contained, and self-directed, but not without sophistication in terms of (1) asserting identity and difference within the nutritive self, and (2) offering a place to openness and thus to the "external" world in terms of food. In addition, a third factor needs to be added, which (3) places the meaning of this nutritive and affective process in terms of the *preservation* of the self. For, Aristotle argues that the aim of food (*trophē*) is that it lays the groundwork "for activity (*energein*)," namely, activity of the soul "to preserve (*sōdzein*) that which has it as such" (*DA* II.4, 416b18–20).

The language of "preservation" that is key to the affective process of nutrition finds resonance in Aristotle's account of *pathos* and *paschein* in the context of sensation (*aisthēsis*) in *DA* II.5.[56] In the following passage, Aristotle argues that there is a form of *paschein* that is not destructive, but positive, namely, in enabling the preservation (*sōtēria*) of a certain disposition and nature:

> Being affected (*paschein*) is not used in a single sense; it sometimes signifies a kind of destruction (*phthora*) of something by its contrary, and sometimes rather a preservation (*sōtēria*) of that which has a potency by that which is in fulfillment (*entelecheia*) and which is like it. (*DA* II.5, 417b1–2)[57]

Aristotle argues that *aisthēsis* is a form of affectivity (*paschein*) that enables the preservation of the perceptive process and activates its nature. The nutritive process is to be understood similarly in that its affective process enables enactment of nutrition's potencies while also preserving and enabling a living being's nature (*physis*).

Thus, the processes of nutrition and sensation share commonality in being characterized as affective processes (including the language of *paschein* and *pathos*) that harken back to the potencies of each living being to enact and preserve itself. The end-results, the *ergon/pathos* of feeding/being fed, and the *ergon/pathos* of sensing/being sensed, are not incidental, external, or harmful to living beings, but in fact bring about an enactment or self-realization of that living being.[58]

Still, feeding and being fed, and similarly sensing and being sensed, can only come together to preserve and actualize (*energein*) the self through insertion of a *mediating third*. In the case of *aisthēsis*, this mediating "third" is the (elusive) *medium*, which complicates claims of "perfect mirroring" between that which senses and what is sensed, and which constitutes, formulated in more contemporary phenomenological language, an ever-withdrawing unsensible (untouchable) space that is the condition of the possibility for any *aisthēsis*.[59] Accordingly, in terms of the sensing animal at least, this means that *aisthēsis* acquires a fundamental openness since the medium complicates any identification with boundaries or with confining *aisthēsis* to either side of the active and passive bifurcation. Consequently, due to its "irreducible spacing," a sensing animal is indebted to, yet radically separated from, alterity, and what emerges is a mediated space of affective co-creation of the sensing animal.

Similarly, the "mediating third" in the process of nutrition offers a comparable space of complexity and withdrawal for the nutritional self, and thereby complicates situating the nutritional being on either side of the active or passive divide. Continuing the comparison with the sensing animal, what emerges in the case of nutrition is a similarly mediated space of affective co-creation, where the active and the passive never purely *match*, but are marked by distance, both temporal and locational.

In Aristotle, the first indication of the *temporal* distantiation implied in nutrition is in the following passage:

> Now it makes a difference whether "food" (*trophē*) means the last or the first of what is added. If both are food, the one undigested (*apeptos*) and the other digested (*pepemmenē*), we might speak of food in both the ways referred to above; for when the food is undigested (*apeptos*), contrary feeds on contrary, but when it is digested (*pepemmenē*), like feeds on like. (*DA* II.4, 416b3–8)

What food *is* is ambiguous, and must be thought along a temporal arc. If we are conceiving food in the present tense (as indicated by the present active participle *apeptos*), then food is completely *different* from that which is fed. However, if we conceive of food in the past middle/active participle (*pepemmenē*), then food is *identical* to that which is fed. In the latter case, the body (that which is fed) is affected by "like" (the digested food, i.e., food in the past tense).

This may sound straightforward, but it is anything but so. In this affective nutritive process of which food is the *medium*, food goes through a temporal assimilation process, which ultimately makes it *like* the body. *Is* food then the body? *Are* we what we eat? In food's undigested state, the answer is no. In fact, the opposite is true: in its undigested state, food is the radical other, the *opposite* (*enantion*) of the living self. However, in a digested state, the answer seems to be an unhesitating yes. In the latter case, this implies that we are adding yet *another* affective component to the process of nutrition, insofar as the active voice and the passive voice of nutrition are now linked by another *quasi-self* (food in its digested state) that allows for preservation of the concrete self.

Summarily, then, the *mediating third* occupies a space of temporal withdrawal, where its existence as *medium* is contested once it finds itself in the past: once food *is like* the body, it thereby gives up its autonomy as medium. Only in the present tense does it occupy foreign territory—albeit as part of a dichotomy where opposites are linked to each other and thus dependent on each other. As a result, the active voice (of feeding) and the passive voice (of being fed) encroach on the third, seeking to assimilate it, but food's true alterity withdraws with its loss of its present state. What is left to witness in digestion is the space of the disappearing third, which the past tense can no longer capture. This implies that the active and passive never truly match, but are marked by a temporal zone of affective indeterminacy.

In addition to temporal withdrawing, the *mediating third* is also prone to further ambiguity in the form of *spatial dislocation*:

> But 'that by which is it fed' is ambiguous, just like the phrase 'that by which the helmsman steers,' meaning either his hand or the rudder, the latter both moving (*kinoun*) and being moved (*kinoumenon*), and the former only moving. Now all food needs to be digested (*peptesthai*), and that which enables digestion (*pepsin*) is heat; on account of this every ensouled being has heat. (*DA* II.4, 416b28–31)

The *mediating third*, which thus far had been considered only as food, encounters ambiguity and doubling in requiring yet another medium enabling its digestion: the mediating fourth—that is, heat.[60] This proliferation of the medium means that we schematically encounter something like the following:

[A-agent] soul (unmoved) moves
    [intermediary] bodily heat (moved) moves
    [intermediary] food (moved) but does not move
[B-patient] body (moved, is fed)

By adding another intermediary (moved/mover) to the process of digestion, the process of nutrition again acquires expansion by including another factor involving the self—that is, heat (or *pneuma*)[61]—but also acquires further complication, by finding itself dislocated. From heat to undigested food to digested food, the question of *where* food is cannot be easily answered, as a dazzling series of movers and moveds takes over and cannot easily be contained. If bodily heat is not merely moved but also a mover, then arguably the same thought could be duly extended to food itself, especially if food serves a further function in processes of "growth, nourishment and reproduction." What food is and contributes to thus acquires further complexity.[62]

Similar to the temporal evaporation of food's present tense announcing a temporal zone of affective indeterminacy, the ongoing proliferation and dislocation of food's multiple active and passive processes testifies to nutrition's spatial zone of affective indeterminacy. The indeterminacy does not lie so much in the chain of movers and moveds as in the indeterminacy of place and time where one moves from being fed to feeding. Where and when exactly does externality transform to internality? Can we clearly and markedly distinguish where and when a plant feeds on its own processes versus where and when it relies on diffuse and external processes that enable its feeding?

From Aristotle's Account of Nutrition Back to the Middle Voice and Plants

Given the above reading of two zones of affective indeterminacy in Aristotle's account of nutrition, it is time to return to the language of the middle voice and discern its relevance specifically for the nutritive lives of plants. For if our reading of Aristotle is correct in discerning nutrition as an all-encompassing affective process taking place in zones of temporal and spatial indeterminacy, and if this makes it impossible to base nutrition on one dominant *subject* of control or on one easily determinable and delimited external *object* of action, then the middle voice offers an attractive alternative to the dualistic form of thinking distinguishing activity from passivity.

If it is the case that the middle voice offers us a subject "that achieves something which is being achieved in him,"[63] then the process of nutrition, as analyzed above in a deconstructive reading of Aristotle, offers a clear embodied example of such a middle-voiced existence, specifically by drawing attention to the process of internal hetero-affection that includes zones of temporal and spatial indeterminacy between subject and object. In these zones, what is active and what is passive seek to meet, but find themselves suspended in an undecidable space and time where affective processes endlessly overlap and withdraw. This is exactly the indeterminacy that the middle voice seeks to capture, allowing us to envision the processual nature of nutrition far more clearly without unnecessarily focusing on *who* is doing *what* to *whom*. Nutrition pulls us both outward toward externality and food, while also pulling us inward toward the process of nutrition, where the active and passive voice of the organism find each other connected yet separated by the medium.

Provocatively, Aristotle argues in *Parts of Animals* that "plants get their food from the earth by their roots [. . .] they use the earth and the heat in it instead of a stomach,"[64] thus giving extra weight to the thought that plants live a middle-voiced existence, with their "external stomachs" being found in the medium—the soil—itself. Where, when, and how does this process of nutrition take place? If nutrition takes place through the external stomach, surely there must also be an "internal" stomach that digests this food so that it turns in to the plants' homoeomerous and anhomoeomerous parts? Again, the middle voice's presence makes itself powerfully felt by holding those questions open and pointing at a fundamental indeterminacy that rules the process of nutrition.

The characterization of nutrition as a middle-voiced process, and specifically as an affective process with temporal and spatial indeterminacy, works par excellence for plants because they are the *exemplary masters of nutritional transformation*. Since nutrition is by definition a middle-voiced activity, and since plants' existence turns on nutrition and plants are first and foremost experts on transforming nutrition, the middle voice with its emphasis on process, participation, and nontransitivity offers multiple ways to grasp and anchor plant existence accordingly in firm and complex affective terrain. Describing plants in terms of the active and the passive will never fit: plants *live* the open-ended, participatory, futural, nontransitive existence of the middle voice.

A fluid, localized, and temporalized affective ontology takes its place, and alongside it we find a subject that is "deposed of its action." Even more radically, and beyond simply being internal to its action, the subject in the middle voice of Agamben's conception is "exposed and put in question together with it."[65] This *deposition and exposition* of the subject speaks to the existence of plants, where processes take center stage and where the question regarding a central subject or "locus" of control seems misguided and misplaced: "deposed." Yet, this is not to say that the existence of plants is not *their* individuated existence, but perhaps such existence has to be rethought from central to decentralized, from singular to plural,[66] and from identity (of the subject) to a network of individuations.[67]

The "logic" of its distribution system is a case in point: it relies on three distinct communication systems (hydraulic, electrical, and chemical) that at times complement each other.[68] Signals may move and be distributed through the vascular, hydraulic system that transports water, sugars, and minerals from "the roots to the crown" and from the "leaves to the fruits and roots."[69] Additionally, information may be carried across directly from *cell to cell* (as in electrical signals), allowing plants to "communicate not only from their roots to their crown and vice versa, but also from one root or leaf to another."[70] The efficient, two-directional nature of its hydraulic system of nutrition without a designated center points at the success of *decentered*, perhaps liminal, vegetative coordination, and the *direct* inner communication from root to root, and from leaf to leaf, proves the plant's remarkable "distributive," anarchic emergent coordination of selves.[71] Thus, while dependent on middle-voiced zones of vacuous, liminal mediation, vegetative nutritional existence is all but lacking sophisticated coordination, choice and voice. However, this choice and voice needs to be cast in a peculiar—decentered, distributive—vegetative way. If we follow Mancuso's research of the signals of the root apex of plans closely, and grasp that most plants have millions of such roots, then vegetative choice, for instance to pursue or not pursue certain nutrients in the soil, is located within this network structure composed by those million tiny computing structures.[72] This is a distributed, yet highly coordinated, form of choice.

In short, nutritional processes in plants benefit from being grasped through the lens of the middle voice, as this allows due focus on process, participation, and nontransitivity, something that is seemingly "lost" in the misleading biological language of vegetative "autotrophy." Simultaneously, the middle voice opens up to testify to the unique voice and choice that each plant has in this process, which is dependent on a complex and sophisticated "logic" for coordination (e.g., absorption, production, and evaporation) of nutrients such as water, sugars, and minerals.

Plants, Growth and Withering, and the Middle Voice

Perhaps by following the trajectory of *growth* in plants, these ideas on the middle voice can find even more stable ground and sharper articulation. Notably, growth is especially significant when it comes to plants, because, in contrast to most animals,[73] plants keep growing all their lives. In fact, as research indicates, if plants stop growing, they perish. In this regard, "a steel band around the trunk of a plane tree" does not only stop its growth, but also leads to its death.[74] Further, one could argue that growth is *the* form of movement that plants engage in,[75] although this movement is often too slow—in terms of the scale of human time—to be captured by the human eye.[76]

Crucially, not only do plants keep growing, the development of growth is "indeterminate, undefined, or open,"[77] which is in contrast to the rather homogenous (*homotopic*) development of animals.[78] Aristotle addresses the indeterminate and open growth in plants in the following way:

> All plants as well seem to be alive, since they clearly have within themselves a potency and a governing principle through which they continue growing and withering in *opposite directions*—for it is not the case that they grow only up and not down, but those that continue to be nourished and live toward their ends grow in both (and indeed all) directions, as long as they are able to obtain nourishment. (*DA* II.2, 413a28–34)[79]

The characterization of the growth (and decay) of plants as happening *in opposite* directions is another key factor in grasping plant life from the perspective of the middle voice. Where up and down are determining destinations for the elements, plants are not bound to any particular static location, but they find their existence literally in the midst of all these opposite directions. In fact, in growing in *all* directions, plants exhibit a nonbinary disposition that allows them to be altered constantly, and yet remain and become themselves. Plants are remarkable for not being "torn asunder" by this growth—somehow they are held together and even flourish—although their elemental composition would seem to tear them apart.[80] According to Aristotle,[81] it is the organizing principle of the soul that provides the plant such unification.[82]

The plant's ability to hold itself together among abundant and all-directional growth makes apparent the almost "banal" fact of a plant's double extension, so poignantly described by Marder:

> One of the most compelling reasons for wishing to be in the place of the seed is, it seems to me, that germination commences in the middle, in the space of the in-between. That is

to say: it begins without originating and turns the root and the flower alike into variegated extensions of the middle, in marked contrast to the idealist insistence on the spirituality of the blossom and the materialist privileging of the root.[83]

The above suggests that a seed's growth *physically* represents the middle voice: it extends from the middle in both (and indeed all) directions, and still is able to keep itself whole. In growing from the middle and extending, a plant truly finds itself suspended in a middle-voiced activity: it grows through its own enactment in all directions without an externally or internally discernible "who" that stands *over* or *beyond* these activities. In fact, while plants, in being sessile, seem tied to the *where* of their activities, this locality is undergoing continuous change in the process of growth and is thus made unstable. The association by which growth thrives (for instance, in terms of fungal association) and the potentiality it harbors direct us to grasp the locality of vegetative growth less in terms of stable grounding, and more in terms of messy, soil-infused, creative un-grounding.[84]

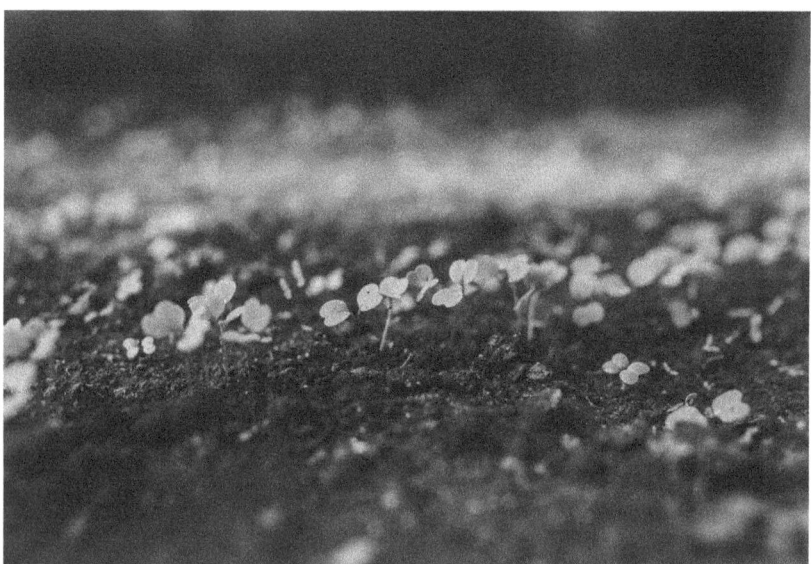

Figure 1.1. Arugula plants in the stage of seedling, when the roots develop and spread and rapid growth occurs.

Moreover, in both growing toward the light and digging into darkness, the plantal location of the middle voice is qualitatively different and yet finds "itself" *in* or *through* these radically different activities that the plant is. In other words, insofar as the middle voice highlights the immediate involvement of the subject in action, the open and indeterminate growth of plants indicates that such involvement is plural, constantly changing, and qualitatively different for each part and open-ended in all directions.

These ideas on the middle voice find further amplification by investigating the particular divisibility and growth of plants, which puts to the test ordinary notions of "self." Aristotle already remarks on the fact that a plant is potentially divisible, and that its parts may adopt an independent life. He speaks in this regard of one actuality (*mia entelecheia*) of the plant soul, which harbors a *potential multiplicity* (*dunamei de pleionōn*, *DA* II.2, 413b19), "since each divided part has a whole soul"[85] (cf. 409a9–10, 411b19–30).

This is to say that a plant such as a spider plant may harbor within itself other plants, and even other genomes,[86] and that it has ways to both incorporate and host potentially independent plants but also ways to accommodate their separation and actual independence without suffering. While many animal beings (with the exception of starfish and lizards, for instance)[87] cannot regrow body parts or would be partially disabled by losing parts of themselves, the voluminous and open-ended growth of plants may easily accommodate such losses of body parts and may not even suffer or be worse off due to it. Process philosopher Whitehead casts the plant accordingly in terms of the political model of a democracy, arguing that the plant—unlike the more centralized and hierarchical "monarchic" model of the animal—"can be subdivided into minor democracies which easily survive without much apparent loss of functional expression."[88]

The success of spin-offs of spider plants and other plants should not be surprising if we ponder the particular growth and architecture of plants. Eighty percent of plants are described as colonial, which means they depend on *reiteration* for their architectural structure and growth.[89] Reiteration describes how a plant that originally starts with a single architecture can add architectural units—reiterations—to the first, ultimately accumulating all such reiterated units.[90] Most trees can accordingly be described as "colony trees," with its iterations becoming more numerous over time, but also smaller (in size). Ultimately, the form of these reiterations "is simplified to the point that they end up reduced to a leafy stem with flowers."[91]

The reiterations that are constitutive of many plants have their own root system, which makes them self-sufficient, and "capable of leading an independent life."[92] This means that the growth of many (and at least all colonial) plants defies assumptions of a "center" that organizes and keeps the plant whole, thus leading some theorists to speak of a "free and open association" of units. Mancuso and Viola speak of "numerous 'command centers' and a network structure not unlike the Internet's."[93] Accordingly, the French poet Michel Luneau writes that the various elements of a plant "obey nobody but themselves and ask their followers a simple and essential agreement: growth. Each organ is free in the means by which it attains this growth."[94]

The potential multiplicity that Aristotle so early on recognized thus finds evidence in modern science, which does not only diagnose *potential* multiplicity of plants within the same unit, but also *actual* multiplicity and independence of plantal parts within the same unit through the concept of "colonial growth." Thus, there is both a remarkable (potential and actual) freedom of each part of a plant, as well as a remarkable ability to keep together or holistically integrate remarkably different parts within a flexible yet unified whole.

What keeps this relational whole "together" in terms of making choices and coordination has recently been described as "swarm intelligence." Mancuso and Viola discuss the coordinated action that root tips—hundreds of millions for trees, or tens of millions in small plants—make together: "each root tip maintains a preset distance from the root tips around it." Plants, like birds in swarms, "display so-called emergent behaviors, which don't exist in individual organisms."[95] In animals, "swarms are formed by great numbers of people, mammals, insects, or birds. But in plants, these dynamics actually come into play inside one plant, between its roots. In short, every single plant is a swarm."[96] This is compared to "a network capable of functioning collectively."[97]

The *middle voice* again makes itself strongly apparent here, since colonial plant growth shows that plant life is composed of reiterated multiples that nonetheless function collectively. Agamben's idea that the middle voice confronts us with the *deposition* of the subject thereby also resurfaces,[98] especially since such deposition may allow us the conceptual freedom to move from the singular to the plural, and reiteration allows us to deny ideas of originality versus copy, and priority versus posteriority. Since the middle voice does not depend on or assume a centralized, reflexive, and intentional subject that stands apart from its affections and activities, but instead focuses on the inner participation and localization of a subject in a process, it can easily accommodate a shift toward decentralized affectivities that are plural but nonetheless cohere together through collective commitment to the same processes of nutrition and growth. In this way, each plant becomes part of a communal life, composed of symbiotic lives.

That plants take into account communal factors, such as genetic heredity, for their growth has recently been proven through new botanic research: plants from the same mother "produced many fewer roots, advantaging the plants' aerial growth," illustrating that plants do not just act based on a "stereotypical and repetitive mechanism" of defense and competition, but may exhibit a "noncompetitive activity linked to their genetic proximity."[99] This proves that plants have not only "a more complex estimation that takes into account different factors, including genetic kinship,"[100] but a way to foster community beyond their own—communally composed—individuated being. Thus, the explanatory power of the middle voice in plant growth lies in laying out, explaining and integrating, to inflex Whitehead's account differently, the *anarchic community of affective lives* that is one plant.

Thus, similar to our account of nutrition, our examination of vegetative growth confirms the idea that the actions and passions central to plant life escape ramification in terms of the division between agent-patient, inner-outer, or subject-object. The subject engaged in nutrition and growth is not one, but consists of many reiterations where originality and priority cannot be asserted.[101] In addition, plants "need each other and the elements"[102] to grow, and both temporal and spatial zones of indeterminacy destabilize identification and closure. In other words, the flexible nature of processes such as nutrition and growth offer us a vision on plants as qualitatively different, quantitatively multiple, flexible in position and direction, and temporally open.[103]

Within the context of growth, we also need to address the diminution of plants—either "natural" or "enforced." The diminution of plants need *not* be counter to the ultimate natural development, and may actually be part of the natural affective self-actualizing process of the plant. This is also the way that Aristotle approaches it, since he includes not only growth, but also diminution or withering (*phthisis*)[104] as key to the natural, nutritive life: "nothing withers or grows naturally without being nourished" (*DA* II.4, 415b30). He defines growth as making additions to "every part of its figure and form" (*GC* I.5, 321b28)[105] and argues that withering entails shedding such additions: it is a uniform *contraction* of the animated matter,[106] and specifically of the "scheme of proportions."[107]

If we translate these insights into a more contemporary discourse on plants, Aristotle's ideas hold significant promise. Plants—like animals—can diminish in size (over time), or particular parts may atrophy, but that does not necessarily mean that they are moving toward destruction. The very opposite can be true: perhaps a "return" to a smaller size will make a plant more successful in the long run, or allow it to *preserve* itself while going through seasonal changes.

The radical nature of this return to a smaller size is particularly visible in annual plants, which "perform their entire life cycle from seed to flower to seed within a single growing season."[108] The cyclical nature of growth and withering that plants undergo, and their remarkable possibility to become dormant for many months, offers a powerful testimony to the extraordinary strategies that plants have to protect themselves against, and may even benefit from, potentially harmful *pathos*.[109]

So far I have mostly discussed the plant as successfully negotiating natural, seasonal change. What about changes that artificially impose itself on a plant's growth and that might negatively affect its growth? Here we can think of humanly built obstacles such as walls, fences, roads, and foundations that block the growth of plants. Perhaps with enough force and adaptability, plants may pierce through such walls, fences, roads, and foundations, or may find ways around such obstacles, but if no nutriments, sunlight, or place to anchor its roots are found, a plant might consequently wither. Further, if even more access to nutriments is limited, not only quantitative but also qualitative, substantial change may occur, and such a plant may die.

If, as current botanical research has discovered, touch may influence or even inhibit growth, and thus supports the thesis that "[a] plant feels what kind of environment it is in,"[110] and if, as research shows, many plants ultimately perish if they stop growing,[111] then we need to be careful in thinking through the artificial boundaries and environments we impose on plants. In a world where space is limited, where natural resources are increasingly exploited and depleted,[112] and where climate change radically alters conditions and habitat, how could we, accurately and sensibly, conceptualize the nature of affectivity in plants, and specifically that which results from impositions on vegetative growth and natural withering?

The examples are numerous and the details are complex, for sure. We can think of trees budding earlier or later than usual and then being caught up in freezing temperatures, thereby losing opportunities to bloom, grow, and prosper the following year.[113] We can think of climate change–induced droughts and plants consequently withering and possibly dying—with "brown being the new green" a helpful slogan to encourage more sustainable use of resources, but with potential and actual harm done to plants.[114] We could go on with numerous other examples. We can also think of climate change–induced rainfalls, rising water levels, and shifting fog levels, where some species such as extremely slow-growing redwood trees, must "chase" the fog to stay alive.

What is clear on the basis of even these limited examples is that, despite the wide-ranging adaptability, flexibility, and endurance of plants, there are certain limits to what plants can endure—where withering surpasses the realm of common resilience and where growth and preservation are no longer possible. In the next section I explore these limits more thoroughly, with a focus on finitude and community. I will try to show that both radical openness toward others in combination with an ability to integrate death in their midst is crucial to grasping the remarkable resilience that plants have. In this analysis, the middle voice has a special occasion to make itself heard as the vegetative voice of radical openness and hospitality, as well as the vegetative voice of resilience and endurance.

The Integration of Finitude and the Meaning of Community in Plants: The Middle Voice as the Voice of Openness and Resilience

The above discussion of withering in plants brings up the point of existential limits, and the consequent need to address finitude in plants. Here, again, plants may surprise us in terms of the depth and complexity of their adaptability: plants may "live and die at the same time."[115] And some plants take this to an extreme: some are hardy enough to even tolerate the trauma of being ground up: plants such as the water hyacinth (*Eichhornia crassipes*) can reproduce a new plant out of each piece.[116]

The term "endurance" seems particularly well equipped to address plants' resilience in the face of death. For, plants literally *harden* in time[117]—as is visible in the dead wood that is reinforcing the sturdy structure of a tree.[118] Relatedly, in plants the process of preparing for winters is called *hardening off*.[119] Thus, the woody appearance of many trees expresses both a future-oriented disposition reflecting support of current and future growth, and simultaneously entails in its dead wood a direct material memorization of its past.

Further, not only in its dead wood, but also in the vacant spots[120] where branches have broken or dropped off, the current architecture reminds us of the plant's lifeless past. Hallé points out this remarkable ability to integrate both death and life,[121] and while referring to colonial trees such as oak and eucalyptus and to clonal plants such as date palm and buttercup, he writes, "Their structures weakly integrated, their reiterations relatively independent from each other, these plants have the capacity simultaneously to die and to live without our noticing a behavior so different from ours."[122]

The integration of dead cells into its living structure manifests the open, medial nature of plants. For if part of itself is dead and yet structurally supporting the present and the future, then the middle voice in discerning an elusive, exposed, or even deposed subject—to speak with Agamben—literally applies to the dead vegetative subject that still materially reinforces the living plant without taking up actual new space or time.

Where our discussion of nutrition discerned a zone of temporal and spatial withdrawing, then certainly here in the case of hardening off we find a similar zone of temporal and spatial indeterminacy, whereby past and future easily intermingle without being able to point to agency or patiency, or to ask *who* is doing *what* to *whom*. For, if dead wood strengthens a plant and protects it against frost and disease, then *who* is actually doing this? If dead cells intermingle with the living, then what kind of present-yet-absent vegetative being are we addressing? In this hybrid life of absence and presence, the plant can truly grow, wither, and flourish. Thus, the middle voice is not only successful in capturing the undecided division between agent and patient in plant life, but also the *unimaginable hybridization of life and death that is a plant*.

In its ability to rewrite its future in the face of (ongoing) death and possible threats, a plant does not operate alone but clearly stands in community with others. This is apparent from the example of a forest ecosystem, where the symbiosis of rotting wood, molds, and wood-inhabiting fungi provide new growth for plants, insects, and birds alike.[123] Four types of community may be discerned as we consider the relationship between time, finitude, and community in plants: (1) vegetative communities such as pioneer plants that prepare the soil, die, and leave a diachronic trace; (2) ancestral vegetative communities that leave internal diachronic traces through epigenetic changes; (3) contemporary vegetative communities with

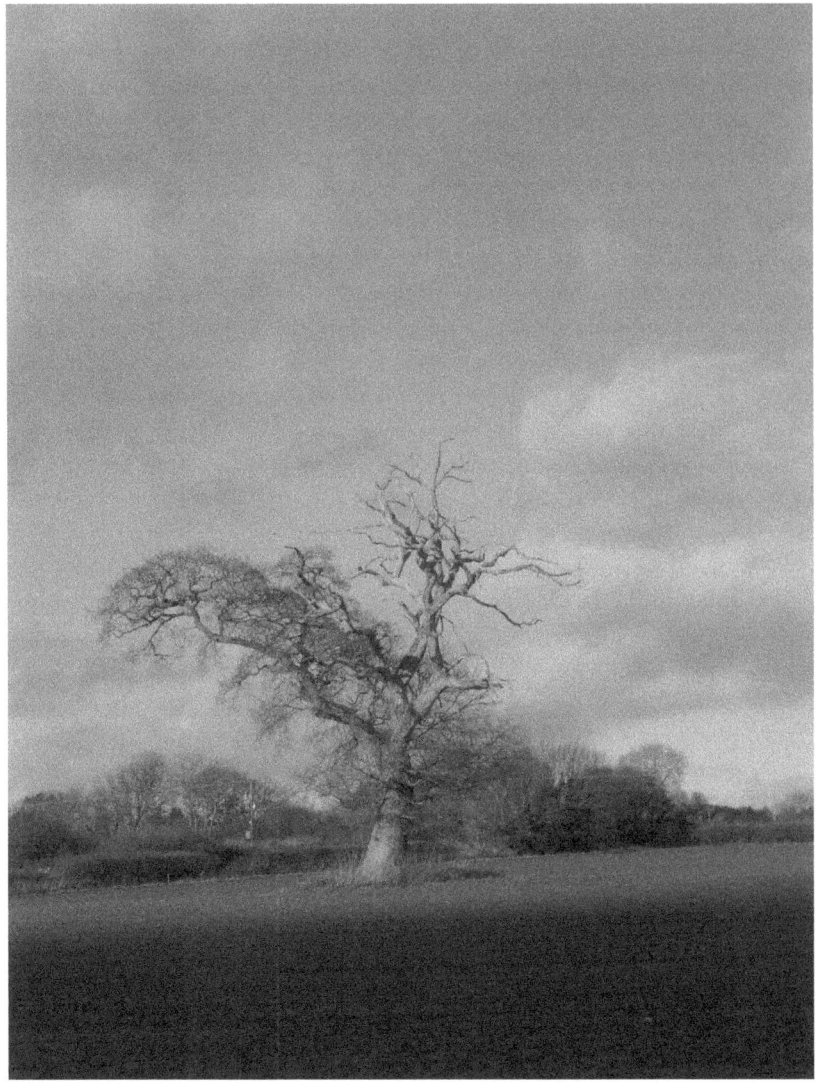

Figure 1.2. Half-Alive Oak Tree.

whom plants live in symbiosis; and (4) nonvegetative communities (such as fungi) with whom plants form a living partnership. All these kinds of communities reverberate through each other—through leaving a diachronic ("vertical") trail, or through leaving a synchronous ("horizontal") trail, or by doing both. I will briefly index the four types of community below, without pretending to be complete in my descriptions.

The first kind of vegetative community that enables through their death the life of current plants may be exemplified through the role that "pioneer plants" play in terms of preparing the soil and thus allowing the emergence of a diverse range of other plants in the present and the future. "Pioneer plants," also known as "pioneer species," of which nettles, thistles, and dandelions are examples, can grow in types of soil that are virtually deplete of minerals.[124] With their deep roots, they dig down deep looking for minerals, and in that process work the soil and "prepare" it for other kinds of plants who grow more superficially and need a richer soil. Moreover, the *death* of these pioneer plants enables the growth of further plant life. As they decompose, they leave behind pockets of oxygen and nitrogen and further nutriments in the soil, thus offering an example of vegetative *sacrifice*[125] as well as evidence of a material trace that prefigures the currently and futural living.

A second type of a vegetative community that leaves a diachronic trail may be found in the community that leaves an *internal* diachronic trail: that of the ancestors of the current plant population. This type of vegetative community has come to the fore through epigenetic research. What is remarkable about epigenetic research is that it shows that plants (like other living beings) do not only pass along their "form" (as Aristotle would have it) or "their genes" (as current discourse would say) but also transmit their memory for both flourishing and environmental or physical stress. The flourishing or stress that plants experience can cause changes in the epigenes—the protein-rich "support structure" of the DNA-helix—resulting in changes to gene activity. Those epigenetic changes can be inherited, thus allowing for transgenerational memory in reaction to environmental or physical stress.[126] Thus, although plants may themselves not have been *directly* exposed to stress, they "behave as if they had been stressed" based on the epigenetic changes that have been passed along. In other words, a plant's inheritance does not only concern the so-called "positive" factors allowing it to sustain itself and grow, but also its "negative" moments and its ability to resist or cope with it.

In showing how traces of vegetative experiences through generations leave their marks on present and futural lives of plants (both in positive and in negative ways), epigenetic research clarifies, in conjunction with research on pioneer plants, that the community of plants is to be viewed beyond simply that of their contemporaneous others: individuated plants emerge as products of complex diachronic relations with both their direct ancestors and the broader vegetative community that has made them possible. The communal lives and deaths of these prior communities undergird their existence and propel them forward toward new ways of living.

The vegetative ability to be susceptible to grafting is an example of how a third type of community, that of a *synchronous* plant-to-plant community, may be assembled and garner resilience through fostering hybridity. The horticultural technique of grafting[127] builds on the ability of plants to unite a rootstock with a scion, which can usually only happen between "plants of the same species and closely related plants."[128] What is fascinating about grafting is that it reveals the dynamic ability of plants to be co-affected and co-emerge jointly, in a newly assembled hybrid form. In this regard, Garner speaks aptly of graft union as "the healing in common of wounds."[129]

Grafting may play a powerful role in building resilience and protecting plants against disease. Rootstocks that are resistant or tolerant "to soil-borne problems such as fungi and nematodes, different soil types, drought and waterlogging"[130] may be used to help scion plants to battle disease and difficult circumstances. One famous example is how rootstock selected from a North American (Texan) species offered immunity against the insect disease Phylloxera and thus was able to protect scion vines that otherwise could not have lived in Phylloxera-infested regions in Europe.[131] This illustrates how plants by directly *mixing* "in the present time" can propel each other into another present and another future—one where they may overcome illness through helping one another—by literally and physically reinforcing resilience through mixing.[132]

The final type of—contemporaneous—community is that composed of plants with nonvegetative others. We can think in this regard of the community that is built with fungi in the soil, with which plants form an intricate symbiosis: "In certain cases, the fungus forms a sort of sleeve around the plant, penetrating into its cells. This kind of symbiotic association is called 'mutualistic' because it's useful to both living organisms: the fungus provides the roots with mineral elements, including phosphorus [. . .], and in exchange receives some of the sugars produced by the plant through photosynthesis, which it uses as a source of energy."[133] Another example is that of symbiotic nitrogen-fixing bacteria: they "invade the root hairs of host plants, where they multiply and stimulate formation of root nodules, enlargements of plant cells and bacteria in intimate association."[134] As these examples show, the relational milieu in which plants dwell is not

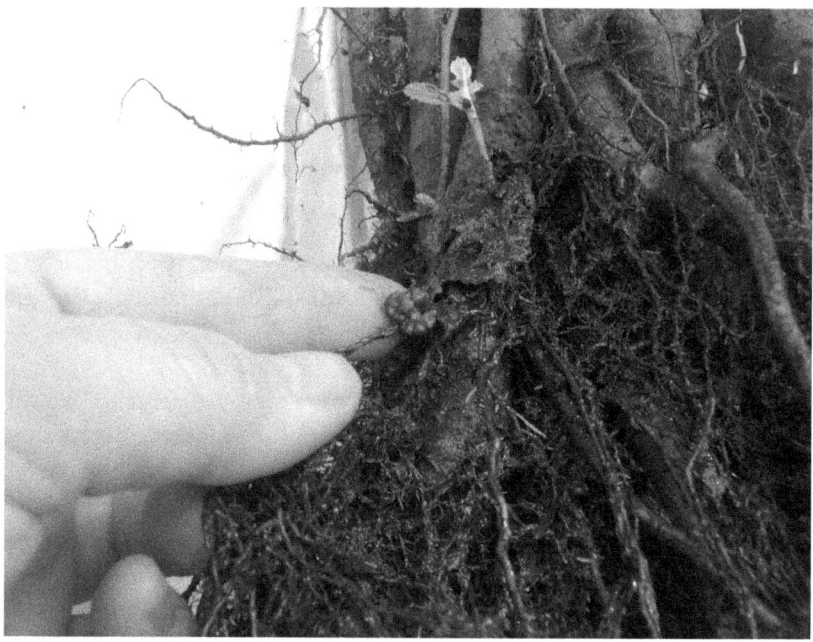

Figure 1.3. Nitrogen-fixing nodule: A root nodule that lives in symbiosis with nitogren-fixing bacteria.

just extraneous to them; through profound interaction in the interface, plants *become* the nourishing, growing, withering beings that they are.

In summary, this section on finitude and diachronic and contemporaneous communities has shown, first, that plants have remarkable ways to *physically* integrate death and dead structures meaningfully in their lives, testifying to a past that lives on through them, well beyond the past and the present. Second, vegetative processes of nutrition and growth, as well as ways of responding to stress, deprivation, and illness, are the products and living manifestations of their relationship to *trans-generational, trans-species, and hybrid vegetative communities.*

The ancestral path carved by pioneer plants adds on to the remarkable ability of plants to integrate death in their midst: it testifies to the power of trans-species and trans-generational communities, since the underlying possibility of their growth is the material death of their predecessors; thus, vegetative traces of the past reinforce present species. And the inheritance of epigenetic changes in current generations of plants proves that plants embody the (successful or traumatic) past of their parental predecessors, and will consequently *live out of this past*: their lives are not (just) their own but an assemblage of the past, present, and future. Finally, artificial and natural grafting practices in plants show the power of contemporaneously mixed assemblages, where, through junction in the present, one plant may reinforce the other's adaptability and strength, preparing it for an altered future.

The vegetative response to changes such as deprivation, illness, and trauma indicates an emphasis on *process* versus subject-object, and an emphasis on *participation* versus externality, which are all so typical for the middle voice. Especially given the role of the community in reacting to stress, vegetative life fully *participates* in processes that constantly transform and alter each other: *horizontally* in terms of contemporaneous assemblages such as grafting, and *vertically* in diachronically transforming its own life and being informed by the vegetative traces of its predecessors in the past, which drive it into the future. Since these communal predecessors have died, but are materially informing a plant's vegetative life, the middle voice's subject finds itself exposed and deposed, *withdrawing in indeterminate zones of temporality and positionality* that enable a remarkable, future-oriented, resilient existence. The vegetative resilience that emerges is not belonging to one or the other, but something that permeates and transforms all and that is materially instantiated in odors, epigenetic changes, rootstock/scion hybrids, and more.

Thus, the middle voice comes into play on the vegetative communal level, addressing finitude, as the voice of radical openness and the voice of resilience. Through deep diachronic traces with other plants as well as concrete contemporaneous relations of symbiosis with the soil, with fungi, with other plants, and more, plants—both individuated and in collectivity with others—prove themselves intricate ongoing products of the "'in-between' space of becoming."[135]

Conclusion

> Might we imagine that relations come first and not the extremities of these relationships? We are only ever in the intervals between intervals—and so, we exist like *glissandi* in our own aleatory music.
>
> —David Scott, *Gilbert Simondon's "Psychic and Collective Individuation": A Critical Introduction and Guide* (2014, 42)

The middle voice opens up an alternative and promising stance to contemplate the affectivity at the heart of plant life. If it is the case that the middle voice offers us a subject that is "inside the process of which it is an agent,"[136] and provides us a vision of life that grows from the middle, without origin or end, then plant life *par excellence* offers us an instance of middle-voiced life. First, plant life is nutritionally caught in zones of affective indeterminacy where externality and internality seek to meet but are infinitely separated in time and place. Second, plant life literally grows and withers *from the middle*, and produces numerous reiterations without originality, integrating death in its living structure, securing and enabling the future through endurance. Third, pathologically speaking, in responding to disease and deprivation, plant life manifests the middle voice as it "achieves something which is being achieved" in it.[137] Plants emerge and become who they are as products of a polyphonic, communal space. In this space, they result from hybrid, trans-species and trans-generational partnerships, which both sensitize and protect plants in numerous assemblages and through numerous means—as hybrids, as epigenetic residue, as traumatic memory,[138] exuding and responding to alarming gasses, parasites, stressful circumstances, and other factors.

Still, while plants have a remarkable ability to integrate death into their lives and to *endure* many changes that would otherwise be fatal, there is a critical threshold to such changes. While plants over time have successfully adapted to changes in their environment and habitat, at the current moment they are facing numerous threats, such as genetic engineering, the rise of monocultures, the domineering of invasive species, and climate change. If we focus on climate change, it is not only the global nature of this phenomenon, but also the *rate* of change, that can do remarkable damage to plants, especially given their slow rate of growth. The "winners" of climate change will likely be weeds and adaptable invasive species; the "losers" in terms of plant life will likely be native species "that are highly specialized in what they eat or where they live, especially those whose habitats disappear completely."[139] The consequence of this will not only be less diversity of species, but also "a less productive species."[140]

In other words, the riches of the plant world, with its polyphonic communal spaces and temporalities and its diverse, unique choices, is at risk of losing its diversity and heterogeneity, and rapid species extinction is at stake, and already happening, especially for those who cannot adapt quickly enough, or whose life is based on a close symbiosis with a disappearing habitat (especially native species). In the concluding chapter of this book I will speak more extensively on this, and on what kind of e-co-affective response is needed to address the dangers of the anthropocene, which is threatening and already transforming plant life and the inherent ambiguity, complexity, sophistication, and depth of its characteristic *polyphonic, middle voice*. Not only plant life, but all life stands to suffer as a consequence.

Chapter 2

Animals and Affectivity

Aisthēsis, Touch, Trauma, and Bird Feathers

The tangible is received, perceived prior to the dichotomies of active and passive. It is received like a bath that affects without and within, in fluidity.

—Luce Irigaray, *An Ethics of Sexual Difference* (1993, 164)

There is something alive in a feather. The power of it is perhaps in its dream of sky, currents of air, and the silence of its creation. It knows the insides of clouds. It carries our needs and desires, the stories of our brokenness. It rises and falls down elemental space, one part of the elaborate world of life where fish swim against gravity, where eels turn silver as moon to breed.

—Linda Hogan, *Dwellings: A Spiritual History of the Living World* (1995, 19)[1]

The sense of touch, far from making the living organism into a mere spectator, pledges it to the world through and through, exposes it to the world and protects it from the world. Touch bears life to its fateful, or felicitous day.

—Jean-Louis Chrétien, *The Call and the Response* (2004, 86)

Introduction

He is a young boy, scanning the skies and the orchards, tracing birds to what will become their empty nests. All alone in the fields, he walks and runs under a broad and expansive sky, with birds as his only companions. Far away from the sounds of the world, they share the fleeting daylight, and find a common home in the dark clay soil, the silhouettes of the trees, the wind bristling in the hedges. He will still watch birds ninety years later, but then from the confines of his comfortable home—sometimes through glass sliding doors or sometimes through the glowing television screen casting their projections.

I wonder: what is it like to have such a deep connection, to experience its evolution? To connect through different media, in different places and times, in the presence of ever-changing substitutes? And then: what will be lost, with his death, by their death, by the final reconfiguration of that shared sphere that I will bear with me in writing this?

In its attempt to think beyond and before the classical active-passive binary, the previous chapter discerned the importance of the middle voice, which enables an account of process and movement in terms of locality and participation rather than a strict divide between inner-outer, subject-object, and ultimately agent-patient. As I argued, the middle voice is particularly well suited to capture the life of plants, as it allows us to bring to the fore the remarkable—seemingly hidden—processes in which plants engage, such as photosynthesis and growing-from-the-middle. In addition, focus on the middle voice grasps the reluctantly heard voice of plants in terms of communication and protection against disease, and allows us to grasp their *community* less in terms of one centered around independent selves-in-communication, but rather in terms of an anarchic community of mimetic "selves" that seem both bound to and independent from each other.

In exploring the middle voice, the previous chapter has accomplished two important tasks: (1) conceptually and ontologically, to think beyond the active-passive divide, and (2) biologically, ontologically, and ethically, to provide affective ontologies that are central to plant life.

This second chapter seeks, similarly, to accomplish these tasks, but now regarding animal beings. The chapter clarifies yet another way to think beyond the active-passive divide, and to bear witness to and give a voice to another group of living beings—animal beings, and specifically birds—whose specific affective ontology needs philosophical articulation. The focus on *touch* that I provide in this chapter is strategic in that it brings into view the constitutive role of the sensitive, affective, material interface for animal life. The material interface of touch, I argue, does not extend only to include the relationship between the individuated animal body that is touched with that which touches it, but *constitutes and generates* the individual animal body, recalls and informs particular species patterns, and creates communal experiences.

Here, I first promote a reading of *aisthēsis* that sees it as part of a productive form of *categorical contamination*. In my view, and opposite to Aristotle, *aisthēsis* can ultimately not be separated from other categories of affective change; instead, by affirming categorical contamination, *aisthēsis* can emerge as the primal force for the signification of animal life that it is, including references to generation, qualitative change, trauma, and demise. Based on a deconstructive reading of Aristotle, I argue for the significance of the untouchable medium that makes touch and animal life possible. The untouchable medium disrupts identification between that which is touched and that which touches it,[2] and gestures toward a view of the aisthetic animal whose temporal and spatial horizon is always still becoming, ever different, and ever anew.

I consequently focus on birds and their sense of touch to give the discourse on touch the particularity, complexity, and depth it needs in line with its affective materiality.[3] Thus, in opposition to the idealistic contours of freedom and transcendence within which bird life is often thematized, I focus on the very materiality of avian feathery interfaces, moved by the wind, reacting to stress and trauma, and opened up by and interwoven with avian others through practices such as allopreening.

Aisthēsis, Categorical Contamination and the Need for a Metaphysics of Fluidity

I begin with Aristotle's account of *aisthēsis*, as his account is helpful in signaling the conceptual terrain within which the discussion of *aisthēsis* takes place (that of *paschein* or being affected), even if I ultimately disagree with his static categorical division of affectivity and want to replace it with a theory of *categorical contamination* that allows *aisthēsis* to emerge as a primal force for the signification of animal life. While the overarching trend in Aristotle scholarship has been to read Aristotle in line with a strict commitment to categories of substance and limiting change accordingly to categories such as quality, quantity, and place, much has been done in continental philosophy, specifically following Heidegger's reading of Aristotle, to interpret Aristotle as a thinker of life-in-motion,[4] and to open up his categorical distinctions accordingly. For instance, in his summer 1924 lecture course *Basic Concepts of Aristotelian Philosophy*, Heidegger encourages us to trace the meaning of Aristotelian concepts back to their "indigenous ground" (their *Bodenständigkeit*), which allows us to move Aristotle's philosophy in the direction of a more fluid ontogenetic metaphysics. As for Heidegger's understanding of *aisthēsis*, which will guide the following analysis, I will follow his idea that "*aesthanesthai* is not used in the narrow sense of perception, but as awareness in the sense of having-there the world. It is not theoretical considering, but being-open for something that is around me."[5]

In *De anima*, Aristotle devotes many chapters to *aisthēsis*, discussing the various specifics of the senses of vision, hearing, touch, taste, and smell. *Aisthēsis* is a term notoriously difficult to translate, first because *aisthēsis* has such a wide range of meanings in the Greek language,[6] making the concept hard to capture in English.[7] In addition to its broad meaning, the Greek term *aisthēsis* confronts the modern reader with a classificatory either/or: either to classify it along the lines of activity and translate it as perception, or along the lines of passivity and translate it as sensation.[8] This is ironic, as Aristotle himself locates *aisthēsis* along the full range of the active-passive axis and warns against simply understanding the concept as one or the other.

The conceptual terrain within which Aristotle places *aisthēsis* is that of *paschein* (being affected):

> *Aisthēsis* entails, as has been said, being moved (*kineisthai*) and being affected (*paschein*); for it is thought to be some sort of change. (*alloiōsis tis*, *DA* II.5, 416b33–35)[9]

The passive voice (being moved, being affected) that characterizes the process of *aisthēsis* directs us to its *dependence* on that which is sensed. Thus, Aristotle's formulation "gives prominence to the sense objects throughout,"[10] analyzing each sense by way of its corresponding objects.[11] Still, the passive voice of *aisthēsis* should not obscure the very *active* nature of *aisthēsis*, as this passage shows:

> Being affected (*paschein*) is not used in a single sense; it sometimes signifies a kind of destruction (*phthora*) of something by its contrary, and sometimes rather a preservation (*sōtēria*) of that which has a potency by that which is in fulfillment (*entelecheia*) and which is like it. (*DA* II.5, 417b1–2)[12]

Aisthēsis is to be categorized according to the second form of affectivity listed here, in that it entails preservation and fulfillment (417b1) of a living being's potency, and harkens back to a being's disposition and nature (417b14–15).

What is important for our endeavor here is the conceptual emphasis of founding the process of *aisthēsis* both on its dependence on the world, and on the active, inner dynamic founded on one's nature (*physis*) and disposition (*hexis*).

It is precisely this ambiguous passive-and-active dynamic of *aisthēsis* that, ultimately, makes Aristotle pause to call *aisthēsis* a form of *paschein*. For, in his general theory of alteration and qualitative change (*alloiōsis*), which he often phrases in terms of *paschein*,[13] focus on exchange of (opposite) qualities stands central.[14] What, then, should he do with the process of sensation, where, similar to the process of acquiring knowledge, we do *change* and are affected, but do not exchange qualities? A process that invokes and evokes something that was, somehow, always already, part of our nature? A process of change that, even more poignantly, activates and advances one's sense, one's nature, and allows us to fulfill and become ourselves? To address these concerns, Aristotle declares that both *aisthēsis* and the process of acquiring and expressing knowledge need to be excluded from the conceptual terrain of affectivity or *paschein* proper (417b14) or, if included, need to be qualified as very *peculiar* forms of it.

While Aristotle's approach to *aisthēsis* is praiseworthy in terms of integrating passivity and activity into one, the rigorous "border control" he employs to keep the various categories of affectivity (*paschein*) apart is a source of unease. To recap, he distinguishes qualitative, incidental change (what he generally calls *alloiōsis*) from another form of change, that is, substantial change (which he does not call affectivity or *paschein* unless it pertains to the generation and corruption of elements[15]), and excludes *aisthēsis* from being part of either, or, if included in qualitative change, then only marginally so, as a form of fulfilling (and thus not *changing*) our nature.

The source of unease lies in the *artificiality* of the boundaries being drawn. Isn't it the case that *aisthēsis* really underpins animal being and should be counted among the forms of substantial change that make animal lives possible or impossible? Certainly, Aristotle would agree with this in light of his account of touch, writing, as he does, that *aisthēsis* in the form of touch makes life possible (*DA* III.12, 434b23–25). Additionally, he writes that excess of qualities (such as heat, cold, and hardness) does not just destroy the sense organs, but "destroys the animal" (*DA* III.13, 435a13–14). When *aisthēsis* is successful, we live, and when it fails, it may have disastrous consequences for our being.[16]

A further objection may be formulated on basis of the fact that *aisthēsis* may very well *include and imply* qualitative change. For instance, if skin is touched by a warm surface, not only does it perceive warmth, it also *becomes* warm. While we may conceptually distinguish the two, the phenomenon of touch both implies the sensation and the process of the skin's altered temperature. And, further, as Aristotle cordons off *aisthēsis* to the terrain of the "fulfillment" of our nature, is it not the case that some forms of *aisthēsis* do this more substantially, such as touch, while other forms at other times are neither noticeable nor even effective?

All of this demonstrates that the strategic exclusion of *aisthēsis* from various other categories of change—qualitative change and substantial change—is highly problematic. The arduous border protection Aristotle practices is in fact undone by the porous borders themselves and the fact that, in asserting various categories of change, they acquire their meaning in opposition to what is excluded and thus *include* these other forms of change. And Aristotle's remarks about the *embodiment, vulnerability, and danger* of touch speak to the existential consequences of what I call the categorical contamination of *aisthēsis* with other forms of change.[17]

In addition to categorical contamination, a second, more dangerous, source of unease lies in Aristotle's underlying commitment to hold on to the notion of a static identity, specifically on the level of substances that are natural and unchangeable. Aristotle's model seems only to allow for flexibility and change on the level of qualitative change or on the level of the *unfolding, adapting and fulfillment* of one's nature vis-à-vis one's interaction. The form of change he argues for is, as Battersby would say, mostly one of *flexibility*, that is, "an adaptation of 'the same.'"[18] In other words, based on his categorical divisions, he seems committed to a metaphysics of flexibility that holds on to the idea of a preexistent identity that consequently "flexibly 'responds' to or 'reacts' to changes acting within and without."[19]

Aristotle's account of *aisthēsis* predominantly appears to confirm Battersby's definition of a metaphysics of flexibility, since Aristotle seems to align with a system of categorical distinctions and the assumptions of an underlying substance that remains similar, if flexible, through the changes that occur. Still, Aristotle's conceptual account of *aisthēsis*, and particularly his account of touch, arguably has elements indicative of the alternative model for which Battersby pleads: that of a Heraclitean model of *fluidity*, if fluidity is understood here not just as flux but as ontogenesis. Evidence for this may be found in those elements of Aristotle's account of *aisthēsis* which, as I have argued earlier, (1) indicate categorical contamination between the various forms of change, parenthesizing the notion of an independent subject untainted by the changes, and which (2) develop the idea that the *aisthetic* experience belongs both to subject and world.

If the *aisthetic* experience belongs both to subject and world and enables their becoming, and if there is room for difference and rupture in this account, Elizabeth Grosz's ideas on the role of the accidental and the undetermined may come to resonate. She writes about the importance to "acknowledge the capacity of any future eruption, any event, any reading, to rewrite, re-signify, reframe the present, to accept the role that the accidental, chance, or the undetermined plays in the unfolding of time."[20] The *unfolding* of time is, for Grosz, not an abstract unfolding of a purely conceptual matrix, but an unfolding of time that instantiates the unfolding of the embodied, *aisthetic animal*, whose body is the sediment of the history and memory of previous generations, and who lives life in view of a temporal horizon that is always still becoming, ever different and ever anew.[21] This temporal horizon involves thus both the individual and the species, and offers ways to expand the discussion of *aisthēsis* from the individual to its community and its species.

To make this more precise, the next section brings into view an account of *aisthēsis* that emphasizes the *synergy* of the emergence of self and world, and an account of touch that focuses both on the *constitutive* nature of this sense, and the fact that touch presupposes an untouchable medium and an irreducible openness to the event of touching. Grasping this untouchable precondition of touch enables an understanding of the creative place of *aisthēsis* that precedes the dichotomies of active and passive. Consequently, we may acquire a view on animal life as affectively dependent on and emerging along with the world; and what allows for this dependence, response, and co-emergence is, what I call, the mediated space of (pres)absence.

The Touching Animal: Touching, Being Touched, and the Untouchable Medium of Touch

Aristotle's account of *aisthēsis*, and particularly touch, is pivotal in that it shows that the co-emergence and co-constitution of animal and world is based not simply on correspondence, but on difference as well. In my deconstructive reading, I will put special emphasis on the notion of rupture and difference, as I see this as integral to the work that the medial interface of touch accomplishes in generating new possibilities.

For Aristotle, *aisthēsis* is a *synergistic* process in the strong sense: *aisthēsis* could not be had if it were not for *externalities* that affect us, yet bring into action and connect to the very potentialities that living beings as such are. In this regard, *paschein* indicates the *transitive*[22] nature of *aisthēsis* insofar as the process of sensing happens in collaboration with that which is sensed. It is for this reason also, as the beginning of *DA* II.5 indicates, that there is no *aisthēsis* of the sense organs themselves: they "give no sensation apart from externals" (*DA* II.5, 417a4–5). This means that we need to situate the affective motion that is *aisthēsis* in the middle of the fluidity of life, and need to address the *aisthetic* self not as pre-formed, but as emerging as part of a mutual becoming of self and world. In other words, as Elberfeld also notes, *aisthēsis* emerges as a *middle-voiced* phenomenon:

> Why does it make sense to render the process of perception exclusively in the middle voice? In conventional explanations, perception is understood either as something purely passive in the sense of a mere taking-in of data or, in more modern times, as a purely active comportment, in which data is constructed by and as the perspective of the subject. If one pursues perception in its fullness more precisely, it indicates that it is neither a purely passive nor a purely active process. It is on the contrary the *founding of a relationship* between the perceiving and the perceived, in which both sides are as active as they are passive. For the perceived is always reflected in the perceiving and the perceiver takes it up and associates it with its context. A place of perception arises here, out of which both the perceiving as well as the perceived come to the fore in the subtlest interplay in the sense of the middle voice.[23]

More specifically, for Aristotle the *synergy* at stake in any process of *aisthēsis* brings together the activity (*energeia*) of the sensible object (*aisthēton*) acting upon the sensible subject, and the activity (*energeia*) of the sensible organ (*aisthētikon*) being affected. Accordingly, Aristotle writes:

> If then the movement (*kinēsis*), i.e. the acting (*poiēsis*) and the being acted upon (*pathos*), takes place in that which is acted

upon (*poioumenōi*), then the sound and the hearing in their activity (*energeian*) must reside in the potency of hearing: for the activity (*energeia*) of what is moving and active (*tou poiētikou kai kinētikou*) takes place in what is being affected (*en tōi paschonti*). (*DA* III.2, 426a2–6)

Aristotle draws a parallel between movement—which includes acting and being acted upon—and *aisthēsis*, which is a particular instance of movement. Similar to how movement, generally speaking, brings together the *energeia* of acting and being affected, in the same way *aisthēsis* brings together sound and hearing. Moreover, the additional point that Aristotle is making in this passage in *DA* III.2 is that this activity is happening only in *one* substrate or subject, and that is the *aisthetic* animal. While sound and hearing are different in meaning and definition, the *factual, immanent* process of *aisthēsis* is one only, and finds its embodiment in the living sensitive animal.

If we approach this idea with an eye on the promise of a metaphysics of affective fluidity, what Aristotle is saying echoes much of what Erwin Straus describes in *The Primary World of the Senses:*

> The sensing subject does not have sensations, but, rather, in his sensing he has first himself. In sensory experience, there unfolds both the becoming of the subject and the happening of the world. I become insofar as something happens, and something happens (for me) insofar as I become. The Now of sensing belongs neither to objectivity nor to subjectivity alone, but necessarily to both together. In sensing, both self and world unfold simultaneously for the sensing subject; the sensing being experiences himself and the world, himself in the world, himself with the world.[24]

As Straus sees it, the *mutual becoming* of both subject and world happens through the experience of *aisthēsis*. In terms of temporality, the *aisthetic* experience belongs to both subject and world and enables their becoming. Put more in Aristotle's terms, in being affected in *aisthēsis*, in actively sensing and expressing one's *physis*, the world and the subject emerge—for one moment—as one and identical.

Still, while Aristotle might accede to this unification of *aisthetic* subject and world through momentary unification, his account also allows room for difference and rupture. For instance, he emphasizes that initially the perceptible thing and the perceptive power are different:

> The *aisthetic* power is potentially such as the sensory thing already is in fulfillment, as has been said. So then it gets affected when it is not like, but once it has been affected it has been likened and is such as that thing is. (*DA* II.5, 418a5–6)

Aristotle points to several differences between the aisthetic subject and the world. First, the *aisthetic* subject initially lacks the particular form, which arrives with sensation. Second, the aisthetic subject will, in perception, receive the form of that which is to be perceived, but will not *materially* be similar to its perception.[25] Third, in line with the discussion of acting and being affected in *Physics* III.3, the third difference between *aisthetic* subject and the world as it is perceived consists in a difference of meaning and being: while processes of acting and being affected may connect and be embodied in *one* place or time, their meaning (*logos*) and being (*einai*) are still fundamentally different (*Physics* III.3 202b16–22). This would mean that while aisthetic processes, such as sound and hearing, connect up in one place, these processes themselves—while intersecting—have different meanings.

This implies that the phenomenon of *aisthēsis* is placed in a unique time and place: indebted to both subject and world, it is neither identifiable with, or reducible to, either,[26] because it generates new possibilities in the sensate and new possibilities in the sensible. Thus, through the experience of *aisthēsis*, the *aisthetic* animal is able to derive meaning from, and emerge along with, its other and vice versa.

Aisthēsis is never an experience of "neutral" mechanics, but involves us through and through, and is thus an experience of pleasure or pain, or both. In other words, the discernment that *aisthēsis* brings in terms of seeing, touching, hearing, etcetera is not just a distantiated "seeing something red" or "touching a rough surface," but implicates the self through its own bodily flesh and develops and positions it accordingly, pleasurably or painfully or both. In this, there is no question of a preestablished self, and thus we need to move beyond Chrétien's words of feeling "a response to the appeal made by a sensible that is other than myself."[27] Rather, we need to speak here of a painful or pleasurable *becoming of animal being*, emerging in sensitive transitivity and response to what affects it.

This vulnerable emergence of sensitivity is particularly applicable to touch (*haphē*) since touch operates through close proximity and thus "implicates" us directly.[28] In addition, touch for Aristotle is not only analyzed as one of the five senses, but is viewed as the *foundation* of or key to "general sensitivity,"[29] since touch is the most important form of sensitivity that needs to be in place for an animal to *be*:

> So touch and taste are necessary (*anangkaiai*) for an animal, and it is clear that without touch it is impossible for the animal to be, but the other senses are for the sake of well being. (*DA* III.12, 434b23–25)[30]

Rather than an "accessory" sense, touch is *constitutive* for animal life as such, and not only for its life, but also for all the other senses: "without touch there can be no other sense" (*DA* III.13, 435b2–3). This thought also finds profound echoes in contemporary thinkers such as Irigaray, who, following Aristotle, argues that "[the tangible] remains instead the ground that is available for all the senses. A landscape much vaster but never enclosed in a map, the tangible is the matter and memory for all the sensible." For Irigaray, the tangible accordingly "constitutes the very flesh of all things that will be sculpted, sketched, painted, felt, and so on, out of it."[31]

Aristotle argues that touch is constitutive because, in contrast to the other senses, it does not operate through an external medium but is *direct*. And, as Sorabji speculates, Aristotle might have inherited this idea of directness because of the etymology of the word for touch, *haphē*, which originally meant "contact" and which was still often used that way.[32] If an animal would not be able to sense that something is *directly* touching it, it would not be able to avoid some things and seize others, thus making it impossible for the animal to survive (*DA* III.12, 434b18). Additionally, Aristotle argues that touch includes taste (*DA* III.12, 434b19), and if an animal were not able to taste what is harmful or beneficial, this would make nourishment and existence impossible.

Despite the apparently straightforward approach to touch, Aristotle's account of touch has interesting complications. Where he initially emphasizes *directness* between that which touches and that which is touched, Aristotle later inserts that this directness is only seemingly the case. Just as in the case where a body is simultaneously struck as the thin cloth that is covering it (*DA* II.11, 423b8–13) but still allows distinction between the cloth and one's skin, in the same way the *aisthetic* animal seems to be simultaneously touched as its flesh while in fact the medium *intervenes*. The medium, Aristotle argues in the case of touch, is not an external medium as in the case of the other senses (e.g. air or water), but the animal's own body, and particularly its flesh (*DA* II.11, 423b26–27).

Proclaiming flesh to be the medium of touch is daring and productive, and seems to be the result of Aristotle's willingness to both preserve the idea that every form of *aisthēsis* includes a medium, and the idea that touch has a certain directness to it, which precludes an external medium such as air and water.[33] Assigning flesh the task of the medium in question does double duty in keeping touch both direct *and* mediated. Chrétien speaks in this regard of touch's tendency toward proximity, and its drive to *forget* mediation and distance:

> To touch is to approach or to be approached, not to apply a surface against another. Proximity forgets, through contact, what separates it from the thing that it touches.[34]

While every sensation requires distance (cf. *DA* II.7, 419a13–14, 419a28–30), the sense of touch "forgets" this distance and separation. Touch seems to be contact, but through insertion of the internal medium—flesh—it is always only approximating this contact. And perhaps this forgetfulness is made possible because the flesh does not feel itself in touching and thereby paradoxically becomes intangible[35] even while it is so actively involved in *aisthēsis*, namely as a mean that measures (*DA* II.12, 424a32).

Thus, the enigmatic *medium* of flesh creates the intangible space within which touch happens, and is thereby *constitutive* of touch. As Heller-Roazen formulates it: "the truth of the matter is that every touching and touched term solicits and encounters this element, precisely as that 'in which' all contact comes to pass; every grasp, be it forceful or gentle, exerts itself upon it and within it. Despite its structural inaccessibility, the medium of touch is therefore not impassive."[36]

What this untouchable *hiatus* accomplishes is disrupting an identification of the touched with what is touching it and vice versa, and this brings forth an irreducible openness or "irreducible spacing"[37] to the event of touching. Said differently, touch allows the affective animal body to come to the fore in its most remarkable presence *and* absence—as allowing the world to be relatable to it, but only *mediated*, and never direct. While touch *seems* so direct, the immanent materiality enabling it recedes and withdraws. And I speak here of *immanent* materiality, to emphasize that the place for touch is not one of transcendence, but of implicit, non-thematized materiality. What makes touch possible is an embodied spatiality and temporality, which can vary from one situation (body, species, culture, context, captivity vs. wild) to the next, and is open-ended and fluid.

The untouchable *hiatus* provides the animal affective body a sense of *spatial sphere* (or perhaps better: locale) that it would otherwise not have. Due to the nature of its medium, the touching animal body emerges as taking up space, or, better said, as *inhabiting* space.[38] The nonlocalizable and enigmatic space of the medium of touch ensures that the *aisthetic* animal cannot be identified with its boundaries, escapes narrow confinement to either side of the active-passive division, and presents touch as the paradigmatic sense through which the animal shows itself indebted to alterity, while remaining also radically and absolutely separated from it as well.

Birds, Sensation, and Touch

To give the discourse on touch the particularity, complexity, and depth it needs to explore animal affective ontology effectively, it is important to zoom in on a specific form of animal life. I have chosen to focus on birds, and specifically on the role of bird feathers. The attention given to birds provides a unique way to articulate the nature of the untouchable medium due to the presence of feathers, and provides evidence to correct the distorted image of birds as figures of transcendence, namely by highlighting the specific material, immanent features that inform avian existence.

THE PLASTICITY OF AVIAN *AISTHĒSIS*

Birds speak to our imagination, and specifically when it comes to their ability to fly, to sing, and to be perched up high in trees removed from the banalities and worries of everyday life.[39] In this vein, the birds in Aristophanes' *Birds* offer humans disenchanted with the ruthless, imperialist frenzy of humanity a place for "soft and lovely leisure."[40] Perched up high, flying through the sky, it is no surprise that these "winged singers" have been felt to be "intermediaries" between our earthy existence and another dimension:[41] that of the sun and the gods. Accordingly, romantic poets such as Keats speak of the bird with an almost immortal allure, such as in his poem "Ode to a Nightingale":

> Thou wast not born for death, immortal Bird!
> No hungry generations tread thee down;
> The voice I hear this passing night was heard
> In ancient days by emperor and clown:

The bird's removed stance draws us in, and offers a place to speculate about immortality, transcendence, freedom, and leisure. To offer closer identification with the nightingale, the narrator of Keats's poem "flies" toward the bird at night and embraces its "embalmed darkness." However, in doing so this human narrator must abandon its familiar—visual—knowledge of the world and dwell in uncertainty and "guess."

While the romanticism evoked by the flying bird is attractive, and its connection to forms of transcendence almost inevitable,[42] the tendency to romanticize birds in this way speaks to our own perspective, and our wish to transcend our human, all too human, existence. Birds in this regard provide an interesting medium for our own aspirations and desires, but are not provided a space of their own. If we truly want to do justice to the affective life of the bird, we must, in some sense, start anew and recover in the bird those aspects of immanence that solidly ground it in its material existence.

If we follow Aristotle's idea that it is *aisthēsis* that fundamentally grounds an animal's life, then this forms an important first stepping-stone to clarify the bird's immanent materiality. Pursuing, with Sparrow and Malabou, the notion that "the practical or embodied dimension of sensation" includes the "affirmation that it is sensation that delivers the materiality of the world to sensibility,"[43] it is necessary to uncover this materiality of the world as it shapes and forms the animal body. Opposite Merleau-Ponty's idea that the body remains tied to an identity that can evolve, but "remains what it is,"[44] the alternative proposed here is to underline the dynamism of the mutual formation of animal body and material world. The term *plasticity* captures this mutual formation of body and world, and does not only point to the fluidity of this experience, but also to the fact that, as a material, plastic "cannot retrieve its original form once sculpted or molded."[45] Consequently, the interaction at stake in *aisthēsis* has an irreversible quality, and—given the explosive nature of plastic—may also include a level of "destructive violence"[46] that shows the uneasiness of encountering alterity.

In his *Becoming Animal*, Abram seeks to grasp bird life in terms of its embodied intelligence-in-action, and carefully articulates the complexity entailed in flying. He writes: "here [in flight] it is not an isolated mind but rather the *sensate, muscled body itself that is doing the thinking*, its diverse senses and its flexing limbs playing off one another as it feels out fresh solutions to problems posed, adjusting old habits (and ancestral patterns) to present circumstances."[47] The sensate body of the bird is not only an example of embodied thinking, but also an example of a *temporal* unfolding, as its body speaks to ancestral patterns and its "decisions" engage these patterns in ever-new ways. Pondering the dynamism between bird and wind, Abram speaks of the bird relating to the wind as its "unseen and wildly metamorphic partner."[48]

The issue of *partnership* here is crucial, in that it indicates that a bird's flight is not just a solitary experience, but one lived in interaction and collaboration with its surroundings—wind, trees, water, other birds (in pairs, in formation), and more. Pushing this a bit further, and following Straus's idea that in sensory experience "there unfolds both the becoming of the subject and the happening of the world,"[49] we could say that only in the sensate, muscular motion of flying, the bird *and* the wind unfold and *become* such. In sensing "the speed and direction of the airflow over their wings" through delicate pressure-sensitive sensors,[50] birds adjust their feathers, wings, direction, and height and *become* birds; simultaneously, the wind does not remain static, either, but curves and plays off the bird's body to *become* the forceful and intricate power that it is.

Thus, Abram's and Straus's words enable us to see flying as a *transformation*: there is no question here of static, pre-given identities of bird and wind, but both the bird flying and the wind blowing evolve through the radically plastic nature of their interaction. The partnership discussed here with regard to flying gestures at a larger, encompassing meaning of avian life, one where avian aesthetic life is fundamentally open and fluid but yet solidly embedded in its own materiality. This materiality includes a large temporal, spatial and communal horizon, where ancestral patterns, flight routes, breeding grounds, and pair dynamics all offer evidence of the pluriform factors enabling the bird's fluid aisthetic life.

Bird Touch—On Filoplumes, Interstitial Margins, and the Untouchable Hiatus

> A bird's feather is split . . .
>
> —Aristotle, *Parts of Animals* (IV.12, 692b12–13)

Investigating the materiality of the bird body, and specifically its feathers, is crucial to acquiring deeper insights into avian aisthetic affectivity. I aim to show that the specific materiality of bird feathers—in the form of the highly sensitive filoplume, and the seemingly empty spaces between the feathers—underpins the importance of the interstitial medium. Variations in molting patterns in response to stress and other factors prove the intervening and reconfiguring power of the interstitial place of touch. This allows us to grasp *aisthēsis* even more deeply as affective co-creation, producing an avian existence born out of spatial and temporal reconfiguration within the feathery interface.

Focusing on their materiality, feathers are composed of keratin—the same substance that makes up the horns of cows and the nails and hairs of humans.[51] There are various types of feathers, and the most obvious are the contour feathers, which "include the long, strong wing and tail feathers, but also the short feathers that cover the body and rectal bristles around the mouth."[52] The second kind of feather consists of "fluffy, down feathers" that act primarily to insulate the bird.[53] The third type of feathers, called the *filoplume*, demands particular attention for reason of its appearance and function. Filoplumes, or thread-feathers,[54] are usually hidden beneath the contour feathers. They "have an extremely slender, almost invisible stem . . . and usually no vane, unless a terminal tuft of barbs may be held for such. . . . These are the nearest approach to hairs that birds have."[55] In terms of location, filoplumes are "dotted over the entire body surface and always rooted close to the base of a contour feather."[56]

Filoplumes are remarkable for various reasons. To begin with, they "lack muscles within their follicles and cannot be adjusted or moved independently."[57] Thus, their function is that of sensory intermediaries clustered around and connected with the base and shaft of contour feathers, providing a sense of the wind's speed and the bird's own feather position[58] and communicating this accordingly.[59] Additionally, filoplumes are notoriously hidden (at least in most species), and due to their odd, hardly

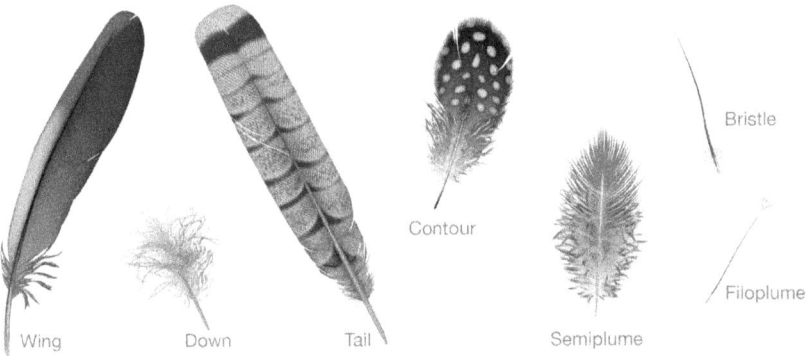

Figure 2.1. Types of bird feathers.

feather-like quality, often overlooked and described—even as recently as the 1960s—as "degenerate, functionless structures."[60]

These two features of filoplumes keenly exemplify and expand Aristotle's ideas on touch. Where Aristotle assigns flesh to be the medium of touch so as to encompass both the mediated nature and seeming directness of touch, the discovery that birds have hidden, highly touch-sensitive filoplumes connected to both skin, wind, and other feathers adds to the enigma and complexity of bodily mediation in animals. These oddly shaped, seemingly only supplemental hair-like feathers actually perform a crucial function in the bird's existence.

Given their function, I contend that filoplumes offer the bird an additional medium to their flesh, or at the very least a sophisticated extension to the medium of flesh. Allowing for this spatial extension is not just a pedestrian act, minimally tweaking biological assertions that feathers are outgrowths of the outer layer of the skin (epidermis), but instead an important philosophical point that argues that the phenomenon of touch in the bird extends beyond the contours of the flesh and takes up space in its interstitial margins. Between the plumes, the downy feathers, and the contour feathers, an intricate layering network of seemingly empty spaces provides sensitivity, insulation, and movement. The spaces *between* the feathers and the *absences* of feather (vane)-structures in the filoplumes enable the sensitive touch of the bird.

This makes it difficult, if not impossible, to discern *where* touch occurs, and this is precisely the point I have been making regarding the nonlocalization of touch. Is it the wind moving the contour feathers, which then move the downy feathers, which then move the filoplumes? Is it the direct pressure of the wind on the filoplumes through openings in between the contour feathers? The nonlocalizable nature of touch in the feathers underlines the fact that an animal takes up its own space, has its own sphere,[61] and cannot be identified with its physical boundaries: it is, as in the words of Plessner, "everywhere and nowhere."[62] To speak of the animal as having a sphere, means that an animal must creatively *mediate* its space in the world, and incorporates what Goldner might call "a latent and perhaps inexpressible knowledge of its own space, place and motion."[63] The bird has its own place, relative to that which we can speak of far and near. As Chrétien argues, "things do not touch each other but are there only for a nearby third party."[64]

Moreover, filoplumes suggest that the interstitial places where avian touch happens "do not give themselves to sensation as a distinct object," similarly to how Chrétien argues that an external sensuous medium does not give itself to sensation.[65] If this is the case, then the *distance* provided by the birds' interstitial feather-spaces is nothing but crucial to the experientially *proximate* nature of touch. It is the tendency of touch to make things proximate, but, as Chrétien points out, touching includes approaching and retreating and distance:

> For proximity to remain proximity, it must always replenish itself with new distance, yet the zealous linearity of its open-ended advance, focused on what we approach, occults all mediation. What allows touch to exercise its function remains untouchable. There is thus indeed an internal veiling of the phenomenon.[66]

In other words, there is *no adequatio* between touch and what it touches. Thus, the interstitial spaces between feathers and the seemingly nonfunctional filoplumes are not just spaces of absence indicating lack of function, but in fact indices of the *untouchable hiatus* that makes any kind of touch possible. For the bird, that which touches thus always remains at a distance, even while it is so close.

The intricate, interstitial layering web of feathers in birds demonstrates clearly that *aisthēsis* goes beyond direct contact and thereby undermines the stereotypical distinctions between active and passive, interiority and exteriority. Locating animal *aisthēsis* in the space of affective co-creation, the overlayered feathery space of absence becomes the immanent meeting ground of affectivity, a mediated space where animal identity is born, not out of similarity, but out of difference.

Interestingly, the process of molting in birds offers a concrete demonstration of the spatial and temporal reconfiguration of the feathery space of affectivity, and specifically offers ways to reflect on how a bird's affective feathery identity is (re)created again and again. Molting allows a bird to replace its old feathers by producing new ones (and most birds molt approximately once a year). While the process of molting in some birds is sequential, with parts of the plumage being renewed one after the other, in other birds, such as ducks and geese, the process is one of simultaneous molting of the entire plumage, leaving such birds temporarily unable to fly.

Since molting happens episodically and repetitively, it allows us to discern the concrete marks that temporality makes on the embodied feathery existence of the bird. Since molting requires significant energy from the animal, it ideally occurs only during periods when there is ample food and no high-energy demands, such as breeding or migration, are expected. Thus, molting marks the affectivity of the avian feather body in its natural, ideal, episodic patterns, with molting as a process of being affected that reconstitutes and preserves the bird, as opposed to a sense of being affected that marks destruction and harm.

Still, because molting sometimes prevents a bird body from being airborne, there is a fine line between the sense of being affected as preservation and the sense of being affected in terms of danger and trauma. For, if molting prevents flight, and prevents a solid protection of the feathery space of (pres)absence and also makes a bird more dependent on larger amounts of food, then it leaves the body open to danger, making it vulnerable. Even when a bird does not lose all its feathers, but only its tail feathers, the distinct "clumsiness in flight"[67] allows potential harm to the avian body.

Thus, molting denotes the marks that temporal, natural patterns make on the avian body, allowing it to reconstitute itself but also, simultaneously, open it up to possible trauma. Reflecting on the intersection of trauma and molting, it is worth noting that some birds have a remarkable "*plasticity* of response"[68] in terms of their molting patterns when it comes to trauma. Katherine McKeever, a researcher of owls, reports in this regard the following: "There is no doubt at all that stress—whether metabolic (starvation, poison) or psychological (continuous anxiety in unsuitable captivity with irresponsible and frequent handling) can utterly defeat the normal molt pattern—even preventing it altogether."[69] Thus, some birds, such as owls, may have protective mechanisms in place in order to *mediate* their submission to the patterns of molting.

In short, the avian body appears capable of a *plastic* temporal reinvention of its feathery space of touch, dynamically reconstituting itself according to the needs of the seasons and other demands. In the next section I will look closer at trauma and how it literally leaves its traces in the bird's feathers.

Avian Vulnerability—On Fault Bars and the (Re)allocation of Trauma

Whereas the previous section explained the interstitial spaces between feathers in terms of the untouchability that makes touch possible, this section draws the space of intangibility wider and deeper, not only in an attempt to do justice to the wider social and natural atmosphere of birds, but also to provide room for the cross-contamination of categories of affective change that involve the *aisthetic* animal in temporal and episodic moments of change (such as molting), as well as moments of trauma and rescue (such as hunger and stress and the release thereof).

The first place to look at in discerning a traumatic place of touch in birds is the concept of fault bars. Fault bars may be found in contour feathers, and are defined as "translucent bands or more rarely spots in feathers, produced by stressful and adverse conditions during feather formation and caused by defective barbule formation."[70] While previous investigations mostly defined these bands or spots as "hunger traces," more recent research indicates that hunger is only one factor among many, and that other causes may include stressful experiences, human handling, noise from traffic, and changes in the weather.[71] When the feather is damaged substantially, it may "tear, lose portions of the vane, or break away entirely."[72]

If we zoom in on the barbules of healthy contour feathers, they emerge as miniscule "projections" at the edge of the barbs of feathers, allowing for interconnection between the barbs. By contrast, fault bars appear through the lack of such barbules, and thus appear as "a thin, translucent line across the feather vane."[73] Thus, fault bars are literally traumatic openings, physical extensions of absence that do not only testify to past trauma, but may also indicate susceptibility to future trauma. For, as Erritzøe describes, "the feather structure becomes weaker with many

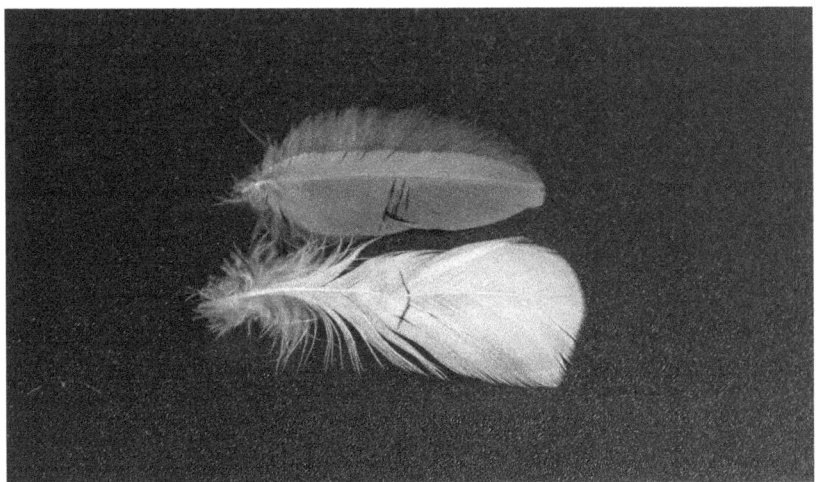

Figure 2.2. Faultbars in the feathers of a grey heron (*Ardea cinerea*) and white cockatoo (*Cacatua alba*).

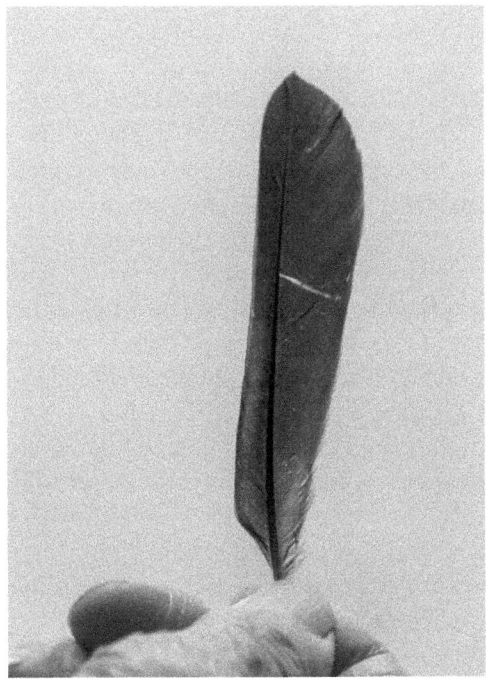

Figure 2.3. Faultbars in the feathers of a European blackbird (*Turdus merula*).

fault bars,"⁷⁴ and when the feather breaks, "the feather will not be renewed before the next molt."⁷⁵ Erritzøe therefore argues that to have many of these fault bars is a great handicap for a bird, because it decreases the animal's maneuverability, therefore making in an "easier target for a predator."⁷⁶

The etymology of the term "fault bar" offers further clues to its philosophical relevance in the context of affectivity, suffering, and *aisthēsis*. With the Middle English "fault" deriving from the common Latin *fallita*—"a failing, coming short"⁷⁷—the emphasis turns to being or becoming deficient and *absent* (and which might, in some of the connotations of "fault," be a blamable quality or feature). In other words, with the fault bar we acquire insight into the absent space of trauma, of a trauma that seemingly leaves nothing behind, but in fact, literally speaking, constitutes a truly absent untouchable space: a space where barbules do *not* extend and do *not* touch, a space where inner corporeality and solidarity is left wanting. For growing feathers, trauma intervenes in the interstitial space of possibility and *enlarges* this space to facilitate increased exposure and vulnerability to demise, predatory or otherwise.

Thus, fault bars clarify and magnify (in a perverse direction) what avian touch usually is successful in, in terms of flourishing: co-creating and interconnecting the body with itself while remaining open to the other. In trauma, the fault bars represent a different kind of untouchable space, namely, one where, due to increased *absence*, the space of mediation literally and figuratively thins out, possibly foreclosing on *aisthetic* opportunities, successful flights, and a flourishing avian life.

What fault bars clarify (through the absence of barbules) is that feathers are not solitary but that each feather is a community of parts, and that trauma gives rise to a split in this community, which in turn might predict harm to the entire being's existence. A feather is not just a feather, simply used for flight or touch; rather, each feather is a community of connected projections into space, with each space crossed over and interlinked from one side to the next. This is a space of protection and openness, and too much openness in its "membranes" will predict danger and cause it harm. The potential harm associated with such fault bars might be temporary, for if an animal survives until the next molt, then (given absence of current stressful experiences or nutritional deficiencies) healthy feathers might grow in.

But, if multiple feathers show fault bars and if the bird has too many broken feathers, this predicts badly for the bird. Here, the avian feathers may literally *remember* in their structure past trauma and accordingly project the individual and the species into a vulnerable future.[78] This makes us wonder whether there is a parallel to the reaction of plants to trauma and whether the embodied "memory" that plants have for trauma has echoes in avian embodied life. As discussed in chapter 1, damage to apical buds in a plant may result in suppressed growth in areas close to this damaged area, even while these adjacent areas themselves still have full potential and are not themselves directly traumatized. In addition, through epigenetic changes, plants may "communicate" trauma and its corresponding reaction to trauma to future generations. Might there be ways where trauma to feathers is still visible in the feathers or adjacent areas even after molting, or is there a way to communicate and transfer such trauma (and the reaction to such trauma) to future generations?

As Erritzøe reports, based on research in the American Kestrel: "from year to year the same individual produced the same number of fault bars."[79] Might this indicate that signs of *trauma* may be continuously mimetically reproduced, even years after the initial exposure to stress? Or do these continuous fault bars over the years indicate the ongoing nature of stress in the bird, indicating the existence of high or low stress tolerances?[80] And what is the genetic and epigenetic story of fault bars?[81] If it is the case, as Erritzøe indicates, that a bird species that was disproportionately targeted as prey of the Sparrowhawk has *fewer* fault bars than in the general population, then what does this say about the power of memory, as embodied by genetic and epigenetic patterns, and its ability to change the vulnerability and susceptibility of birds to trauma and fault bars?

Remarkably, a new theory suggests that birds have fascinating ways to *mediate* the location of feathers with fault bars and thus may allocate spaces of absence to less vulnerable spots. This theory, called the "fault bar allocation hypothesis," argues that a bird "can develop adjustment mechanisms that reduce fault bars on feathers that are important for flying."[82] To explain this theory, Erritzøe cites a study of white storks where the fault bars were mostly located on the inner-wing feathers rather than at the outer wing, making them less susceptible to flight problems than they otherwise might have.[83] If this study of white storks is representative of a general avian strategy in response to harm, then their reallocation of fault bars offers additional evidence that animals can reorder and restructure their own affective space of touch, including their place of traumatization.

The idea that the "sediment" of trauma can be reallocated, literally and physically, to a different embodied space where it might be less destructive, offers powerful proof of the embodied negotiation and mediation between the animal body itself and its emergence in the world. The bird body is not what it is, and its failure to identify both with itself and the world, even in trauma, is a powerful testament to the avian mechanisms that enable the possibility to rewrite and re-signify present and future trauma. If trauma may be minimized by literally dis-placing and reordering it, then this indicates (1) that the avian body as such is always already shifting and dynamic, and never identical to itself and the world, and (2) that its future is both informed by sediments of the past as much as lived in light of a temporal horizon that is always already still becoming. In its dependence on the past, it will remain dependent and constrained, but in its capability to re-signify the meaning of events, an avian future also indicates the promise of being open-ended and ambivalent.[84] The *material* reinvention of space in trauma signifies the reimagining of the meaning of trauma, and needs to be distinguished from a sheer psychological space of traumatic unfolding.

Bird Bonding—On Allopreening, *Synaisthēsis*, and Community

The previous section focused on avian vulnerability and indicated that the untouchable condition of the possibility of touch may leave visible traces in the case of trauma (in the form of fault bars) but also enables a reinvention of embodied space and a rewriting of the meaning of trauma. However, in rethinking the place and meaning of avian trauma, our investigation hovered more or less on the level of the individual bird and the interstitial spaces of its feathers. In this section, I seek to expand the meaning of the untouchable condition of touch more broadly by including a discussion of avian allopreening, that is, birds tending to the feathers of another bird. By expanding the untouchable hiatus to include a bird's social context, I hope to achieve not only a further deepening of the place and meaning of affect and touch, but also to acquire more clarity about the meaning of bird identity in relationship to its avian other.

It is well known that a bird may preen itself, that is, "tend its feathers with its beak, arranging, cleaning, and generally maintaining them."[85] It is less well known that birds may also engage in allopreening, which is tending to—preening—the feathers of another (*allo*). Such behavior may sound familiar in primates such as monkeys, who allopreen to socialize and remove parasites off each other, but its occurrence in birds is far more rare. Still, as Birkhead argues, socially living birds "have much in common with primates,"[86] and allopreening in birds is an indicator of shared affective terrain.

In his account of owls engaged in allopreening, Marzluff describes how staring at a partner and cooing low may solicit such behavior. In case of a positive response, the partner stares back. Edging up and sitting next to the other, birds usually face the same direction, close their eyes, and groom each other "by picking through the feathers."[87] In the spotted owls that Forsman and Wight discuss, allopreening occurred most often after the young were fledged and the adults had time to themselves. For some pairs, it was almost a daily activity.[88]

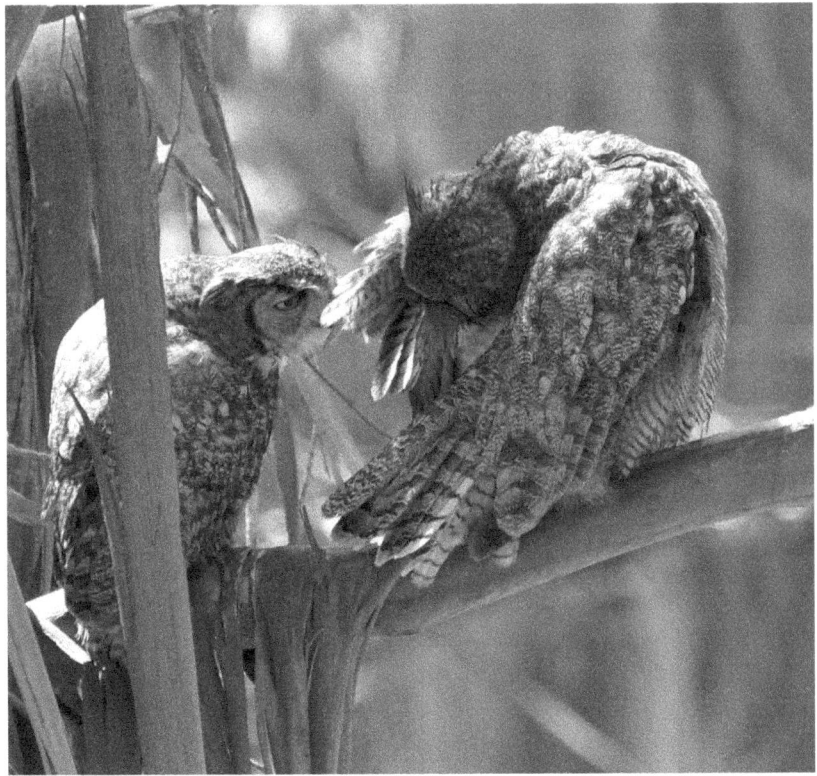

Figure 2.4. Two horned owls allopreening: the owl on the left is assisting the other owl with preening.

Allopreening consolidates bonds[89] and facilitates the removal of dirt and parasites, with beneficial effects thus extending beyond one's kin[90] to permeate the community at large.[91] Especially since allopreening is predominantly oriented at the bird's head and neck, which it cannot reach itself, the benefits of mutual allopreening may include a double orientation to oneself and the other within the wider community.[92]

Given the proximity of birds in allopreening, birds expose themselves to the possibly powerful but also delicate touch of the other's beak. Since the bird beak is extremely touch-sensitive yet simultaneously hard, sharp, and forceful,[93] allopreening is indicative of the remarkable vulnerability and openness of the bird body as it emerges through and with others as part of the avian community.

Allopreening in many ways emphasizes and magnifies the crucial insights that Chrétien's reading of touch in Aristotle's *De anima* presents. In Chrétien's account, touch pledges the organism to the world, "exposes it to the world and protects it from the world. Touch bears life to its fateful, or felicitous way."[94] Allopreening in birds deepens these insights, since it indicates that the emergence of the avian body is not only in dependence and response to the (natural) world, but also crucially a response to its avian other, who through touch exposes it to, and protects it from, the world.

With that, the interstitial space of touch draws wider and deeper. Where touch is made possible by the physical and metaphysical space of the in-between,[95] that is, the *lacuna* between the feathers and the untouchable *hiatus* as such, respectively, allopreening extends this space. In the first place, quite literally, the interstitial space between feathers is physically further opened up in allopreening as a bird exposes its feathers and skin to the other. Simultaneously, the new space opened up is immediately interwoven and intersected by the presence of the other—its beak, its feathers, and so on. Thus, as the beak of the other carefully and diligently cleans out and thus empties the affective space of touch, it simultaneously creates a new affective space where self and other are intertwined. Further, in cleaning and bonding, allopreening renews and co-creates the feathers in their protective, sensitive, and insulating function. In other words, allopreening affords us a glance at the sensitive, social side of touch, as birds together create space and meaning for each other by literally recreating their plumage.

The interstitial space between feathers thus draws wider and deeper in that the bird body emerges in its dependence on the bird other. In the case of trauma and fault bars, our discussion earlier indicated the possibility of birds rewriting and reorganizing the meaning of trauma in the reallocation of their traumatized feathers. Here, with allopreening, the possibility to rewrite the meaning of bird life and bird trauma from a social perspective affords more complex possibilities, in that allopreening may prevent or alleviate trauma in others, maintain and strengthen the affinity and affection for each other, and afford refined pleasure in life. In its most positive expression, what may emerge from allopreening are lifelong friendships, as in the case of guillemots, whose friendships develop over twenty years in intense allopreening practices.[96]

Focusing on the more negative reasons for allopreening, the need to prevent and alleviate suffering for each other may extend beyond the pair bond, as Birkhead recounts in the case of the enormous oil spill of the super tanker *Torry Canyon* along the coast of Cornwall in 1967, the UK's worst oil spill. Birkhead reports how a tick-infested guillemot prompted the other birds in the group to fall "over themselves to preen the infested individual."[97] The guillemots he describes sense trauma *en masse* and seek to prevent further suffering, gathering as a group to remove the ticks from the affected bird and seeking to protect the community from being infested by parasites. Allopreening here serves to protect both the individual and the group, and in opening up and interconnecting anew the space between feathers, the social fabric of communal avian being is also being rewoven.[98] Sadly, such behavior may be potentially harmful to the group, too, because in allopreening especially oil-infested birds, the preening birds may ingest oil, which can lead to life-threatening conditions such as "ulcers, pneumonia and liver damage."[99] In other words, trauma may be alleviated through allopreening, but allopreening may also physically and socially endanger the avian community.

Notably, the trauma at stake need not be purely physical to solicit allopreening. As Birkhead notes, allopreening often occurs after stressful social interaction, as a way to soothe each other. If the stress is intense, such as in woodhoopoes' battle with their neighbors, the allopreening afterward is equally intense, leading ornithologists to emphasize the correlation between allopreening and stress reduction.[100] The correlation between allopreening and stress reduction speaks to the meaning of reassigning and restructuring avian meaning through embodied, affective, social practices.

As Aristotle writes, the life of friendship (*philia*) is that of association or community (*koinōnia*) (*NE* IX.12, 1171b32–1172a1), and implies living together (*sudzēn*). Notably, this communal life is one in which the friend emerges as a second self (IX.9, 1170b7). Crucially important, in the *Nicomachean Ethics*, Aristotle states that such a communal life participates in *sensing-together*: *synaisthanesthai* (*NE* IX.9, 1170b4, b10).[101]

Even if Aristotle's analysis is geared at *human* friendship, his focus on *synaisthanesthai* may render much. For, if our analysis of touch in birds so far has been correct, then by extending Aristotle's account of friendship to include *synaisthanesthai* in birds, we may learn that avian touch at its apex involves nothing but a crucial restructuring of the meaning of *aisthēsis* through community, where the *aisthēsis* of one individual is made possible and informed by the *aisthēsis* of yet another individual. Here, *synaisthēsis* is not simply the sum of its constitutive parts but signifies a recreated meaning of existence, similar to how cohabitation or shared living (*sudzēn*) does not simply mean the addition of another person in one's home, but the reevaluation and co-creation of a new shared space and a new shared sense of temporality. Said differently, the action of adding the prefix "syn" or "co" to the front of verbs that represent the constitutive activities of living and sensing radically alters the meaning of those activities in light of the value of a bigger community in which they take part.

When these newly established affective, *aisthetic* communities face trauma, death, and finitude, birds may be radically affected. In this regard, Birkhead in *Bird Sense* recounts the story of a goose who died, and whose partner goose remained next to its dead partner for an entire week.[102] Here, it is hard not to suggest mourning, specifically in the face of a description of a behavior that so poignantly seems to embody loss. Still, we need to be careful to universalize this claim about mourning to all birds in similar situations, since in some cases birds seemingly easily get over such loss, as in the case of a male crow who, having been with his female partner for thirteen years, within days of her death found another female partner.[103]

What the above examples show is a range of affective behaviors solicited by trauma, finitude, and death. None of this behavior, I argue, would have been possible had it not been for the affective, embodied, social practices that make up the world of meaning of avian life. At its center stands touching and being touched and what enables it: the absent yet not impassive physical and metaphysical space of the untouchable. Crucially, affective touching offers a place for community formation, and the implementation and emergence of new and different senses of spatiality and temporality.

Conclusion

This chapter has argued that Aristotle provides us with an account of *aisthēsis* that—despite assertions to the contrary—depends for its meaning and function on other categories of change (qualitative change and substantial change). The consequence of this categorical contamination is that *aisthēsis* is fully immersed in the whole range of affective changes, including not only sensibility, but forms of qualitative change, trauma, coming-to-be, and demise. Beyond categorical contamination, the generative and synergistic nature of *aisthēsis* points at a prominent metaphysics of affective fluidity, which brings into view an *aisthetic* animal whose being and affectivity are not only indebted to the other, but who emerges and becomes along with the other through interaction.

In its focus on birds and bird feathers, this chapter contends that the condition of the possibility for avian touch lies in the untouchable interstitial space between the feathers. This untouchable space of absence is the immanent meeting ground of affectivity, a mediated space in which animal identity is born out of difference, and where flourishing, pain, trauma, and demise literally leave their traces. Interestingly, as new research on fault bars shows, birds may allocate and consequently re-signify this place of trauma, proving the embodied mediation of the animal body with itself and the world. Powerfully, the example of allopreening serves to explain how the re-signification of avian life is also indebted to the social fabric of avian life, which can accordingly explain powerful ways of preventing and diminishing trauma in others and lead to lifelong bird friendships.

As we have seen, the untouchable space between feathers can be opened up in several ways: as a consequence of molting or trauma, for instance, or due to allopreening. Still, the opening-up of this space goes hand in hand with powerful mechanisms to close it off again, so as to regrow new feathers, re-allocate traumatized feathers, or to re-signify the meaning of intimate friendships. All of this proves avian life to be part of a metaphysics of affective fluidity.

The next chapter continues this metaphysics of affective fluidity, but with a focus on the mammalian, human placenta. The placenta, as we will see, brings along with it yet another form of affective embodiment, and specifically one that *mediates* between the coming into being of two lives: baby and mother. Physically located in-between, it offers us a *medial* space to rethink boundaries on a concrete level, and the language of immunity and hospitality will serve to clarify the continuous border-opening-and-protection that is at stake in this special "organ."

Chapter 3

Generative Human Affectivity

The Placenta as Place-and-Time-Making In-Between

It was the feather that took me to the baby's umbilical cord. The feather, that element of bird, so formed, so groomed to catch the wind and lift, that one-time part of a whole flying.

—Linda Hogan, *Dwellings: A Spiritual History of the Living World* (1995, 19)

Nature itself provides us with some teachings about what hospitality could be in our time. For example, if a woman can give birth to a child, and even to a child of another gender, this is possible because, thanks to the two, a place in her is produced—one could say in Greek *gignestai*—that does not belong to the one or to the other, but permits their coexistence: the placenta. Neither the woman nor the fetus could survive without this organ that secures both the existence of each and the relation between the two.

—Luce Irigaray, "Toward a Mutual Hospitality" (2013, 44–45)

[T]he place coincides (*hama*) with the thing, for the boundaries (*ta perata*) coincide with the bounded (*peperasmenōi*).

—Aristotle, *Physics* (IV.4, 212a30)

Introduction

No. I did not insist to keep it—not even a part. Presented to me in a clinical plastic bowl, I saw it as an afterthought to the birth of my baby. Yet, somehow intrigued by it, I urged that a picture be taken of it. Of it? The neutral, abstract term I use chills and surprises me. For, somehow, I have felt all along that an injustice has been committed to this being, these beings, that have sustained me, my (and in fact: all) children in utero.

The previous two chapters explored the affective existence of plants and animals. Chapter 1 discerned the conceptual importance of the middle voice for grasping nutrition, growth and diminution, and trauma and illness in plants, and chapter 2 analyzed *aisthēsis*, and specifically touch, in birds, arguing that the untouchable space of absence—located predominantly in the interstitial space between feathers—should be understood as the place of affective mediation where animal identity is born out of difference, and where flourishing, pain, trauma, and demise leave their traces.

This third chapter is devoted to grasping the inner logic and affectivity of the human placenta. My goal is to engage the placenta before and beyond the unobtrusiveness and lifelessness with which it ends after birth,[1] and to demonstrate its generative, affective power as much as possible *on its own terms*. What needs rethinking is the fixation on the placenta as an *after*thought or *after*birth: even when assessed as extra-fetal-organ with a functional embryological role, it is still considered of lower ordinal importance and thereby easily cast aside as no longer part of an ontology of childbirth. But must we accept this subordination of the placenta to the merely *after*, or point instead to the placenta's enduring ecstatic and material trace of the co-emergence of self and other that persists in mother,[2] child, and species?

The placenta, I argue, is more than what the neutral and almost pejorative term *extra-fetal organ*[3] conveys: physically located in-between mother and child and generating their identities, the term "maternal-fetal organ"[4] is insufficient as well. While the placenta had been previously considered as merely a static "inert" barrier, keeping the circulation of mother and child apart, new research shows the placenta has far more permeability and plays a key generative role, actively synthesizing, secreting, and transporting molecules affecting both mother and child.[5] Given its generative role in affectivity,[6] I speak of the placenta as a fetal and maternal place-and-time-making boundary.

Importantly, if the placenta is to be thought in both material and ontogenetic terms, namely both as a formative anatomic organ and as a place for ontogenetic invention, we must ask how this generative place-making, this hospitality, becomes materially constitutive of mother, child, and placenta alike.[7] This generative affectivity could be what Elizabeth Grosz calls the "unlivable memory of the species, the inaudible themes that make and regulate living bodies, [which] are the directions or orders, the temporality, of formation and functioning that enable the individual members of species to form themselves and once formed, to act, and to do so in the distinctive ways that represent the actions, potentially all of them, of their species."[8]

In this, to focus on the place and role of the human placenta affords us a deeper look at human affectivity *as it is generated*. Here, we find no fully developed, independent human selves (since even becoming a mother is what is to be developed), but rather early conditions for human lives and what makes them come into being. Foregrounding more intricate, social, human relationships, this place of generative human affectivity involves a complex and profound negotiation of "the difference between the 'self' and 'other.'"[9] The placenta as medial boundary constitutes a place and time for the encounter and becoming of mother and child, not only as sapient beings, but in their very nature. Before and beyond the difference between self and other, the placenta offers a model of *affective symbiogenesis* where selves come into existence in and through the very materiality of one another, contradicting the presumed "immunitary logic of self-preservation."[10] Moreover, even after its factual "demise," the human placenta's residue in the form of microchimeric, ritualized, and social traces reminds us that organisms are all but static, but rather, thoroughly mixed, prone to change, and full of specters of future possibilities.

In this chapter, Aristotle's and Heidegger's notions of *topos* and *physis* will provide further philosophical grounding to this conception of the placenta as place-making boundary, specifically in allowing us to think of pregnancy in general and the placenta in particular as the place-and-identity-making boundary of intertwined and unfolding lives. Where in the previous chapter the openness of the bird feathers was deemed crucial to the bird's touch, both in terms of vulnerability and protection, here the placenta as generative boundary is folded inside, unfolding, creating and constituting various forms of life. With an eye to such ontogenetic development and growth, this chapter will also address the various forms of temporality that are secreted by the placenta, left by contact with both mother and child. Traces of such contact are present in the form of microchimeric cells left in the bodies of both mother and child, which may have harmful or beneficial effects for their future lives.

My account of pregnancy, as analyzed with and through the placenta, focuses on this organ of the in-between that builds, constitutes, and regulates the (emergent) living conditions for the pregnant milieu.

My analysis does not deny that, before or after pregnancy, other semantic, emotional, logical, and social dimensions intersect with this phenomenon. In this regard, I do not reject the idea that there was a pre-pregnant self or that there will be a post-pregnant self (nor that these selves may be at odds) and that there may be a self that in some way endures.[11] Relatedly, from a more ethical and political angle, my project does not argue that pregnancy—as a reproductive phenomenon—needs to be the prescriptive norm for leading meaningful human lives. Rather, my reading has a different focus: it emphasizes the material, affective forces of the placenta and the embodied pregnant milieu these forces give rise to. And, instead of being prescriptively the norm, it argues, factually and retrospectively, that any human life as we know it owes its existence to this in-between organ that ensured a pregnant milieu. Moreover, as Hill also articulates, focusing on the placenta as in-between, as "interval between woman and fetus is to articulate pregnancy as a function of her body rather than as woman's sole purpose."[12] How exactly this material phenomenon and its enduring trace (in the form of microchimerism) informs the semantic, emotional, logical, and social strata of the pregnant woman and the future child, and how this intersects with the different "selves" of the pre- and post-pregnant woman, lies beyond the confines of this chapter.

As I emphasize the materiality of the affective forces that the placenta institutes, I will also highlight the importance of the pregnant community as it emerges, which I will cast in Plato's language of city-state (*polis*), thus resulting in my chosen term "pregnant city." I will draw attention to the fact that, interestingly, this community or city does not disappear once pregnancy ends and the placenta—as organ—dies. Instead, this community is spatiotemporally implaced in the biological lives of those who, so-called "independently," remain (mother and child). This, in turn, underlines the importance of rethinking community as it underpins not only the formation, but also the continuation, and future, of our lives.

The Placenta: An Initial Encounter

My own reaction to the placenta as a new mother, with which I started this chapter, is not my only direct experience with this organ. Years before I became a mother, I was assigned, as a medical intern, to collect placentas after childbirth, to briefly examine them for ruptures and abnormalities, to check the umbilical cord for abnormalities in vessels, and then to

Generative Human Affectivity 83

store them in a large freezer destined for research.[13] Holding them in my latex-gloved hands, the placentas were still warm, full of blood, but, oddly removed from their functionality, they seemed *out of place*: lifeless, heavy, dense, yet deflated compositions of flesh and blood that had completely lost their connection to both the living being that suddenly could survive "on its own" and the mother, within whom it had dwelled all its life.

My own impressions—as a mother, and as a medical intern—both speak to a similar, underlying issue: namely, surprise and even shock at the fact that the placenta can undergo such radical transformation from serving as life's most crucial underpinning to cast-aside, superfluous waste. And even with recent developments such as placental dietary supplements or cord blood banking that place the placenta squarely within the sphere of biomedical, biopolitical, and capitalist power structures,[14] what it values (even when it comes to harvesting stem cells) still betrays the remarkable unique co-generative and co-constituting affectivity that is internal to the placenta. Hence, I seek to contest the subordination of the placenta to

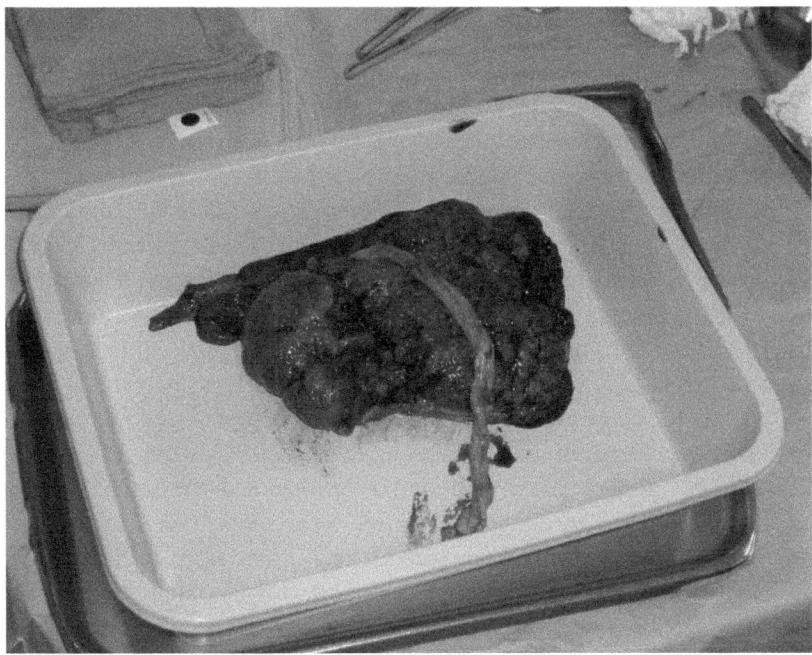

Figure 3.1. Placenta post-partum in clinical hospital setting.

the merely *after*. Integral to the dynamic process of ontogenesis that I am sketching are the enduring places and temporalities that the placenta creates in co-affectivity. Accordingly, I seek to emphasize the placenta's generative and constitutive affectivity and its enduring ecstatic and material trace of the communal bond between self and other that is not only a mark of a past sublated, but also its material condition of possibility.

In the next section, I will discuss the complex and profound negotiation of the difference between "self" and "other" through the topic of *mimesis*. I will do so to craft a *placentology* that accounts for the possibility of ontogenetic becoming in the mother-child-placenta triad, a becoming that breaks with a linear genetic history of origin and authenticity to shape, with a nod to Plato's building of a city (*polis*), what I shall call the *pregnant city*.

Placental (Re)presentation: *Mimesis*, Self, and Other

The placement, origin, and function of the placenta encourage us to revise our thinking about the generation of selfhood and difference. First of all, the placenta's location elucidates much about its being, and offers a helpful starting place for rethinking of identity and difference. In Loke's words: "the placenta spends its entire life outside the baby, but within another individual, the mother, where it is intimately attached to her womb."[15] Loke emphasizes here the in-between placement of the placenta, externally connected to the baby, and internally harbored within the mother's uterus. Its anatomical placement has previously been considered to underpin its presumed "barrier" function, keeping the circulation of mother and child apart. However, as new research has shown, the placenta is far more "active" than previously thought, as it creates and synthesizes molecules for nutritional and metabolic support, regulates hormonal "information" systems, and is heavily involved in immunology.[16]

Thus, its placement "on the border" is deceptive insofar as the placenta does not serve merely as an inert passageway or passive border but actually "sends signals to both the mother and the fetus."[17] Here the term "conduit for information" might seem appropriate, were it not that the placenta is even more powerful than that: "in many cases it is the *originator* of the signals."[18] The "molecules of life" that it produces indicate its active role: it creates nutrients, enzymes, hormones (such as growth hormones and estrogen), and cytokines—"small secreted proteins released by cells [that] have a specific effect on the interactions and communications between cells"[19] and that play an important role in immune responses, inflammation, and other processes.[20] Some of these molecules "have structural functions, others function in metabolic processes, some in information signaling and regulation, and some in immune function."[21] In short, the placenta offers concrete nutritional and metabolic support, creates and regulates hormonal "information" systems, and plays a key immunological role allowing for and sustaining pregnancy.[22]

Given these functions, we could argue in more philosophical terms that it is the placenta's task to offer the ontological and physical conditions of the possibility of making the growth and development of both mother and child possible. And when we focus more specifically on the representative role of the placenta in relationship to the fetus, the placenta's function might be comparable to that of Plato's ideal guardians fostering the youth.

The comparison of the placenta with Plato's guardians, and the comparison of pregnancy with Plato's building of an ideal city (*polis*) in *logos*, may seem odd. However, for multiple reasons, appealing to Plato's *Republic* offers analogical strengths. First, my reading of Plato's "model city" seeks to hold onto Plato's conception of unity and community building, as well as to his idea that a cohesive community stands or falls by the dedication of its leadership to the whole of the community. This implies, for my interpretation of the pregnant city, that I grasp the phenomenon of pregnancy as the emergence of a community, which is dependent on the higher order logic of supervision represented by the placenta.[23] And, where Plato's philosophical guardians rule their city from out of a specific hierarchy and encampment, with dedication to the city and sacrifice with regard to their happiness,[24] I similarly cast the placenta as situated in a specific zone, generating and ruling the pregnant city not so much from a top-down position or by holding property in common with its own cells, but by giving rise to the pregnant city from out of a nonoriginating beginning (the in-between), sharing its life-generating products with the city, while sacrificing, ultimately, its own life (as an organ) to the pregnant city and the emerging lives of mother and child.

Moreover, Plato's account of guardianship is particularly apt because his ideal guardians watch, test, approve, and deny what crosses the borders of the *polis*,[25] and create the proper nourishing grounds for the educational, psychological, and athletic trajectories of the community's youth. Similarly, in producing and metabolizing nutriments, in selecting and denying damaging materials, and in carefully opening the borders where needed, the placenta plays a "border" function analogous to that of the guardians in Plato's *polis*, ultimately fostering growth and development of new human life.[26]

Simultaneously, despite embracing certain aspects of Plato's "ideal city" in the *Republic*, I strongly reject Plato's account of philosophical leadership and his idea that reproductive labor needs to be ruled and regimented by philosophical guardians.[27] In fact, I argue for a strategic subversion of Plato's city and his ideas of reproductive labor, in that I seek to replace his idea of philosophical leadership with that of the material leadership and logic of the placenta. Thus, while holding onto the idea of community building as well as dedicated leadership, I replace Plato's notion of rational guardians—who emulate and desire an immutable form and live their lives following a metaphysical logic—with the fully physical and embodied logic of the placenta that produces emerging and changing forms.[28] The result of this is to present an account of biological community building that is not built from a top-down idealism of pure, immutable forms or rational paradigms, but is, conversely, a generative logic that secretes changing, emerging forms from out of its material basis. And, notably, this generative logic does not simply *allow* the other parts of the city to emerge, but also regulates and connects them, similar to Plato's ideal guardians who watch, test, approve, and deny what crosses the borders of the *polis*.

My reasoning thus subverts Plato's thinking and simultaneously shows us that Plato's metaphor of building a city is helpful in a very different context, namely as applied to thinking about (1) the genesis of a pregnant milieu, (2) its unity and the relationship to its three main parts, (3) the sacrifice of some of its parts, and (4) the mimetic representation across the various parts. In making this argument, I push Plato's ideas strategically beyond his problematic appropriation of reproductive labor for his own account of philosophy, and, instead, by appropriating parts of Plato's account, sketch an alternative story of biological community with full attention for the material, and ontogenetic, components of our emerging-together.

While I will address the issue of placental place-and-community building in the next section of this chapter, it is important to first address here the topic of placental mimetic (re)presentation, in that it speaks to the issue of "identity and difference" and seeks to disrupt the original-copy distinction that guides much of the common discourse on the placenta-embryo relationship. Sloterdijk, in *Bubbles*, zooms in on the unique, unconditional, irreplaceable commitment of the placenta to the child, and calls the placenta the child's "placental double,"[29] or its "innermost second element."[30] Sloterdijk's choice to name the placenta the "second" or the "double" of the baby with whom it forms a holistic bubble sparks reflection on the nature of the mimetic relationship between child and placenta. Whereas traditionally the baby is considered to be *first*, and the placenta as merely its material "copy," Sloterdijk's words encourage us to see the baby and the placenta as fully engaged in a holistic alliance. By understanding the placenta as "catalyst and mediator"[31] of our generative existence, our human existence would be judged incomplete or false were we to deny the placenta's constitutive role.[32]

This raises the interesting issue of originality, identity, and difference. If the potential baby is not the "first" and the placenta is not the "second," how could we better understand their relationship within the logic of the mimetic as much as possibly exceeding it? If we look at the scientific, embryological aspects of the story, even the commonly expressed idea that the placenta is "derived entirely from the baby"[33] and is thus "genetically part of the fetus"[34] encounters complication. For, in the very early stages of human development, after conception, there is only *one* type of cell—blastomeric cells—and nothing seems to differentiate those cells to commit toward either trophectoderm (the precursor cells to the placenta) or inner cell mass (the precursor cells to become the embryo). What will define their cell lineage specification is simply their *location*: when they are externally located, these blastomeric cells will turn to placenta-forming cells, and when they are internally located, they will become embryonic cells.[35] If we follow through on this thought, we could argue that the pre-existing spherical whole of blastomeric cells acquires qualitative distinction by differentiating into the inside and outside of a whole.

Thus, we can speak at the very early stage of the pre-embryo and the pre-placenta of an identical grounding—with difference created by placement over against each other, and specifically by the determination of cells that are *outer versus inner*. No essential difference delineates what will become placenta and child, simply placement relative to each other. Philosophically, this reveals an almost unfathomable unifying identity between precursor-placenta and precursor-child with placement as the determinant of each one's fate.

Beyond this initial stage of identity, the blastomeric cells consequently split up into two cell lineages that give rise to the existence and respective "autonomy"[36] of child and placenta.[37] Here, at least initially, measured in sheer size[38] and autonomy, the placenta seems to have a stronger presence than that of the child, since the placenta could survive even if the embryo were not able to,[39] which is certainly not the case the other way around, at least not until a much later stage.[40] Added evidence for the importance of the placenta is that as its cells further grow and develop, it starts to produce all the key "molecules to life" and thereby grows into the kind of self that *represents* the embryonic self on an almost "higher" and "more primordial" level given its higher-order materiality and oversight. As Loke writes: "Indeed, the placenta dominates the life of the baby, rather than the other way round."[41] If we relate this back to Plato's concept of guardianship in the *Republic*, then his account also seems to emphasize that the class of guardians have a strong and essential function in *constituting* the lives of citizens as they emerge; arguably, the role of the placenta in dominating and constituting the life of the fetus/baby is similar.

Said more strongly and directly: from an earlier purely identical relationship between pre-placenta and pre-embryo cells, the placenta grows into the kind of complex being that at least initially appears to be more autonomous (both qualitatively and quantitatively) than the other being (child) it is said to represent. Would this mean that we would need to see the placenta after the initial holistic mirroring stage as the then more independent and initiating self who becomes a role model for the baby's self? Not only conceptually, but also experientially, this reversal might encounter revolt. Why? Appearance has much to do with it: for who would prefer to call the amorphous, bloody fleshy mass without elegant proportions (lacking head, rump, and limbs), sense-organs (in the traditional sense), and a conventional "brain" the *primary self* of the two selves? Additionally, its apparently temporary[42] and ultimately expendable function may also explain why we would prefer to grasp the placenta as "secondary" to the other "self."

We need to grasp the relationship between placenta and embryo beyond that of pure identity (as in the first stage where they share similarity by being composed of the same blastomeric cells) and beyond that of a mirroring model (which seems at least superficially to apply to the second stage). Instead, the changing relationship between placenta and child over time may best be grasped through the German term *Darstellung*, which is often used in the context of discussing mimesis. *Darstellung* means to present, and specifically to present something to someone: it is the act of "placing (*Stellung*) there (*Da*)."[43] In aesthetics, it accordingly signifies "that which an art work *presents* or *offers* up."[44] This means that *mimesis* does not mean the sheer doubling of an original reality that is already there, but rather indicates the expression, interpretation, presentation, and putting-into-place of a reality. As Gadamer writes in *Truth and Method*:

> The situation basic to imitation that we are discussing not only implies that what is represented is there (*das Dargestellte da ist*), but also that it has come into the There more authentically (*eigentlicher ins Da gekommen ist*). Imitation and representation are not merely a repetition, a copy, but knowledge of the being (*Wesen*).[45]

If it is the case that the relationship between placenta and baby pivots around this complex form of mimesis, then the placenta is not simply a double or substitute for the baby, nor is the baby simply a double for the placenta, but the placenta brings about, knowledgeably, through *Darstellung*, a *mediated instantiation, localization, and presentation of the meaning and being of the new, emerging life*. And when Gadamer is using the term "authentic" (*eigentlich*) for the process of *Darstellung*, he refers to the fact that it is not the original that is truer or more authentic, but precisely the representation that installs the truth of the process. For the process of *Darstellung* as I seek to analyze it, related to the placenta, Gadamer's interpretation entails that in the representation that is the placenta, a particular meaning of the baby-to-be emerges and presents itself that would otherwise not exist.

Following Gadamer's interpretation of artworks in terms of *Darstellung*, Lotz emphasizes that "what presents itself in the representation is not something static that could be immediately identified; rather, it comes into being and remains 'fluid' throughout."[46] Additionally, following Lotz's Gadamerian interpretation of *Darstellung* in the form of a performance of a play, in which "the being of the character is indeed *constituted* throughout the performance,"[47] I seek to signal that *Darstellung* not only includes fluidity, but also the *establishment* of emerging being within a relationship. For the interpretation of the placenta, this means that placental representation will establish itself in meaning and embodiment according to its relational engagement with itself, the baby, and the mother.

Summarily, then, the *placentology* presented here stimulates us to revise conceptions of originality regarding ontogenesis and to rethink the meaning of selfhood and alterity in the triad mother-placenta-fetus. Genetically, in being derived from the same cells of which the fetus will be composed, the placenta initially emerges as the mirroring double of the fetus. However, functionally, over time, the placenta emerges as the (re)presentation of the baby's self. Not appealing to a "truth" that it represents, it instead functions as a Dar-steller, that is, as *installer and presenter* of what it is to be a self.

These ideas regarding mimesis and *Darstellung* encounter further depth and complexity when we examine the relationship between placenta and mother. For the placenta also changes the woman's physiology by producing and taking over functions of her biological system, such as growth-hormone production, which is otherwise produced by the woman's pituitary. Already in decline in the second trimester, the production of growth hormone by the maternal central nervous system ends completely in the third trimester and is then taken over entirely by the placenta. It is surmised that this leads, among other things, to certain effects such as "inducing relative maternal insulin resistance" and reliance on lipolysis, thereby effectively "sparing glucose for maternal brain and fetal/placental metabolism."[48]

This act of placental substitution is philosophically significant. In the case of growth hormone takeover, the act of substitution signifies the placenta as designated (re)presentative and originator of change of maternal physiology during pregnancy. Whereas the woman's physiology prior to pregnancy may have engaged in homeostasis ("maintaining an internal state in support of viability"[49]), the placenta is involved in changing this state to the new physiological state of allostasis ("changing an internal state in support of viability"[50]). The fact that the placenta does so not by just adding factors to physiology, but by changing its metabolism from the inside out is thought provoking. For we have here an organ that hijacks a system's principles from the inside out/from the outside in in order to bring about an altered state of being. Provocatively, we could speak here of the placenta as extra-maternal organ (instead of extra-fetal organ).

The act of placental substitution that transforms the potential mother's state from homeostasis to allostasis allows the potential mother to function differently during pregnancy, and her altered state also benefits the placenta's and the child's functioning. For instance, due to changed maternal metabolism, a sufficient flow of glucose can be ensured.

Combining the above insights, placental substitution is in fact not a singular act of substitution, but a substitution, presentation, and *Darstellung* on behalf of *three* lives. The placenta offers the ground for the possibility of existence, and also allows different, material, spatial beings to come into existence. It is a *presentation* rather than a representation in that it brings into place—following Gadamer's ideas—and instantiates "knowledge of being"[51] in both offering regulatory insight and material instantiation and direct material excretion of its knowledge. The act of placental substitution in the case of growth-hormone takeover is astounding: this is an organ that not just "knows" what needs to be altered, but also puts it into place. The placenta can thus be the regulating organ as well as the actual material pituitary replacement and instantiation as well.

Thus, with a nod to Plato's *Republic*, we could argue that the placenta offers a subversive notion of Plato's guardianship. Similar to Plato's guardians, the placenta offers regulatory knowledge; however, the placenta is different in that it does not offer guidance through emulation of transcendent ideas, but through material instantiation and direct material excretion of its knowledge. Moreover, where Plato's guardians seek guidance in a transcendent ideal, the placenta allows, through *Darstellung*, for the meaning of itself, the baby-to-be and the mother-to-be to emerge fluidly. And finally, where Plato's city depends for its location upon the tilling and working of the interface of soil,[52] the beginning of the pregnant city is built on the interstitial organ of the placenta: it thus builds community out of the in-between as much as it gives rise to individual, differentiated existences that have their own function and being, yet depend on each other for their existence. The placenta generates by enforcing maternal change in the form of *allostasis* and enables on the side of the fetus and itself *allogenesis:* the growth and creation of a whole new other life.

Similar to Plato's ideal city that prioritizes the well-being and unity of the city over its individual components,[53] the placenta equally represents the well-being of the pregnant city as a whole, which might be detrimental to some of its parts. For instance, pregnancy can have very dangerous, and even deathly, consequences for the pregnant woman, such as preeclampsia and severe bleeding. Overall, the placenta's mimetic relationship to both mother and child indicates a stage beyond mere doubling, genetic repetition, or simple co-existence: what is at stake is an originary ground that allows beings to come into existence in and through the very materiality of one another. Integral to this dynamic process of ontogenesis is the place and time the placenta creates in co-affectivity.

The Placenta as Boundary and the Establishment of Place

The previous section discussed *Darstellung* without a focus on the actual issue of place connected with the *Da* ("there") that is crucial to grasping the role of the placenta. The placenta's place and its place-making capacities are remarkable as they speak not just to place, but to the underlying *physis* (nature) that emerges alongside with this coming-into-place. Loke's words speak to the placenta's location and its corresponding function:

> In the uterus, the placenta occupies a position midway between the baby and mother, in a kind of "no-man's land." . . . From this position the placenta is well placed to monitor and regulate all communications between mother and baby. It effectively acts as a gateway controlling what passes through . . .[54]

It could be argued that the placenta does not just determine what crosses the border, but is the actual border between mother and child. What is helpful in Loke's remark is the focus given to the placenta monitoring, regulating, and controlling communication. This demonstrates the higher-order logic of supervision that the placenta embodies. Moreover, the fact that the placenta offers regulation from its *medial* position, inserting itself in-between mother and child, simultaneously indicates a nonhierarchical, nonoriginating beginning,[55] reminiscent of Marder's words regarding the place of germination of plant seed, which, in his words, "commences in the middle, in the space of the in-between. That is to say: it begins without originating and turns the root and the flower alike into variegated extensions of the middle . . ."[56]

Undoubtedly, the placenta is unlike plant seed due to its spatial placement *between* mother and child (vs. being caught up in-between the growth of the plant itself in terms of roots and flower), but nonetheless it evokes a similar notion of mediality and nonoriginality where it concerns the growth and development of mother, child, and placenta alike, and allows mother and child not just to be "the originators" to which it is simply the hardly apparent in-between, but, to apply Marder's words in a different context, prove mother and child to be "variegated extensions of the middle,"[57] that is, products and extensions of the placenta.

With this thought—namely, seeing the placenta not just as by-product but as in-between nonoriginating beginning that brings into place a "new physiology" (*allostasis*) of the future mother as well as "new life" (*allogenesis*) that is the future child—we are also well positioned to see the weakness in Loke's quote above, since the placenta is more than just a gatekeeper between two beings, located in a "no man's land." The placenta in fact *creates a place* and is thereby not located in the vacuous zone of negative space, but precisely the opposite: in a zone of emergence. More than a gatekeeper, its material conditions allow mother and child and itself to emerge as this place unfolds. The placenta is not the bridge that connects what had already been asserted before. Rather, the placenta brings into place the emergent realities of motherhood and child.

Heidegger's account of place in *Building Dwelling Thinking* further deepens this thought: for him, *things must themselves be places*.[58] As Mugerauer clarifies, for Heidegger, "the primal scene does not begin with fixed, pre-given objects in a containing pre-given space which then are arranged into a desired or intended design."[59] Heidegger's example of the bridge as place is telling:

> it [the bridge] does not just connect banks that are already there. The banks emerge as banks only as the bridge crosses the stream. The bridge expressly causes them to lie across from each other. One side is set off against the other by the bridge.[60]

The bridge that Heidegger talks about is not inserted into an empty space outlined beforehand. Rather, the bridge allows "a place to come into existence."[61] If we extend this way of thinking to the placenta, then the placenta is not the bridge that connects what has already been there (mother and child), nor is it being placed in the no-space, that abstract space[62] without actual space of place,[63] the "no man's land" that Loke speaks of. Rather, the placenta brings into existence a place. Like the banks of a river, mother and child emerge as connected yet differentiated beings because of the place-making presence of the placenta. Various cultures pay homage to the placenta's place-making presence, for instance by burying the placenta under a fruit tree in the ground,[64] or by using one word—such as in the Maori language—to indicate both place and placenta: "whenua."[65] In both ritual and language, the placenta is regarded as the ultimate place-maker that not only generates place and life for the born, but can also establish a new connection for the born to the earth and all life that grows there.

Perhaps surprising, Heidegger's account of place is actually quite close to Aristotle's definition of place,[66] particularly in that place, for Aristotle, is coincident with the thing, and is defined by way of its boundaries:

> Further, the place coincides (*hama*) with the thing, for the boundaries (*ta perata*) coincide with the bounded (*peperasmenōi*). (*Physics* IV.4, 212a30)

The notion of "thing" here is slightly deceptive, if only because for Aristotle place is primarily connected and dependent on the motion and rest of *natural* beings, that is, beings that are by nature (*physis*).[67] In this regard, his rejection of the void depends on the fact that the void could not serve to explain the motion or rest of such natural beings. Thus, his account of place as "concrete place"[68] is intimately and primarily grounded in his account of nature, and specifically in defining what the concrete place of a natural being is, so that it would account for its motion and rest.[69]

This stipulation is important, as it clarifies Aristotle's account of place and offers a particular, productive edge for our analysis of the placenta. If it is the case, as Aristotle argues, that place is coincident with a natural being, and if place is defined by the boundaries from which a natural being unfolds, then the placenta emerges as the natural boundary and place-maker of human life.

Before we unpack this further, let us turn toward clarifying the meaning of the boundary in clearing and freeing place, as worded by Heidegger:

> A space is something that been made room for, something that has been freed, namely, within a boundary, Greek *peras*. A boundary is not that at which something stops but, as the Greeks recognized, the boundary is that from which something *begins its unfolding*. That is why the concept is that of *horismos*, that is, the horizon, the boundary.[70]

With this clarification of Heidegger on the role of the boundary as "that from which something begins its being"—that is, unfolds—we find a way to sharpen our definition of the placenta, namely as the natural boundary from which both mother and child begin their unfolding and encounter their place. Notice here the shift from Heidegger's singular to my plural: the placenta is unique in providing the boundary and thus the place not for one being, but for two (and perhaps three, if we include the placenta itself).

Further complexity can be brought in once we take Aristotle's idea into account that place, as a *where*, is essentially "a mode of being-in,"[71] that is, "being in something else" (*en allōi einai*; Physics IV.2, 210b24) and what is bounded "should not be thought of as contained by another body; rather, it is immediately in the limit, i.e. place."[72] This means that the limit is not *another* place, but in fact is different insofar as it is *constitutive of place*.[73]

Should we translate this back to our account of the placenta, then the placenta emerges as the natural boundary and constitutive principle of the place of both mother and fetus, both of which are defined by this boundary that encloses them and yet lets them emerge and makes them possible.[74] The place-making capacity of the placenta finds further etymological support in the Ancient Greek language: the Greek word for the vessel holding liquid that Aristotle uses to illustrate place in the *Physics* is *angeion* (208b2–23, 210a24), which does not just designate vessel, but also *afterbirth*.[75]

Perhaps it sounds odd to think of the pregnant mother here as being bound by the placenta. If we are thinking through the spatial, Euclidean dimensions, then we find the fetus bounded by the *inner* boundary of the placenta, which then finds an *outer* boundary in the uterus wall, which is then enveloped and carried by the mother. However, this more traditional and "mathematical" placement of the mother as the container within which another container (her uterus) envelops placenta and child in fact does *not* contradict the alternative and more primordial account of place, boundary, and place-making provided above. For, in Aristotle's and Heidegger's interpretation of place, the limit or boundary is a constitutive principle that *grounds* a being and provides it its concrete place. Principles that "normally" would define inside and outside are thereby shifted. Accordingly, the placenta can be thought of as both the material and ontogenetic principle that allows a pregnancy to unfold: from the mother's perspective, as an outer limit, internally connecting her to new life, and as an inner limit establishing an altered physiology and a new state of being within herself. From the fetus' perspective, the placenta provides also both the *inner and outer* limit, externally providing connection to the mother, and internally mediating itself with itself and mirroring what it may become.

Insofar as pregnancy involves multiple beings, we could argue that both the mother and the child are determined by this larger process as such and thereby find themselves *placed and part of, enfolded by* this larger boundary of the placenta as place-maker as such. As Jeffrey Malpas writes,

> One of the features of place is the way in which it establishes relations of inside and outside—relations that are directly tied

> to the essential connection between place and boundary or limit. Already this indicates some of the directions in which any thinking of place must move—towards ideas of opening and closing, of concealing and revealing, of focus and horizon, of finitude and "transcendence," of limit and possibility, of mutual relationality and co-constitution.[76]

This idea of mutual relationality and co-constitutionality is particularly applicable to the placenta's role in pregnancy. The placenta's existence and growth and changing function over time in dialogue with the fetus and mother make it hard to talk of the co-existence of mother, child, and placenta. The issue here is not co-existence, but rather co-constitution of identities *in and through one another*. Life does not live nor unfold and grow within a container, autonomous and fenced off, but rather is determined by the boundaries between inside and outside that limit and enable it. In other words, "places always implicate other places . . . they extend out to be inclusive."[77]

While Aristotle's account—supplemented with Heidegger's reading—is very helpful in discerning the placenta's role as place-making boundary, his account of place also leaves room for the kind of criticism leveled at him by Irigaray. Irigaray argues that any account of place needs to include embodiment, and that the interval (*diastema*) between bodies that Aristotle rejects is in fact present and "must be thought of as extensive and embodied."[78]

Although I disagree with Irigaray's critical assessment of Aristotle's account as one centered on the notion of "containers" in light of my foregoing argument stressing the notion of *natural and concrete place* in Aristotle versus that of abstract space, the force of her argument lies in critiquing the empty, disembodied limit that would constitute a being's place. This account of the limit denies that place is always embodied, and that its boundary is both in physical and metaphysical community with that which is inside and outside of it. The same problem prompts Irigaray to reject Plato's concept of the *chōra*: in Irigaray's reading, the *chōra* stands for a nonintelligible, empty, inscriptional space.[79]

As Irigaray reads Aristotle's own *aporia* regarding the question whether place may grow along with the growing thing whose place it is (*Physics* IV.1. 209a28), she writes:

> at issue is the extension of place, of places, and of the relation of that extension to the development of the body and bodies.

An issue either forgotten or ignored in the junction of physics and metaphysics, since these two dimensions have been set aside or dislocated, but an issue still alive today.[80]

Irigaray's critique is poignant, in thinking through the *material* embodiment of a thing's place in light of its growth and development.[81] In addition, woman, in Irigaray's view, has so far been supposed "only to be a container for the child, according to one moral position. She may be a container for the man. But not for herself."[82] What Irigaray seeks is a definition of place that grants that "each of us (male or female) has a place—this place that envelops only his or her body, the first envelope of our bodies, the corporeal identity, the boundary, that which delineates us from other bodies."[83] Only when both female and male *is* a place can a meeting between male and female occur.[84]

But what would happen with Irigaray's criticism if we provide the factual physical embodiment to the limit and interval that she is seeking with the physical and conceptual notion of the placenta that envelops both mother and child? Here in fact Irigaray's most recent thinking of the placenta as the natural "third" that mediates between mother and child[85] could be used to provide an account of our own most unique natural boundary and serve as an argument against her earlier argument that it is the mother that is necessarily to be seen as the obvious container. To quote from her recent article on mutual hospitality:

> Nature itself provides us with some teachings about what hospitality could be in our time. For example, if a woman can give birth to a child, and even to a child of another gender, this is possible because, thanks to the two, a place in her is produced—one could say in Greek *gignestai*—that does not belong to the one or to the other, but permits their coexistence: the placenta. Neither the woman nor the fetus could survive without this organ that secures both the existence of each and the relation between the two.[86]

If we rethink the position of the boundary with the placenta, we acquire a significantly positive notion of place, namely (1) as horizon and limit, committing ourselves to look both beyond and inside ourselves, (2) as an embodied, concrete interval, emphasizing our embodied interaction with ourselves and the world, (3) as a medium and a mediator between different lives, where the natural space of the placenta can co-constitute identities and let them grow alongside each other, (4) as opening up the possibility of growth and enabling growth both inside and alongside the border, and (5) as enabling an interval that both presents future possibilities, confronts us with our past and mortality, and does not hold us captive within the present.

In other words, given Irigaray's positive appreciation of the placenta (as a mediator between identities) in her recent writing, we could argue that the placenta as place-maker offers the position of a unique, corporeal boundary that allows both male and female its own, concrete place. And perhaps we could even contend that the placenta as place-maker finds a positive precursor in Aristotle, insofar as he (versus Irigaray's own earlier interpretation of *topos* in the *Physics*) provides for a notion of *topos* that is based concretely on the motion and rest of beings that emerge by nature, and specifically with regard to their boundaries.

When we fill in what concretely constitutes the most initial, unique, and primordial boundary of our lives, we find an ambiguous body—the placenta—that in its functioning and regulating grounds not just one life, or two lives, but mammalian life as such. Thus, the placenta provides a form of "originary granting"[87] that is key to *how* places may come about. The placenta's granting is the concrete manifestation of this nonarchical, participatory happening of human place.

Placental Mediation: Immunology and Hospitality

> Childbirth isn't only an offer of life, but it is the effective site in which a life makes itself two, in which it opens itself to the difference with itself according to a movement that in essence contradicts the immunitary logic of self-preservation. Against every presupposed interiorization, it exposes the body to the split that always traverses it as an outside of its inside, the exterior of the interior, the common of the immune. This holds true for the individual body, but also for the collective body, which emerges as naturally challenged, infiltrated, and hybridized by a diversity that isn't only external, but also internal.
>
> —Roberto Esposito, *Bios: Biopolitics and Philosophy* (2008, 108)

Placental place-making can also be grasped from the perspective of immunology and hospitality. The medial place of the placenta, in-between mother and child, allows the placenta to function as the immunological "face" of the child, insofar as it offers the closest (re)presentation of the child with which the mother stands in contact. In Loke's words: "It is the placenta that connects the baby to the mother at the site of implantation so how the mother 'sees' her placenta rather than her baby is what determines the outcome of her pregnancy . . . the placenta lies in between."[88]

Maternal hospitality cannot be understood without the role of the placenta, and in fact is made possible through it. In principle, the maternal immune system would reject the embryo since it consists of foreign, "not-self" material[89]—or, if we are precise—it consists of "semi-not-self" or "semi-self" material since the embryo is genetically half-maternal.[90] Hence, in order to host a pregnancy, some kind of "protective mechanism"[91] must be in place. The placenta plays a key role in this, and one of the ways it can take root is by *not* producing tissue antigens (such as HLA-A, -B, -C complexes) that would spark a defensive maternal reaction.[92] In more philosophical terms, by making itself immunologically neutral or invisible, the placenta makes itself the *faceless* (unrecognized) face of the other (the baby), and thereby is allowed to live in symbiosis with the mother. We might call this technique one of forcing hospitality upon another—based on appearing to be more neutral or similar than might be the case. The faceless face of the other here is notably not transcendent to the process, but materially part of it.

However, this is only a small part of the placental-maternal immunological story. For successful placental implantation and growth depends on a constant negotiation between invasion into the uterus and restraining this growth. An embryo's genetic material is half due to paternal genetic contribution, and half due to maternal genetic contribution; the maternal immune system accordingly negotiates between two genetic forces: one force that seeks to invade into the uterus due to "paternal genes [that] promote growth of the placenta"[93]) and one force that restrains this growth (due to maternal genes).[94] And this negotiation—between promoting and restraining growth into the uterine wall—can be made possible only if the maternal immune system *does recognize* self versus nonself.[95]

Still other biological mechanisms are in place to facilitate the hosting relationship. For one, the placenta is also very *active* in fending off the mother's defense mechanism.[96] Moreover, by producing progesterone, which is (among other things) needed for the mucus lining of the uterus to maintain pregnancy[97] and has an immunosuppressive effect,[98] the placenta has another way of protecting itself and the baby. And, most interestingly and provocatively, through pregnancy the mother's immune system is partly encouraged to *reverse* its defense mechanisms, and turn them into acts of hospitality: the natural killer (NK) cells (i.e., a type of white blood cell that is part of the immune system) that in the case of a transplant would be activated to reject—and kill—tissue, instead produce substances that *promote* the growth of particular placental cells.[99]

This latter mechanism involves perhaps not only a remarkable shift of the immune system, but also a backtracking, re-constitution, and evolvement of the maternal immune system. The philosophical significance of this is astounding: a system that is aimed at protection (of "self") can actually reverse its function, and instead of protecting itself turn toward collaborating with the growth of the other. Since recognition of the placenta/baby as *other* is necessary to host it, Esposito in *Immunitas* writes that "what allows the child to be preserved by the mother is not their 'resemblance,' but rather their diversity transmitted hereditarily from the father. Only as a stranger can the child become 'proper.'"[100] From the perspective of the placenta, this means that its possibility to create a home for baby and mother lies in presenting and negotiating difference and self, and offering a re-constituted notion of home where immunity is not the opposite, but the condition of the possibility for community.[101]

And here is where the story of maternal-placental immunology in dialogue with the narrative of hospitality becomes even more interesting. While it is the case that some autoimmune diseases, such as systemic sclerosis, may actually flare up or develop during pregnancy or post-partum,[102] studies indicate that other autoimmune diseases, such as rheumatoid arthritis, actually improve or even vanish completely during and after pregnancy.[103] This would mean that increased maternal recognition and hospitality of the baby through pregnancy might not only create a place to meet the other, but also *oneself*.[104] Somehow, through placental mediation, the mother's self can better realize herself through better recognizing herself *as* self instead of mistaking herself for another.[105]

In other words, placental mediation not only offers a home to baby and placenta, but may also offer the mother a more refined home to encounter herself. In this regard, Irigaray's interesting thoughts on auto-affection acquire a whole new meaning: she speaks of the need to "discover, and in part rediscover, a relation of intimacy with ourselves that allows us to stay in ourselves when relating with the other."[106] Pregnancy offers yet another way for auto-affection to prove its meaning, since it provides a physical and metaphysical encounter of the female body with itself, and may provide the point of departure for an altered and respectful coexistent becoming.

Toward a Genuine Sense of Hospitality: Place-Making, Temporality, and Microchimerism

The placenta's medial existence and function promote a rethinking of the primacy of originality and copy, of self and other, of boundary and place, and of hospitality and immunology. If we zoom in on the hospitality offered by pregnancy, room must be created for an alternative model to the current one, which far too simplistically views the mother's hospitality as one in which pregnancy is merely the filling of a hollow container, similar to thoughts that view hospitality as a form of receiving that "fills up a void with an alien presence."[107]

Gabriel Marcel defines authentic hospitality as a practice that means "to admit in or welcome an outsider into one's home."[108] He concludes that hospitality involves the other to *participate* in one's home; consequently, he speaks of hospitality as "a gift of what is one's own, i.e. of oneself."[109] And Esposito reminds us that pregnancy is only possible by welcoming the child as radical "other" and encouraging the maternal immune system to develop the needed factors to offer this "outsider" a place within one's self.[110] This would mean that pregnancy is an ultimate act of offering hospitality to the other who becomes part of the self.

However, the hospitality that I seek to address here is even more far-reaching in that it goes beyond this act of maternal hospitality, or even the hospitality that the child affords to the mother by providing her a new place in pregnancy to encounter herself."[111] Placental mediation namely grants a constitutive kind of hospitality that allows us to rethink and redefine what home as generative place-making might mean. As a physical and metaphysical place where different lives can become who they are through dialectical opposition and mediation with the other(s), the placenta breaks through "the immunitary logic of self-preservation"[112] and transcends ordinary conceptions of self and other by redefining "home."

If we ourselves have been made possible by such an original place-and-being-making entity as the placenta, then current studies of *microchimerism* assure us that the placenta's radical place-making abilities still live on as material traces in our bodies. Microchimerism is the condition where genetically diverse cell populations co-exist within one individual (constituting less than 1 percent of the total number of cells).[113] The most common form of natural microchimerism is through placental exchange of cells in pregnancy, but it can also happen in spontaneous abortion, in the case of transfer between twins, and possibly in cell transfer "from an older sibling or previous pregnancy of the mother" to the fetus.[114]

Maternal microchimerism designates the presence of maternal cells in her children, and fetal microchimerism indicates the presence of fetal cells in the mother.[115] Interestingly, the maternal body is more susceptible to embracing such microchimeric changes in pregnancy, as research shows that the blood-brain barrier may also be affected in pregnancy, allowing more permeability.[116]

What is fascinating about microchimerism is its pervasive range (for instance, fetal cells have been found in the brain, thyroid, heart, lungs, liver, kidney, and skin of mothers many years after childbirth),[117] its duration (with fetal cells found recently in the brain of a ninety-four-year-old woman),[118] and the fact that women who have been pregnant may host various generations of cells due to their own pregnancies, that is, they accommodate "multigenerational microchimerism."[119] This demonstrates that different genetic populations with different timelines pervasively and enduringly encode our bodies.

However, the medically and philosophically most intriguing aspect of microchimerism is that fetal or maternal cell populations are firmly integrated into our bodies, generating cells and actively mediating our physiology and pathology. With a versatility that has been compared to stem cells,[120] fetal cells for instance may repair maternal tissues such as the brain or heart, may halt or promote growth of tumors,[121] or may offer benefit in cases of autoimmune diseases such as rheumatoid arthritis; they may also impose risks, such as in systemic sclerosis.[122] Conversely, maternal cells found in children may offer them protection (as in the case of children with diabetes type I)[123] or may be potentially harmful, as maternal cells have been found in the hearts of neonates born with neonatal lupus who died from heart block.[124]

The ambiguity of the physiological and pathological meaning of the long-term residential "immigrant" microchimeric cells that inhabit our bodies is in my view firmly connected to the pre-originary hospitality that the placenta represents. The placenta's place- and homemaking qualities are not committed to one being solely, but to the creation of multiple identities through one another. Consequently, the cells that pass through its permeable border and take up residence "elsewhere" may reflect a similar commitment to fostering the "whole," without necessarily contemplating whether such mixing of cells is physiologically beneficial, neutral, or pathological for the *specific* individuals emerging from what I have previously called the "pregnant city."

Plato's ideal city—which I have used before as a template for the "pregnant" city—explicitly prioritizes the well-being of the whole of the city over its individual parts or groups.[125] Likewise, we could argue, the placental remnants and traces of the pregnant city after birth signify an equal commitment to the well-being of the whole but not necessarily to its individualized parts. Thus, an ambiguity may result where mothers and children alike may either suffer or benefit from the placental mediation that made them possible. In fact, emerging identities of the pregnant city after birth may *both* ultimately suffer, but in different ways, as in the case of infants with trisomy 21 who might suffer from severe cardiac abnormalities, and whose mothers have a "fivefold increased risk of Alzheimer's disease."[126] In leaving microchimeric traces, the placenta proves enduring commitment to the broader community, as the microchimeric cells it leaves behind are mixed throughout various bodies. Thus, the traces left behind by the placenta as organ of the in-between map collective time onto individual time and project beings accordingly into the future. This placental process of community making allows for various forms of life to emerge, and resists to see generation solely as discrete and individuated, but as co-affective, relational, and communal.

As microchimeric traces of the pregnant city shape our bodies, the "verdict" of harm versus benefit need not be one-sided or static, as its physiological or pathological assessment will be prone to temporal changes. A sign of the temporal fluidity of microchimerism is that healthy *trans-generational* microchimeric shifts are needed to support a successful pregnancy.[127] This means, for instance, that "maternal cells acquired during fetal/neonatal life seem to be replaced by fetal-derived cells when females enter the reproductive phases."[128] Moreover, during pregnancy older cell lines—of the pregnant woman's mother (so, cells of the current fetus' maternal grandmother)—may increasingly *re-emerge* in the mother's blood.[129] An additional sign of temporal change affecting the future is that fetal cells, when housed in maternal bodies, will *age* over time and affect their function, and the same applies to aging maternal microchimeric cells, prompting questions as to whether their aging will make them more prone to malignant transformation.[130]

Thus, we could argue that, as human, temporal beings, our pathology and finitude is subject to different timelines encoded by the various kinds and various ages of the genetic populations that we hold. Especially in the case of "multigenerational microchimerism,"[131] such different timelines point at a plurality of differently mixed futures. Such an anarchic, mediated signification of the future may be physiologically ambiguous: it may entail a longer life span for the mother,[132] but may also bring about "an increased risk of Alzheimer's disease with increasing number of pregnancies."[133] Thus, our bodies are not only a microcosmos of our genetic connections, but also residue of multiple timelines mixing, crossing over, and unfolding anarchically and a-linearly within a temporal horizon entailing alternative futural pathologies and finitudes.[134]

Conclusion

This chapter has argued that the placenta is the initial, unique, and primordial boundary that in its functioning, organizing, and place-making capacities grounds not just different emerging material lives (from homeostasis to allostasis for the potential mother, and allogenesis for the potential child), but the pregnant city as such. It is a *Darstellung*—a *presentation* rather than a representation—in that it brings into place, instantiates, and secretes the knowledge to found, sustain, and promote the pregnant city. The placenta—as pivotal in-between—founds anarchically a participatory happening of place, where beings come into existence through the very materiality of each other. The placental boundary grounds place, and as such both limits and opens up to other places. In organizing and constituting the pregnant city, in selecting and denying damaging materials, and in carefully opening the borders where needed, the placenta functions much like the original guardians in Plato's ideal *polis*, ultimately fostering growth and development not just of the youth, but of new life as such.[135]

The placenta's life as *individualized, material living* organ is temporary, and similarly temporary is the material infrastructure of pregnancy.[136] However, the constitutive role of the placenta continues, albeit in different forms, seeping "beyond the present to the past and to the future."[137] First, in cultural rites such as burial rites of the placenta, the placenta is explicitly allowed to continue its existence in emplotting the newborn in the earth and the ground. Second, we could argue, with Broin, that the "residual after" continues on in new social relations that co-constitute and co-develop identities,[138] allowing for yet another (social) *in-between* to reconstitute the life of the placenta. Third, as the phenomenon of microchimerism shows, the placenta's grounding function lives on as the non-messianic, material, microchimeric trace that redirects the futures of mother and child alike by mixing cell populations and inserting itself in ambiguous ways, constantly allowing identity to be born out of difference, by constantly generating new boundaries and new places of contact.[139] The liminal place that is originarily the placenta's thus lives on in the mixed, constantly transforming, natures and futures of our bodies.

The original *chimera* invoked in the term "microchimerism" is in Greek mythology a fire-breathing monster that combined "a lion's head, a goat's body and a serpent's tail."[140] While in mythology this monstrous chimeric being had to be killed by the hero Bellerophon, the phenomenon of microchimerism instead points at one of the life-sustaining traces made possible by the placenta. Instead of death, microchimeric cells, combined with local, earthly reminders as well as social residue, encourage us to rethink the nature of our intertwined identities. These traces of the placental in-between ask us to reinstall the original generative hospitality made possible by the placenta. The exteriority that is part of all of us may serve as an ethical[141] and political reminder to practice the openness and hospitality of which our bodies are the living traces.[142]

Chapter 4

Skin and Human Sapient Affectivity
Skin, Webbed Existence, Temporal Depth, and Trust

Without contestation, the skin defines the interface between the inside and the outside, two worlds that are, by the way, inseparable. What would become of the inside, if it ignored the outside that surrounds it?

—François Dagognet, *La peau découverte* (1993, 17)[1]

Interior and exterior, opaque and transparent, supple or rigid, willful, present or paralyzed, object, subject, soul and world, watcher and guide, a place where the fundamental dialogue with things and others happens and where it is most brilliantly visible, the skin bears Hermes' message and what remains of Argus.

—Michel Serres, *The Five Senses:*
A Philosophy of Mingled Bodies (2008, 52)

Bourgeois-individualist positivism established—against weak resistance from exponents of soul-partnership Romanticism—the radical, imaginary solitary confinement of individuals in the womb, the cot and their own skin throughout society.

—Peter Sloterdijk, *Bubbles: Spheres Volume 1:*
Microspherology (2011, 384)

Introduction

Skin-to-skin, my newborn baby rested on my belly. Smeared with blood, covered in vernix, she was nothing but naked, fragile, soft, and warm. The distinctive closeness of her skin on mine was worlds, and ages, away from the amorphous pressure and movements felt inside until just now. Her placement on the skin made all the difference.

No longer filled out, stretched, or translucent, my skin bulged yet imploded, was left empty, much of it suddenly ridiculously superfluous. By connecting skin-to-skin, a new spatial and temporal configuration of our skins, beings, and togetherness came to be explored. Brought together by the common edge of the skin, one sapient sentient being merged and emerged alongside the other.

Caught in the middle, human *pathos* lets itself predominantly be *felt*. Thus, where the previous chapters focused on the middle voice and plants (chapter 1), sensation and birds (chapter 2), and generative affectivity in the form of the human placenta (chapter 3), in this chapter I will seek to carve out the meaning of human *pathos* in light of its felt—that is, sensitive-sapient—affective terrain. The *affective mediation* I have argued for so far—in terms of the middle voice in plants, feathery mediation in birds, and placental mediation for the generation of human lives—reemerges here in the form of an exploration of the interface of human *skin*.

From surface to depth and identity, from barrier to communicator, from nature to culture, the human skin affords a place for seemingly contradictory concepts to meet each other. Not only that, but the skin also affords a broad look at human affectivity due to its obvious biological aspects (and not only its static presence as organ, but as biologically evolutionary form), its sociological and political dimensions (for instance, as is readily accessed as the social construction and racialization of skin), and its individual underpinnings (e.g., the engineering of one's own skin through the choice of make-up, tattoos, etc.). Instead of a *mere* surface, the skin—much like its evolutionary and embryonic twin, the brain—provides thus the depth, health, meaning, and mooring of our existence.

The human skin provides us a unique and productive lens to grasp and assess human sapient, sentient affectivity, and doing so will offer an important complement to studies that locate human affectivity predominantly in the brain. The advantage of focusing on skin lies in demonstrating how a large part of our human form is not just centrally determined by the inside, nor simply imposed from the outside, but actually materially informed and produced by the inside's exterior. My thesis is that skin provides a novel look at humans' material and ontological affective depth, since skin is as much the site of the interface with (and the product of) the evolution of biology, history, technology and society,[2] as it is the site for individuated and political engineering, where critical and ethical choices and actions can be made and subsequently effect the composition of the very interface's conditions of possibility. Thus, in contrast to a narrow perception of skin that sees it merely as a container geometrically placed in space, I argue that an inquiry into our skin is fundamental to grasp the place of co-emergent creation where humans "can appear as those who they are."[3]

Extending this argument from a more spatially oriented trope to that of time, the skin also affords us new insights regarding the deeper *temporal* structure that underpins human lives. The skin *lives* our age, future, trauma, vulnerability, and finitude, but not merely mimetically so. On the skin, events are not simply stamped and inscribed as they occur, but they are put together, synthesized, according to a deeper temporal order than that of mere chronology. Importantly, I argue that a focus on this deeper temporal order of the skin may reveal how certain forms of engagement with skin (e.g., medical and political) either harm or benefit human beings, confining them merely to repetitions of the same, rather than as dynamic, future-oriented selves.

It is important to envision skin as one of the constitutive principles of human life and action because it (1) shows that sapience and sentience are, from the beginning, intertwined and informed by the interaction of internally emergent and externally emergent factors in the interface, (2) demonstrates that we are ever *changing*, evolving beings due to the dynamic interface of our skin, (3) opens up to the idea that skin is a *surface of choice* and engineering, (4) outwardly rejects a vision of humans as individuals condemned to "solitary confinement" in their skin,[4] without embracing naïve romantic visions of skin, and (5) seeks to make room for alternative epidermal communities based on trust.

To add on to this program: if skin is ultimately a connective co-emergent and co-existent interface—both on a deep, intimate level as in newborns connecting skin-to-skin with their parents,[5] and on a broader, social level in terms of skin politics—then this brings greater perspicuity to the theorization of the harm done by practices that leave our skins untouched (as in solitary confinement) or practices that impose dispositional shame upon the skin and deny us the promise of a living future. To counter such epidermal paralysis, I argue that we need to develop and cultivate a culture that is based on epidermal hospitality and trust.

In my approach, I seek to avoid the Scylla and Charybdis of viewing skin either solely in terms of biological reductionism, or in terms of a sociopolitical construction. Rather, beyond these crude distinctions, I seek to show how the material interface of skin—as a biological, evolutionary dynamic becoming—may inform and open up toward a broader context of cultural semiotics and ontogenesis, ultimately propelling us to embrace altered, more affirming, aesthetic principles of skin to overcome problematic racial politics.

Skin as Place-Maker and as Place of Dialogue: Inner-Outer, Sensibility, Evolution, and the Brain-Skin Parallel

> The skin is a variety of contingency: in it, through it, with it, the world and my body touch each other, the feeling and the felt, it defines their common edge. Contingency means common tangency: in it the world and the body intersect and caress each other.
>
> —Michel Serres, *The Five Senses: A Philosophy of Mingled Bodies* (2008, 80)

From Proto-Animal to Human Animal: The Evolution, Place and Meaning of Human Skin

I argued in the previous chapter that, according to Aristotle, place is coincident with the thing, and is defined by way of its boundaries. To cite Aristotle again: "Further, the place coincides (*hama*) with the thing, for the boundaries (*ta perata*) coincide with the bounded (*peperasmenōi*)" (*Physics* IV.4, 212a30). If it is the case that place is coincident with a natural being, and if place is defined by the boundaries from which a natural being unfolds,[6] then *in utero* the placenta emerges as the *natural boundary and place-maker* of human life. Extending this line of argumentation to human life once born, could we perhaps argue that the *skin* emerges as the biological limit of determination and possibility as much as a place-maker of human life once born?

The conceptual power behind this question and thought lies in the fact that the boundary, as Heidegger articulates, is "that from which something begins its being,"[7] and this limit or boundary is not secondary, but *constitutive* of place and being. Since the skin—as all-expansive and largest and heaviest organ of the human body[8]—is truly *everywhere*, there is room to push the account of place in the previous chapter to a different level: the skin, as boundary, might very well be an all-embracing constitutive principle of our place and being. But what exactly would this mean?

One way to answer this question is by working our way backward and thinking through the evolution from inorganic, to proto-animal and animal life. This is exactly what François Dagognet does in his *La peau découverte*. First, he emphasizes how important it is for living beings to have an inside and an outside. Where inorganic beings have no interior or exterior (i.e., they are homogenously qualified), living beings have both an interior and an exterior: inner and outer are distinct in terms of quality.[9]

Next, Dagognet speaks of "proto-animal" life and how this form of life is "walled under a heavy protecting shell." He argues that the transition of proto-animal to animal life is achieved through a "major act." In becoming animal life, life must turn itself "inside out," and "to place on the surface its sensibility and to replace to the bottom the solid tissue in which it barricaded itself, the spinal column, the bony part from which it will build itself."[10] Dagognet's provocative image of the proto-animal turning itself *inside out* immediately clarifies the nature of the skin's surface—its vulnerability and its sensibility—as well as its deep connection to, and underpinning in, the animal's interiority. Indeed, as Dagognet formulates it, the animal's outside is nothing without its inside and vice versa:

> An outside without its inside is nothing but an absurdity, just as would be an inside refusing to exteriorize itself and escaping any surrounding border or type of fence (even a minimal one). Whether admissible or not, the englobement always requires a frontier or a limitation. No mountain without valley, no place without its other side. No viscera without their skin.[11]

Importantly, the skin as exteriority is thus the exteriority *of* interiority.[12] And Peter Sloterdijk emphasizes that the folding of the surface (or outwardness) *produces* something like an interior or a self:[13] interiority cannot be grasped other than through the skin as (permeable, yet protective) membrane and vice versa. The making and placing of the boundary that skin is implicates thus the process of building an inside, but it also implies the process of connecting to and distinguishing oneself from an outside world. And this outside world is also *produced* in this process: the skin extends and mediates outward and touches and changes what it encounters. Thus, not only is the skin responsible for building an inside, but "the outside [is] built from the inside in the process of building itself as inside."[14] This adds on to Malpas's idea that "places always implicate other places."[15] And with a soft and naked border such as human skin, the outside is felt ever so close and near.

How did the species of *Homo sapiens* acquire its bare, vulnerable skin, and what does the biological history of these practical, material conditions imply for our spatial, sensible engagement? In *Living Color*, biological anthropologist Nina Jablonski explains how our naked skin evolved based on the active lifestyle of our "bipedal human ancestors."[16] The active lifestyle lived brought in its wake the problem of overheating, and human ancestors accordingly underwent important changes in "their digestive system, brain, and skin."[17] Their skin changed to develop a cooling system: the skin lost its hair and acquired an extensive sweat gland system.[18]

Thus, the desire to stay active during the day, under the sun, was made possible and sustained through the development of a hairless and sweaty skin.[19] But because naked skin is vulnerable skin, the skin also needed to increase its barrier function and acquire pigmentation to protect against sun damage.[20] Thus, the "hairless and sweaty skin replete with protective eumelanin," allowed our human precursors to "walk, run, and search for food for long periods under a hot sun without overheating and brain damage."[21] Accordingly, a uniquely human skin came into being, and it is interesting to note that the genes coding for the skin are part of the few areas where the DNA of humans and of chimpanzees differ significantly.[22] This uniquely human skin with its air-conditioning mechanism and protective, colored layer came to provide the ability for active, mobile pursuit and decision making.

The skin's transformation from furry to hairless, and from sweatless to sweaty is a material representation of our sapient-sentient evolution, combining activity and willingness to external (sun, environmental) exposure with an inherent mechanism to cool down and minimize damage (through pigmentation and a thicker epidermis). Thus, we find in the human skin representations of who we are in our engagements—active and sweaty, bare yet protected—that continue to shape our place and our being.

These features speak to the fact that the skin is not just a static, physical barrier between inner and outer world, but a place for transformation: one that allows both inner and outer, self and world, to emerge and respond to each other through its protective yet vulnerable mediation. Thus, where Chrétien speaks of the sense of touch as "pledge" to the world, and how it "exposes it to the world and protects it from the world,"[23] the account of skin as ever transforming place-making boundary wants to take this thought one step further: the skin as (re)generating, sensitive, and biological surface *creates* through its mediation what world and life are and mean. Additionally, what world, self, and skin mean is prone to continuous *change*, which includes shifts of meaning in terms of where the boundaries between world, self, and skin, are drawn.

It is important to envision skin as one of the constitutive principles of human life and action because it (1) shows that sapience and sentience are, from the beginning, intertwined and informed by the interaction of internally emergent and externally emergent factors coming to bear on an interface, and (2) demonstrates that we are ever-changing, evolving beings due to the dynamic interface of our skin.

More polemically, what the skin shows in terms of its emergent evolution and its effects on our human form is that we do not just *relate* to place through our skin, as Casey argues.[24] Rather, skin *creates* the place for both the development and expression of human form that maintains constancy and that is conditioned by the possibilities that may be accessed in the outside and in the inside. In this, skin is the place of appearance of what we call "the outside" as well as "the inside." Moreover, our skin is as much the result of our *species* development as it is the development and creation of our own, individuated space. This idea is partially in line with Sloterdijk's premise, which is articulated as part of his spherology, that "humans are themselves an effect of the space they create."[25] Where my idea of skin as producer of place differs from Sloterdijk's account of spheres is that, in my argument, skin is the place of appearance of both the "inside" and the "outside." Additionally, my account seeks to emphasize the fundamental material and sensitive underpinnings that condition the possibility of such space-making.

SKIN, DEPTH, BRAIN, AND KNOWLEDGE

> The interface constitutes a region of choice. It separates and at the same time mixes the two universes as they meet in it, as they generally bleed onto it. As such the interface in itself becomes fruitful convergence.
>
> —François Dagognet, *Faces, Surfaces, Interfaces* (1982, 49)

The previous section showed that the skin is both a materially constitutive principle for our active lifestyle and the effect of this lifestyle; it offers intertwinement of the living being's exterior and interior, as well as that of our sentience and sapience. The evolutionary development of an active, inquisitive lifestyle in sync with the development of both human skin and brain[26] speaks to the imagination and finds a parallel in their respective ontogenesis: the skin emerges from the same germ layer of ectoderm that gives rise to the lining of the sense organs and to the nervous tissue that will become the brain.[27]

The common cellular origin of skin and brain[28] gives rise to the suggestion of possible parallels between skin and brain in terms of their primacy and function. As Anzieu argues, "The brain and the skin are both surface entities, the internal surface (internal, that is, vis-à-vis the body as a whole) or cortex being in relation with the outside world through the mediation of an external surface or epidermis, and each of these two 'shells' consisting of at least two layers: the outer one protective, and the other, lying beneath it or in its orifices, serving to gather information or to filter exchanges."[29]

Following their co-originary point in embryology, we may point toward certain "knowledge" that the skin harbors in its sensibility, in similarity to the knowledge associated with the brain. Given the primacy of touch for our development, for connecting us and keeping us safe and comfortable—exemplified by the fact that touching and holding are so central to a newborn in surviving, exploring, and situating herself in the world[30]—such knowledge conveyed by the skin is crucial in grounding our existence. Benthien recounts how "it is through the skin that the newborn *learns* where she begins and ends, where the boundaries of her self are. Here, she *learns* the first feelings of pleasure and displeasure."[31]

In a poetic vein, Paul Valéry suggests the brain is conceptually subservient to the skin. He exclaims:

> *the most profound thing in man is his skin.* Our marrow, our brain, everything we need to feel, suffer or think . . . *to be profound* . . . all these are inventions of the skin! . . . However deep we dig, doctor, we are . . . ectoderm.[32]

Whether we fully accept Valéry's claim or not, his main point is persuasive: there is far more depth to what is usually just called the *surface* of the skin: our understanding of the world and our safety and well-being are really at stake at the edge of the skin as we stand in contact.[33] And when we are left untouched—as newborns unattached and neglected, or as adults through cruel penitentiary practices such as solitary confinement—the depth, health, meaning, and mooring of our being falls apart.[34]

Dagognet does not deny depth, but reclaims it from the "shadowy darkness"[35] of nonappearance and relocates depth in the bright light of the surface of the skin. He does this, first, by countering the histophysiologist's tendency to (anatomically) *separate* the skin's three layers (epidermis, dermis, and hypodermis), which would reiterate a tendency to distinguish surface from depth. Instead, he emphasizes holistic (middle-voiced) "dermo-epidermic participation" in the processes in which the skin engages: "circulation, the nervous system, immunological defense, hormonal play, nutrition and the power of vitamins, etc."[36] By showing that all layers of the skin *participate* in these functions, he seeks to undermine a compartmentalized vision of the skin, thus creating room for a holistic, functional understanding of skin as such.

Second, in his account of the various causal factors underlying juvenile acne, Dagognet refuses to view acne's pustules as the mere "external" appearances of a deeper (for instance, endocrine, testosterone-infused) cause. What Dagognet pleads for in its place is to bring into view the skin's own synergy, agitation and "excessive receptivity to stimulation"[37] in interaction with the body's altered sexual hormonal being. He remarks, for instance, on how a hair follicle is not simply a *passive* recipient, but "also works on what modifies it,"[38] and how the skin's metabolization of lipids is characterized by "amplified receptivity,"[39] especially when compared to its stimulus.

Dagognet's explanation of acne inserts the notion of knowledge and choice in the skin, for instance due to the focus on "amplified receptivity" of the hair follicles. Moreover, as he writes, the "span of choice of dramas" connected with burgeoning sexuality "resounds on the skin."[40] Acne "knows" this drama, which involves a complex play of reproductive glands, the pituitary, and the activation of cerebral and psychosocial factors. Acne harbors deep knowledge in its "burning intersection": it is part of and mediates the knowledgeable intersection of the human being with its "physical environment" as well as the interaction between "self and the other."[41]

Thus, while we might not want to make the skin subservient to the brain, as Valéry proposes, there is a fascinating connection between the development of the brain and the skin. First, the skin enables an active, inquisitive human lifestyle, fortifying brainpower and human form. Second, brain and skin find their origin in a similar ontogenetic embryonic layer. And third, both brain and skin entail deep knowledge and "choice," of self and other and their interaction.

We can grasp this knowledge on different levels. For one, this entails a deep, anchoring knowledge—as in the sensitive knowledge and trust of becoming self that is afforded by the skin-to-skin contact of the newborn with her parents. Or it may, more generally, be the knowledge that sensitive skin conveys, thus granting us "an informed life, alert and vivacious."[42] Finally, this may be the knowledge that—on a more material and particular level—the skin harbors, for instance as its hair follicles react knowledgeably to the power of hormones. In all cases, skin appears to complement the brain's knowledge, and to equally stand at the origin of the depth, health, meaning, and mooring of our existence.

To put this more bluntly and clearly: the parallels drawn between skin, brain, and active, inquisitive human lifestyle suggest that the skin is an interface of depth and choice. When Sloterdijk argues that "only in immune structures that form interiors [spheres] can humans continue their generational process and advance their individuations,"[43] my account has shown that the semi-permeable membrane structure of the skin functions on both a physical and metaphysical level. The skin has both been generated by and generates the place and meaning of sapience, sentience, and individuation that we associate with the term *human*.

Skin, Dispositional Synthesis, and the Aristotelian Mean

The notion of *aisthetic synthesis* adds yet more depth to grasp the skin's knowledgeable underpinning for our lives. As Dagognet writes, the skin, as "place of synthesis and biodevelopment," is in this regard very similar to how the brain, "in becoming its organ of the surface (the cortex), [is] responsible for registering."[44] Both brain and skin "are in essence surfaces,"[45] and by that definition must bring together, register, and collect a multiplicity, making it sensible and ordered.

Aristotle's *De anima* clarifies this synthetic, ordering principle of the skin through his account of touch.[46] Since according to Aristotle touch involves not just one pair of "contraries" like the other senses[47] but includes a variety of contrary qualities,[48] its medium must be receptive of a multiplicity. However, what holds this all together as *one* is the organ and medium itself: flesh. This is the one "sub-strate" (*hen to hypokeimenon, DA* II.11, 422b34) that may bring together and allow for receptivity to multiplicity due to its *blending* of various elements within itself (*DA* III.11, 424b24–29). And since Aristotle seems to regard skin, due to its softness and flexibility, as an extension of our flesh and organs,[49] Aristotle's observation about flesh's synthetic power equally applies to the skin.

Thus, the body's own synthetic corporeity—in the form of flesh and skin blending elements—enables the aisthetic encounter of the world.[50] And only by directly "interfacing with and being affected by the differences"[51] can the sense of touch operate and discern that by which it is touched—as that which is always *relatively*, but not absolutely, different. The skin's involvement in what it feels is thus always at play, and what the skin *is* can only be grasped from within a wide terrain of opposites within which it constructs its place.

The synthetic construction of place extends from the skin's and flesh's bodily elements to its aisthetic function. Aristotle writes: "touch exists as a mean (*mesotēs*) of all the tangible qualities, and its sense organ is receptive not just of whatever differences of earth there are, but also of heat and cold and all the other tangibles" (*DA* III.13,435a22–24).[52]

The sensible mean that Aristotle invokes is, as Polansky suggests, indicative of a certain "readiness to be acted upon by the sensible differences so as to discriminate them and as having some standard by which to assess them."[53] This mean, or "standard" of touch, similar to the ethical mean,[54] entails an "appropriate relationship"[55] in that it remains open to the world and notes differences. What is felt is due to a *relationship*, where synergistically the openness to the world is secured through humans' embodied yet open sense of touch. Still, our own embodiment and "mean" often remain "intangible"[56] insofar as it is presumed, but not directly felt: we only feel the "excesses" in relationship to our own skins. However, without the mean, without this ordering "measure," Aristotle argues, we would be directly, materially affected, such as in the case of plants (*DA* II.12, 424a33–424b2). And even with an appropriate mean, the sense of touch always remains at risk.[57]

Deepening this thought about vulnerability and multiplicity, it appears there are limits to touch's embodied synthesis: some intensities surpass the range of the body's balanced mean and concretely untie the synthesis that the body is, thereby producing more multiplicity both in the world and in itself. When Serres writes that "skin intervenes between several things in the world and makes them mingle,"[58] Aristotle would add that this mingling intervention of skin is precisely possible because of skin's own intermingling and ordered mean, and that this intermingling is always at risk of potential damage to the organism as a whole.

In overview, the account of touch and flesh in Aristotle allows us to view the skin in terms of a (material and aisthetic) synthetic ordering principle, where precisely order and balance between extremes allows for openness to multiplicity.[59] The fact that Aristotle formulates touch in terms of *relation* and in terms of balanced multiplicity moves us closer to recognizing the skin's synthetic participation in that which it encounters, while also admitting the skin's need to abstract from that which it encounters. Moreover, the continuum between extremes within which touch operates confirms the extension of the terrain within which touch operates and also the (abstract, composite) construction of this place.

Thus, what Aristotle's account of touch and synthesis adds to our analysis of the skin is its emphasis on disposition, relationship, and place. And we may wonder: does Aristotle's account of touch, as involving a dispositional mean, imply temporal synthesis as much as spatial synthesis? Another question concerns the fact that the skin's (bodily and aisthetic) disposition entails a certain attitude toward difference, which is always in view of the living being's own terrain of extremes. This "dispositional, synthetic" knowledge may very well keep us safe most of the time—on a simple, direct, material level. But, on a more complex, sapient-sentient infused level, we may raise concerns regarding our habitually informed disposition toward difference, and what this implies for trust and hospitality. Is there a way to envision alternative skin reactions, and to engineer our embodied skin to be dispositionally trained to more openness and difference?

One way of envisioning an alternative skin reaction is by following the trajectory of Catherine Malabou's thinking about plasticity. This term, used both as a philosophical and as a (neuro)scientific concept, designates both the capacity to give form, to take on form, and to explode form (e.g., in the use of plastic explosives). Plasticity is *not* elasticity—the resistance inherent in plasticity implies that something plastic "cannot return to its initial form after undergoing a 'deformation.'"[60] Thus, plasticity "designates the definitive character of the imprint, of configuration, or of modification." Malabou's term "plasticity," originally crafted to apply to the brain, fruitfully lines up with the skin. While skin seems far more elastic than plastic, it is similarly elastic in that it "resists endless polymorphism,"[61] and carries the *imprint* of marked changes on its surface (for instance as stretch marks after pregnancy or as sagging skin after losing weight).[62]

The crucial benefit of viewing the skin in terms of plastic is that it avails us not only a look at the skin's adaptation to form in conjunction with its ability to give form, but also the intersection of these modes of motion and the dermato-logics they produce. Moreover, following Malabou's emphasis on the "explosiveness" of plastics, that is, the ability to create resistance to ideology as demonstrated by plastic explosives,[63] our analysis of skin may benefit from an articulation of the plasticity of the skin, in that it may similarly allow for a resistance to form that plastic entails[64] and may afford a dialectic between form and its absence.[65]

Thus, Malabou's account of plasticity crucially complements Aristotle's account of habitual synthesis in that it adds the necessary possibility of breaking through, intervening with, and disrupting the status quo of particular aesthetic skin reactions as enabled by habituation.[66] With Malabou's "plasticity," we find a crucial lynchpin in our search for alternative skin syntheses that move beyond those of habituation. If the skin is plastic in the sense of explosiveness, then it is extremely relevant to think about ways to *transform* the identity politics associated with our skin. This will acquire more emphasis in the final section of this chapter.

Skin and Temporality:
On Temporal Synthesis, Finitude, and Self

> The skin receives the deposit of our memories and stocks the experiences printed on it. It is the bank of our impressions and the geodesic panorama of our frailties. We do not have to look far, or search our memory; the skin is engraved and imprinted to the same extent as the surface of the brain, and perhaps in the same way.
>
> —Michel Serres, *The Five Senses:*
> *A Philosophy of Mingled Bodies* (2008, 75)

Where the previous section highlighted the skin's constitutional contribution to our sapient and sentient evolution and its knowledge and depth, here we seek to explore the temporality housed and enabled by the skin. Both on the "surface of the brain"[67] and on the skin we find the deposit of our memories. More generally, we could argue that temporality makes its marks on the skin (and the brain cortex, too) in a wide variety of ways, for instance in the birthmarks of the newborn, the acne of the adolescent, and the wrinkles of the elderly.

In this vein, Aristotle's *Categories* uses the surface of the skin to describe the temporal palette of various (affective) qualities and *pathē* that may inscribe it. He describes fleeting affections (*pathē*) such as shame that, at least in his mind,[68] leave no permanent mark (on the skin at least), to more enduring affective qualities and permanent conditions, such as having a ruddy constitution:

> when such circumstances have their origin in affections (*pathē*) that are hard to change and permanent they are called qualities. For if pallor or darkness have come about in the natural make-up they are called qualities . . . and if pallor or darkness have resulted from long illness or from sunburn, and do not easily give way—or even last for a life-time—these too are called qualities. . . . But those that result from something that easily disperses and quickly gives way are called affections; for people are not, in virtue of them, said to be qualified somehow. Thus a man who reddens through shame is not called ruddy, nor one who pales in fright pallid; rather he is said to have been affected somehow (*peponthenai ti*). Hence such things are called affections but not qualities. (*Categories* 8, 9b19–33)

The temporal palette of affectivity finds illustration for Aristotle in our skin. In and through the skin, we see the skin's warming and blushing[69] either as mere temporal affect, or as an affective quality brought about through a long-lasting, imposed cause (e.g., sunburn or illness), or as part of a permanent (internal, natural) condition. The categorical, affective distinctions that Aristotle makes are made possible by a combination of "measuring clock-time" (in terms of the coloring of the skin: how long does it stay red?[70]) and distinguishing either an internal or external (natural or unnatural) cause.

Yet, as I outlined in chapter 2, this Aristotelian approach to temporal affectivity runs into the problem of *categorical cross-contamination*, since it is impossible to draw such sharp, clear lines between changes that seem merely temporary happenings (i.e., an occasional sunburn) and the more pervasive and more permanent biological, climatological and cultural constellation to which they belong. A sunburn may be part of leisurely cultural activity and thus indicate a vacation to a sunny touristy destination for those who are well off, or may be part of working long hours outdoors doing manual labor, or may be explainable on the basis of having a certain skin condition (e.g., pale skin) in a certain climate (e.g., California) where sunburns would be more likely. In each case, sunburn acquires different meanings based on the different assemblage of factors influencing it, and accordingly its temporary fleetingness actually turns out to be part of a much larger, more complex and enduring temporal constellation.[71]

If it is indeed the case that such a temporal, complex constellation of affective factors works its way on our skin, and if such factors cannot be neatly divided according to the parameters of chronological time or those of inner-outer, then we might need an alternative account of temporality, and one that specifically does justice to the temporality of our skin and human being.[72] What might this look like?

Serres's poetic language helps out, suggesting the skin "is the bank of our impressions and the geodesic panorama of our frailties."[73] The words "bank" and "panorama" suggest an amassment (bank) and survey (panorama) that presents a sequence of impressions and events in an assembled way: namely as a *synthesis*. When we take the etymology of the Greek word *synthesis* literally—from συντιθέναι to put together, < σύν syn- prefix + τιθέναι (root θε-) to place—we discern clearly that the skin's temporal synthesis must involve something like contraction, and given the history it has contracted, it is both affected—"infected"—by that history and part of "abbreviating" that history.[74]

On the initial embodied level of the living being with its skin, the temporality as we find it is pre-reflective in its abbreviation and affection. In order to touch and receive impressions, a body itself must be passively synthesized[75] (out of elements such as water and carbon, or, in Aristotle's words, out of earth and water and other elements). This passive synthesis, or "contraction," is *temporal*, according to Deleuze, in that it constitutes a *"living present* of the body."[76] The first passive synthesis,[77] to be precise, "contracts the successive independent instants into one another, thereby constituting the lived, or living present."[78] Accordingly, the past and the future emerge as dimensions of this present.[79] Thus, through synthesis of time, the body comes to be "an integral of a plurality of temporal retentions and expectations."[80]

This articulation of the body as an integral of various temporal directions applies directly to the skin in that our skin is also passively synthesized and incorporates all these different temporal directions. For instance, the process of the successful healing of skin abrasions and lesions shows that in the skin, the past is reconstituted in the present and has a futural direction as well, as the healing abrasions provide protection against future wounds. This passive temporal synthesis of the skin is based both on ancestral species and (epi)genetic familial patterns and on contingency and chance, as Serres also indicates in relationship to the patchwork that we call our skin: "our time does not end in a system, but in a rough-cut and patchwork rag."[81]

Temporality not only enables the body's synthesis (and thus the skin's synthesis), but also informs the skin as it embodies the temporal unity of this particular, individuated living being. The skin is in this regard not just a continuous spatial surface but also a surface of temporal continuity and identity. This finds anecdotal evidence in the mesmerizing and enigmatic experience of a parent observing the contradictory "similarity in difference" of a child's growing and changing, yet continuously similar skin.[82]

If memory is the basis for cognition and identity, and constitutes the living present life of an individual in general, and provides it with coherence, similarly we could argue that the "deposit of memories"[83] we find in the skin—as it composes and contracts past experiences in coexistence with the present[84]—truly grounds our present life and provides it with coherence and meaning. On an initial level, this finds itself expressed in the deposit of marks and imprints that condense our past, and simultaneously speaks to the living present and future by changing constantly in nature (e.g., stretching and waning).

Ricoeur's account of identity may prove helpful here to articulate the meaning of temporality for our individuated human existence. He argues that when we speak of the human individual as an "identical," unified self, we should actually split this up into two domains: that of the self as more or less rigid *idem* (the "same") and that of the self as dynamic *ipse* (as "selfhood").[85] The distinction between these two domains emerges clearly, Ricoeur posits, only once we confront the question of the "permanence of time,"[86] in which "idem" refers to constancy (i.e., to what stays the same) and "ipse" articulates the more dynamic, changeable self that nonetheless harbors something that remains constant.

If Ricoeur is correct to articulate that an account of human selves involves the question of "self-constancy over time [and] rests on a complex interplay of sameness and ipseity,"[87] this hints at the need to provide a more thorough account of temporality at work in and on human skin. On the basis of Ricoeur's ideas, and extending them, we could argue that we find in and on the skin a complex temporal interplay between the time of our species (our evolutionary time), the time of our biological and parental ancestors, (epi-genetic time), as well as our *own* time that in itself is a complex interplay between the time of our more constant self and our changing, innovative self.

Thinking about the deeper temporal interplay that informs our epidermal existence requires us to discuss a particular form of human temporality: human finitude. Exploring finitude does not solely bring into perspective our past and our future, but allows us to rethink the relationship between the three temporal modes as lived on the skin. This raises the question: in what way can the temporality of our skins, and of our beings, be harmed or benefited by practices that intervene with this deeper temporal interplay in and on our skins? This question will be explored in the following sections.

Skin and (Shared) Finitude

A possible way to start answering the question about how the temporality of our skins and beings may be harmed or benefited is to zoom in on how certain cultural, technological, and medical practices engage with a specific kind of human temporality: *finitude*. Heidegger's phenomenology is helpful in that it explains how certain ways of cultural engagement may harm us in not allowing us access to possibilities of recognizing our finitude. Simultaneously, as I will argue, Heidegger's account omits discussion of the material and organic underpinnings of death and puts too much emphasis on the isolated nature of the individual experiencing finitude. Thus, while I seek to preserve Heidegger's emphasis on finitude for my account of human, epidermal temporality, I seek to substitute his focus on the fundamental attunement of anxiety, which ultimately singularizes Dasein and brings it to the point of near-epiphany, with an account of *trust* that reveals the power of communal attempts to access new temporal possibilities with and through others.

From a phenomenological, Heideggerian perspective, the time as we live it is unified and has three dimensions: our having-been ("past"), our present being ("present"), and our being-ahead ("future"). Rather than seeing time as a pure sequence of nows, Heidegger sees temporality firmly grounded in our being, with having-been not as an absent past, but as an actual *existence or being* having-been,[88] and the future not a remote possibility, but as our ownmost possibility that we are: Dasein *is* constantly ahead of itself.[89] According to Heidegger, "the primary meaning of existentiality is the future,"[90] because with the future comes the realization of the possibility of our impossibility: death. Only when we truly become aware of our own impending death through the fundamental mood of *angst* can we be opened up to the very possibility that we are. Anticipating death, yet also determining ourselves out of our having-been, we may allow for an authentic present to come to the fore, one where we can resolutely make the present our own.

If we follow Heidegger's argument clearly, but also seek to make it appropriate to our skin and the living, finite biological organism we are, what would follow? In the skin, through aging,[91] we can actually witness and feel our own finitude through increasing lack of elasticity, permanent scarring and what are called "static" wrinkles.[92] Analyzing the skin's histophysiology, Dagognet speaks in this regard of death pushing to the surface: "the death movement of cells that are exfoliated."[93] Thus, the skin presents us with our mortal future, but this future is not simply a future that is unambiguously foreclosed, but part of possibilities, a constant process of regeneration. Dagognet accordingly words this as "the incessant process of renewal."[94]

The encroaching mortality visible in wrinkles, scars, and sagging calls up a looming future as well as a receding past: a past that seems ever so close, yet whose distance seems more pronounced and determined than ever through the lacking elasticity and increasing permanence of the marks it leaves behind. The "recollection" of this past may instill a deep nostalgic longing for the place of youth, and perhaps for eternal youth or "youth itself," as Kant claims.[95] Or it may, as Barbara Cassin emphasizes in her reading of Odysseus, be a nostalgic search to come home to a place where there is no eternal youth, but only a "time that passes."[96] If the scars on my skin similarly grow old and regenerate with me, this is a sign that the past is "with me" yet is constantly able to transform. This means that there is a way of finding a *home* in our skin, insofar as it would allow us to "submit to a common fate: aging, dying."[97]

According to Heidegger, the primary meaning of our existence is disclosed through relating to the future. Only when we relate authentically to the future can we open ourselves up to an authentic present. The moment of vision (*Augenblick*)[98] is a specific mode of the present where Dasein wrestles itself free from an inauthentic present where one simply goes along ("falls") with every day and everyone's objects of concern. In the moment of vision, the present is not cut off from having-been and one's being-ahead, but "in resoluteness, [the present] gets held in the future and in having been."[99]

This account of an authentic present (*Augenblick*) is relevant to our contemplations of skin because it provides an answer to the question about harmful (cultural, technological, medical, political) engagements with our skin that do not allow us access to the skin's deeper temporality and recognition of our finitude. Even if I ultimately reject the transcendent solipsism associated with Heidegger's notion of authenticity, Heidegger's account of an authentic present is fruitful in drawing attention to the power of finitude to liberate us from pure enchantment to the now and opening us up to the broader horizons of our time, where possibilities for contingency and openness may be uncovered and reinscribe us.

Our skin can function as a catalyst for recognizing the temporality that we are, becoming aware of being "ontologically deficient," that is, "intrinsically incomplete and on the way to absence."[100] One consequence of practices that deny and omit wrinkles, whether through facelifts or more temporary techniques such as Botox,[101] and which, in terms of cultural gender norms, affect women more than men, is that it may make time come to standstill,[102] cut off from our having-been and our possibilities. Similar to Heidegger's description of one of the forms of boredom in *Fundamental Concepts of Metaphysics* where Dasein's time is coming to a standstill when Dasein simply goes along with the events taking place in time and place but does not truly *engage* its own being and its temporality,[103] the intervention of practices such as Botox bring our skin-time to a standstill and *freeze* us up quite literally, cutting us off from our past and future and identifying us with a generic, "eternal" present to which we are oppressively tied.

Thus, while seemingly innocent, one of the consequences of wrinkle-removing interventions such as Botox could be that it promotes inauthenticity in installing a *frozen* moment, as it does not allow Dasein's skin its temporal depth and thereby the opportunity to reclaim and truly *insert* itself with all its opportunities in the present. Where the *Augenblick* allows us to be temporalized in the future, and enables us to "being carried away" from that which otherwise traps us, toward possibilities and "resolute rapture,"[104] practices that problematize and remove wrinkles may cut us off from such an ekstasis and temporalize us in the mere present.

If we have been correct to argue, with Dagognet, that the skin is not just the surface, but *is* depth itself, and if the skin offers a milieu within which temporal dimensions may intersect and direct us toward a (more authentic) future becoming, then modifying our skin to identify us solely with our present may limit us access to temporal depth and the possibilities thereby implied. Not only to us, but also to others, this pure identification with the present stands in the way of mortal solidarity.

This has repercussions not only in the sense of what Heidegger calls becoming the "conscience" (*Gewissen*) for others and, thus, the potentiality for us to be authentically together with them in solicitude.[105] Rather, I am thinking here about how recognition of finitude is crucial to experiences of *witnessing* finitude in fragile coexistence. If Sloterdijk, following Levinas, is correct in assuming that death is mostly experienced in terms of the one *witnessing* death, and if death ultimately implies more the dissolution of a shared sphere rather than only the death of an individual being,[106] then the denial of death on the skin precludes the possibility of affectively bonding together in a common skin, with co-fragile aging bodies that have reached "a maximum of interdependence."[107] If the "shared existential risk"[108] of which Sloterdijk speaks is neither touchable nor visible on the skin, how may we together live and face the future on the way toward a radical implosion of togetherness? If vulnerability is invisible, if history makes place for a static present, if uniqueness makes place for a more generic being, how can we trust each other and together face the future?

This latter question is not just of import to personal and interpersonal relationship dynamics, but has broader, political ramifications connected to the social injustices that are tied up intimately with our skin. While skin-engineering practices such as Botox seem politically innocent and thus far removed from the political practices of racializing skin, both practices converge in identifying skin with an (eternal, generic) present and denying skin its temporal depth.[109] Without such depth, there is pure enchainment to the now, and both horizons (of the earlier and of the future) are sealed off—so that neither possibility for contingency nor openness for being reinscribed can occur. Thus, neither can new temporal knots and assemblages be created, nor reciprocal openness that is crucial to building a culture based on trust.

Interestingly, where the practice of Botox has here been shown to bring time to a standstill, it cannot be deduced simply that all practices of skin engineering do so. In fact, I will try to show in the next section that some forms of skin engineering may intervene in the process of ontogenesis to *revive* temporality and reawaken skin in solidarity and compassion. This is particularly important for our cultural and political practices that have allowed for certain epidermal death zones, where a similar temporal logic of the present prevails, but this time perniciously dictated by regimes of power that hold wide swaths of bodies—mostly so-called nonwhite or black bodies—captive in such stasis. Thus, the next and final section of this chapter will discuss both such dangerous occurrences, as well as possibilities for cultural, perceptive, and affective change to happen.

Human Skin, Shame, and (Dis)Trust

Skin will make the world one for all.

—Paul Valéry, *Oeuvres* (824)

An account of human skin would be incomplete without taking up the emotional, cultural, and political atmosphere of the skin. As ongoing reports of police brutality on people racialized as black emphasize time and again, the emotions felt on the skin are part of a wider *polis* and climatological environment that informs and bears witness to our skin. Here we can discern the smaller social sphere of the family with its intimate touch and its "education" of emotions on the skin and the larger, political sphere with its ideological presuppositions that—often based simply on the look of the skin—divides and judges people according to race, class, and gender. Connected to all this is the climatological and ecological environment within which factors such as air pollution, micro-organisms, mosquitos, skin allergens, irritants, and UV radiation are bound to affect the skin, and target specific skins more than others due to issues of inequity and global injustice.

If we want to make an inroad in this discussion, it may be best to start with an evolutionary account of how the human skin is itself the emerging place of an encounter of body, culture, and climate. In her account of the skin of people living near the North Pole, Jablonski focuses on one such intersection.[110] She argues that the UVR-starved conditions of the extreme north necessitated "a combination of biological and cultural adaptations: a depigmented skin and a culture and body of technology structured around the exploitation of vitamin-D-rich foods."[111] Thus, cultural technologies such as fishing and the way our skin looks and functions are directly linked to evolutionary biological and environmental circumstances. In this account, the skin emerges as the body's interface with the physical, chemical, biological, and cultural environment. This interface is not static, but also generates and transforms these physical, chemical, biological, and cultural factors: with a different skin color and function, new technologies may come about, and thus the environment will change as well.

Thus, the skin is not only the product, but also the generating factor in biology, culture, and technology. Simultaneously, on a micro level, the skin is both hosting and transformed by a whole range of microorganisms that become integrated into the skin and our genome. While our skin is "sterile" in utero, as we exit the birth canal it becomes populated with thousands of different kinds of microorganisms (bacteria, viruses, fungi, etc.). Rhodes and colleagues argue that since the microorganisms we live with "exchange genes laterally—that is, within and between various species—the combined human-microbiome self is more dynamic and more interactive than we are used to thinking of ourselves as being (Lederberg, 2003)."[112]

Because of the difficulty to delineate the border between our bodies and the microbiome, and given the intersection of the genomes, Rhodes and colleagues consequently argue, "we are coexistent rather than independent beings."[113] Since these microorganisms may be shared with other species (domesticated and otherwise) as well, our mediated skin inter(sur)

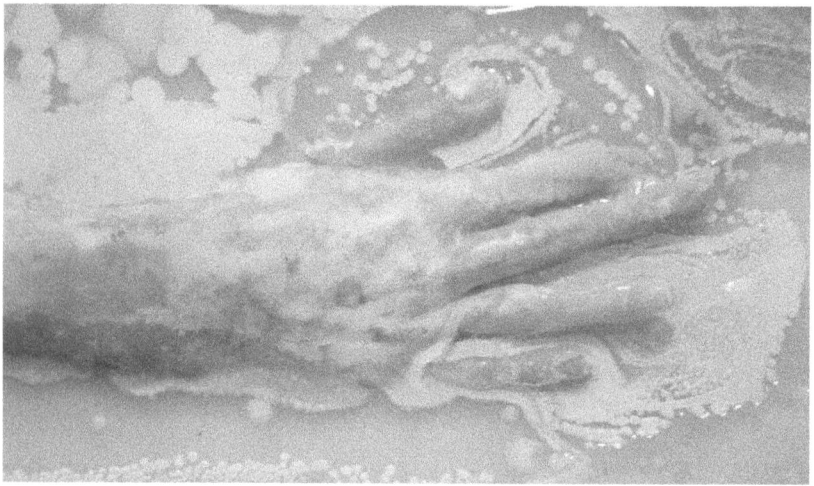

Figure 4.1. "Expanded Self," 2015. Artwork by Sonja Bäumel. Being in the world as an individual really means being a multi-being community in a vital process of permanent exchange.

face encounters more and deeper communal touching-points of what Haraway calls a "webbed" form of existence.[114]

What the account of the evolutionary intersection of nature, culture, and environment shows in conjunction with our microbiotic co-existence is that we are always already emerging co-existent beings and that our skin is not static but in fact culturally, biologically, and environmentally adaptive and dynamic: its evolution thereby co-creates place and time, and not just for us individually, but as a culture located in a specific climatological environment, with specific technologies, ways of providing nutrition, and so on. Yet, the plasticity and historicity of the skin as it speaks to this intersection is often not realized nor admired but made one and the same with its specific presentation in the present, without temporal, cultural, natural, or environmental depth. The skin thereby becomes identified with a stifling, all-encompassing present from which it cannot escape, instead of a contingent interface with past, present, and future. Moreover, in its identification with the present it is valorized on either side of binary *moral* valuations that place one kind of skin over against another. And even when skin is not publicly visible, as in the case of so-called publicly *veiled* skin, such binary valorization may still be at stake.[115] Thus, even when access to (public) skin cannot be assumed, such as in the case of public veiling, the assumptions about valorization—and racialization—of skin, still powerfully apply. The resulting oppression is powerfully *felt*, and one of the emotions that is consequently felt very clearly on the side of the skin is shame, to which I turn next.

SKIN, SHAME, AND DISTRUST

> The skin, a single tissue with localized concentrations, displays sensitivity. It shivers, expresses, breathes, listens, loves and lets itself be loved, receives, refuses, retreats, its hair stands on end with horror, it is covered with fissures, rashes, and the wounds of the soul.
>
> —Michel Serres, *The Five Senses: A Philosophy of Mingled Bodies* (2008, 52)

> But all the *pathē* of the soul seem also to be with (*meta*) the body— spiritedness, gentleness, fear, pity, boldness and joy, as well as loving and hating—for together with these the body undergoes something (*paschei ti to sōma*).
>
> —Aristotle, De anima I.1 (403a17–19)

The skin is the surface of depth, and through it and in it we feel and undergo our emotions and our own depths,[116] from the burning glow of shame to the sweaty, cool, taut surface of fear. Here our feelings do not merely "express" or reflect themselves on the surface, but many of them find precisely their *origin* in this interface, and one such emotion is shame. Aristotle defines shame[117] in the following way:

> Shame (*aidōs*) should not be spoken of as being a virtue, for it resembles a feeling (*pathos*) rather than a disposition (*hexis*). At any rate, it is defined as a sort of fear of a bad reputation and amounts to something which is parallel to fear of danger; for those who are ashamed blush, whereas those who fear death turn pale. So both appear to be in some way affections of the body, and it is in view of this that shame is thought to be a feeling (*pathos*) rather than a disposition (*hexis*). (NE IV.9, 1128b10–16)[118]

According to Aristotle, fear and shame share a number of similarities: shame parallels fear (namely as fear of a bad reputation) and has a clearly visible[119] and palpable bodily affect, as does fear (turning red or turning pale respectively). The very *bodily* nature of the affect[120] provides reason to distinguish it from a disposition, according to Aristotle.

However, here we immediately confront a conundrum and a phenomenon of modern society that radically challenges Aristotle's account of shame. For, in modern culture, many people are *dispositionally* made to feel shame regarding their skin. How can it be, that shame—seen as such a temporal, emotional, and incidental phenomenon by Aristotle—may have acquired the endurance and temporal longevity of something like a disposition? Perhaps we could critique Aristotle—as we have done before—and argue that his categorical distinctions need to allow for categorical cross-contamination. But on top of that, a more pointed political observation needs to be made: that cultural and political praxes may have given rise to a phenomenon of dispositional distrust and shame that is associated with skin.[121] How and why might this be the case?

Aristotle's account of shame brings up the *fear for reputation*, which returns (albeit in a somewhat different form) in many modern and phenomenological accounts of shame: shame is an "interface effect,"[122] in that it indicates our vulnerability when looking at ourselves through a (imagined or not) third-person perspective.[123] Benthien relates how etymologically "shame and skin share the same Indo-Germanic root, meaning: 'to cover.'"[124] In this vein, she speaks of the uncovered skin, as "not only an erotic surface but also the defenseless state of being in its most elemental form."[125]

This close connection between shame, defenselessness, and vulnerability returns in Williams's account, who argues that the root of shame lies in exposure: "in being at a disadvantage," in "loss of power." For Williams, shame is primarily "being in a situation of disadvantage."[126] For Max Scheler, likewise, shame has to do with exposure, but defined in terms of becoming aware of finite (unique) limitations in contrast with an unlimited life.[127]

What happens to us when our skin (its aging, its color, its diseases) makes us feel this sense of exposure, not only incidentally but dispositionally? What happens when regimes of aesthetics dictate that we need to feel vulnerable in our skin? What if shame becomes a dispositional product of ideological force? Then surely it cannot acquire the positive, *transformative* ethical role that Aristotle assigns to it, when he speaks of how fear of disrepute may steer (young) people to do the "right" thing. Similarly, neither can shame in this dispositional sense be self-revelatory and allow for positive reorientation, being "rooted in self love," as Steinbock has it.[128] Instead, dispositional shame makes people feel habitually exposed, vulnerable, and objectified, and consequently vigilant and distrustful.

If dispositional shame is an enforced norm imposed on many skins because they are deemed different than the young, so-called white, healthy standard, and if shame is one of the primary modes of epidermal racialization, then this shapes a culture of expectation that cannot be other than isolating and distrustful.[129] For instance, a violently racial gaze reifies differently skinned people, attempting to turn them into stagnant, merely present objects with whom no *real* interaction is possible. Fanon has explored this phenomenon in *Black Skin, White Masks*, arguing that, in addition to historico-racial schema, racial-epidermal schema inscribe—epidermalize[130]—inferiority and objectification into black skins[131] and solicit shame, self-contempt, and nausea on the part of the racialized subject.[132]

This raises many questions. How does a culture create epidermal inferiorities, dispositional shame, and what may be called epidermal death zones? And how might we alter this? The next section points to our webbed existence and the inherent plasticity and co-generation of our skin that once again can tie us together in a politics of mutual affectivity. In my view, the key emotion, the key *pathos* needed to ensure this new epidermal politics, is trust.

Skin, Webbed Existence, Trust, and Temporal Depth

> The skin insures the liaison between the world and us; the interface is often the first to react; this is what "logic" wants, since it finds itself not on the outside or at the limit, but rather right in its very center.
>
> —Dagognet, *La peau découverte* (1993, 49)

If we truly "listen" to the reality of our skin, we are asked to live up to its webbed, evolutionary, resilient, and plastic nature: politically, ethically, and socially. This web of actual skin connections and spheres is endless, and stands in stark contrast to our current, sterilizing, protective reaction to whatever we touch and specifically to touching other people's skins—where we react in disgust to visible signs of eczema or psoriasis, fear to touch one another, and react with apprehension and anger to other people's skin colors. We have turned to sterilized isolation, and the defensive stance we take finds reflection in the entitlement connected to protecting our own spaces, well branded in terms of titles such as "myspace" and "yourspace."[133] We rather avoid communal spaces such as shared dressing rooms and living quarters for fear of the fungi, viruses, and allergens we might contract. Safely barricaded, we live in what Sloterdijk has called foam bubbles or "foams,"[134]—co-isolated micro-spaces—that in their plurality make up a "foam city."

However, what the account of the evolution of our skin in conjunction with the microbiome living in and with us shows is that we are already co-existent beings and that our skin is not static but in fact dynamic and in its evolution co-creating place and time and ourselves. The skin can show us how to connect, but also how to be resilient, how to adapt to and resist binary oppositions that stifle us. The community that our skin is asks for appropriate communal political and social action, suspending practices that leave us untouched (e.g., solitary confinement) or painfully burdened (e.g., racial profiling). Only when we take Paul Valéry's words literally will humankind make progress and realign itself with the promise and the future of the skin: For him, we can only get along through *accordance of the skin*: "skin will make the world one for all."[135]

What would a new skin politics look like that takes into account our webbed existence and speaks more authentically to the plasticity of the skin that we have and are? In the first place, such a skin politics would need to take seriously the claim that much of our being is at stake in how our skin is being judged and felt—either positively or negatively—and that other than so-called white skins are generally on the negative receiving end of this binary valorization, both in terms of Western nation-state politics and in global politics. Given this, we need to examine how and why it is that such skins carry the brunt of the damaging factors that harm our skin, and thereby our identity and our health and well-being—ranging from racial discrimination to air pollution, from mosquito bites carrying illnesses to skin allergens and toxins, from incarceration and solitary confinement to domestic violence and torture.[136]

Here the *pathos* impacting and living in our skin is not only potentially life threatening but can actually turn deadly, as Achille Mbembe's thoughts on necropower and necropolitics convey. Where Foucault pushed for acknowledging how disciplinary power informs and inscribes living bodies (biopower), Mbembe goes beyond this by articulating how disciplinary power informs and inscribes bodies of the living dead (necropolitics). For Mbembe, the contemporary use of power creates what he calls death-worlds, that is, "new and unique forms of social existence in which vast populations are subjected to conditions of life conferring upon them the status of *living dead*."[137]

Accordingly, we could argue that in some cities and countries, epidermal death zones have been created that sanction death for those in those zones in contradistinction with those living in "normal" society. The lives of those "living" in those segregated zones mimic those of the living, but given diminished economic, educational, and health prospects, such zones are those of diminished, life-like deaths. Placement and zoning is everything, as recent sociological research has also shown in terms of upward mobility, and our politics determines such placement and zoning largely in terms of the identity associated with our skin. The *pathos* that comes with our skin color can be uplifting or diminishing, and the meaning it acquires, as much as the possibilities it is sensitive to, is very much based on the epidermal zone in which we live.[138]

Is there another perspective possible toward such skin politics, one that takes stock of racial politics but also considers alternatives? One that focuses on the resilient nature of skin and takes seriously Malabou's meaning of plastic as *explosive*, thereby enabling a resistance to such political ideologies that simply place one skin color over against another? And what would this look like?

One possible way would be to take the biological genesis and synthesis of the skin as a model for the skin's social genesis and synthesis, re-enactivating on the level of local human community both the variegated evolutionary mixed nature/technology model as well the microbiome that is living with and in our skin. If our skin's microbiome shows the way, a new politics of skin can follow some of its practices, for instance in showing the power of creating life-promoting alliances through hospitality and deep peripheral synthesis.

To establish such life-promoting communal alliances, an affective bond must be created, one forged on trust. Trust is a middle-voiced phenomenon that creates participation and openness. In Adriaan Peperzak's words, "trust creates a kind of participation between you and me, and this changes my life, including my feeling, working, and thinking, at least in some aspect and to a certain extent."[139]

The relationship between those involved in trust is not that of subject and object; rather, linguistically, Peperzak argues we can express their relationship best in terms of the *dative* (a form of the indirect object) to characterize such involvement: "a trusted reality cannot be characterized as a 'direct object' in the accusative: its appearance shows more likeness with the *dative*."[140] By addressing trust in terms of the dative, Peperzak emphasizes that trust is always addressed *to* the other. However, if trust is mutual, it might perhaps be better to speak of trust as a relationship that happens in the *genitive* rather than the dative, insofar as the (non-possessive) genitive emphasizes shared participation in a mutual reality.[141] Emphasis on the genitive here serves a similar function as my earlier grammatical concern with the middle voice, in that both the genitive and the middle voice articulate the participatory and processual nature of the phenomena I seek to describe. In the case of trust, the genitive describes the participatory nonpossessive nature of trust that transforms those involved, and in the case of plants, the middle voice described plant life from the perspective of a dynamic happening, that is, an internally immersed, decentralized, yet coherent and continuous vegetative process.

Even when trust is willingly ignored rather than reciprocally engaged, trust involves both a change in the one who trusts as in the other.[142] Notably, this is not only an issue of cerebral trust, but also includes open, corporeal trust—similar to how touch, in the form of the ethical mean, can only function well through openness to the world.

In trust, one opens oneself up to the other, and with reciprocal trust, this creates a "mutual bond that cannot be broken as long as trust connects our lives."[143] The new affective bond created by trust can—slowly but steadily—undo the harm caused by a racialized ideology that diametrically opposes one kind of skin against another. Still, this can only happen slowly, insofar as the arc of trust is temporally built out from a past towards the future.[144] Additionally, it cannot simply be the task of one individual interfacing with another—for that, the problem is too pervasive and extensive. If what I have argued is correct, namely that ideological skin practices have deprived certain skins systematically of their temporality and assigned them to epidermal death zones where no past nor future can be had, the task would be to create a *political architecture of trust* where such dermatological zones are both faced and undermined. An architecture or structure of trust—what would this look like?

Following Malabou, such structures would be structures of resistance that defy dispositional distrust and isolation. The kind of resistance I am arguing for cannot follow the strategy of "thickening one's skin," a form of resistance that Aristotle already noted to occur in the case of wild boars thickening their skins in preparation for battle.[145] Rather, the structures of trust I plead for need to rebuild and reenact the nature of skin by seeking to bring into place new epidermal knots, assemblages, and communities.[146] Such new assemblages may take multiple forms, but all such forms would converge in the maxim of breaking through dualistic perceptions of skin that place one kind of skin on the side of future and of life, and the other on the side of the present and of death. If Serres is right, and "with cosmetics, our real skin, the skin we experience, becomes visible,"[147] then there is the possibility to engineer and reassemble a new skin, and not only in ways that comply with general culture but in ways that allow for new assemblages that do away with shame and reestablish one's sense of (self-) confidence and trust. The task is to regenerate and *heal* skin in light of a common skin and an open future.[148]

New assemblages can only be had when time and vulnerability move us beyond a reified present and allow for what Heidegger calls a moment of vision: a moment where the present can open up as meaningful and can be reinscribed in light of our past and future. Still, this moment of vision is for the sake of our analysis not a moment tied solely to the individual, but a collectivized moment of vision. While Heidegger helpfully draws our attention to the power of finitude to liberate us from pure enchainment to the now and opening us to broader horizons of temporality, important material changes in our culture and politics need to occur in order that those who have been denied a future so far may collectively see their temporality in terms of an open future rather than a stagnant present.

Overcoming stifling biases of distrust in relation to problematic epidermalizations demands a broader, radical, affective change than that of one individual who then shares with others in solicitude *after* the fact, or *after* one's authentic moment of vision, as Heidegger proclaims.[149] Tracing Dasein, and its moment of vision, back to its "existential 'where'" allows us to parenthesize, as Sloterdijk argues, the "essential loneliness" of Dasein, and returns Dasein to its place-based potential for solidarity: "[Heidegger's] hasty turn to the 'who' question leaves behind a lonely, weak, hysterical-heroic existential subject that thinks it is the first to die, and remains pitifully uncertain of the more hidden aspects of its embeddedness in intimacies and solidarities."[150]

Returning the moment of vision to its co-existence with others allows thus for a collectivized vision, which, in turn, may affectively reorient the content of Heidegger's solipsistic moment of vision (that of solitary anxiety) toward a collectivized moment of vision embedded in solidarity and trust. Speaking of trust in terms of *structures* emphasizes that I see the emergence of trust as an effort of communities and alliances that, embedded in contingency, collaborate to suspend problematic habitual practices and make authentic futures possible.

Conclusion

This chapter has tried to show that human skin is an important affective interface that enables, mediates, and secretes our rational, sensitive, and emotional being. Much more than a simple barrier or superficial surface, its permeability and its co-evolution with our brain, our culture, and our technology speak to the centrality of its existence for our being, which is far deeper interwoven with both human and nonhuman others than could ever have been imagined.

This dermatological interface is not merely passive, but—in a middle-voiced fashion—chooses and (re)generates our time, place, and being. Providing both spatial and temporal synthesis, our skin both reassembles the cohesion between periphery and center and renews synthetic cohesion between our memory, our finite future, and our present. I have ended this chapter on a cautionary political note, speaking of the need to defy what I have called epidermal death zones, zones of pure suffering, and pleading for the establishment of structures of trust.

The next, and final, chapter seeks to take into account all of the forms of affectivity that I have discussed in this and previous chapters (plants, animals, placentas, and human skins), and attempts to extend the analysis of skin to a material interface that encapsulates many forms of life: that of soil—*the skin of the earth*.[151] Moving the middle voice from the interface of one living being to that of the interface where we all connect and meet up, what would follow accordingly? If we follow the analysis of *pathos* as we have traced it so far, where do we end up when we truly admit our metaphysical, biological and sensitive belongingness ("home") while simultaneously recognizing important differences? In the grand scheme of things, might *compassion* be an important conceptual tool to grasp our webbed existence (what I will call our e-co-affectivity), and where does this bring us in terms of ethical and political responsibility?

If I return to where I began this chapter, being inspired by the skin-to-skin contact with my newborn daughter and the new spatial and temporal configuration it brought, I hope that image can guide us to the next chapter, but in an expanded sense. The task would be to reflect on material interfaces more deeply, more expansively, immersing ourselves in thought along the common edges of living beings tied together to the skin of the earth, merging and emerging alongside each other in a world full of contingency.

Chapter 5

E-Co-Affectivity beyond the Anthropocene
On Soil and Soil Pores

and we fight against this depth complex, as if the essential of life unfurls in the shadowy darkness or in the depth of oneself.

—François Dagognet, *La peau découverte* (1993, 54)

I don't think we will ever have a general principle for what sharing suffering means, but it has to be material, practical and consequential, the sort of engagement that keeps the inequality from becoming commonsensical or taken as obviously okay.

—Donna Haraway, *When Species Meet* (2008, 77)

Hospitality is the fundamental virtue of the soil. It makes room. It shares. It neutralizes poisons. And so it heals. This is what the soil teaches: If you want to be remembered, give yourself away.

—William Bryant Logan, *Dirt: The Ecstatic Skin of the Earth* (1995, 19)

Introduction

Standing at the grave, the need to cover my father's body with soil filled me with urgency. For his body to be embedded by the skin of the earth, and return there where new possibilities for life emerge. I dug and shoveled and only slowly covered up a part of the casket. Never was soil so dark, so messy, so dense and heavy, yet so comforting. Only weeks later did I remove the dried-up soil from my boots.

The previous chapters have provided complex accounts of affectivity that are in many ways unique to the very beings discussed: starting with an account of the middle voice in plants, continuing with a discussion of touch and trauma in bird feathers, thinking through the generative in-between that is the placenta, and ultimately analyzing the human (inter)surface that is skin. This fifth and final chapter is different in that it focuses on the interface of soil, and thereby seeks to materially link together many kinds of beings into a new (local-global) community to be. However, before focusing on soil, it is important to understand why we have arrived at soil, and for this reason I will provide here a summary of areas—and themes—of overlap in previous chapters. This will be instrumental to grasping why the argumentative arc of this book bends—for its final chapter—toward soil.

First, we can ascertain similarity in the ways that plants, animals, placentas, and humans live middle-voiced lives: they all participate in processes that encompass themselves with various temporal and spatial zones of indeterminacy. Perhaps the middle voice benefits plants most of all, as its explanatory power truly uncovers the specific, and oft-overlooked, nature of nutrition, growth, and community formation in plants. Still, the middle voice is a helpful conceptual tool for *all* accounts of affectivity discussed in this book, insofar as it draws attention to what Agamben calls the deposition and exposition of the subject, and moves us away from the centralized singular toward polyphonic communal spaces that regenerate meaning.

Another resounding theme has been that of affectivity in terms of location: as generated by the place of the boundary and the in-between. Along these lines, the account of avian touch centered on the untouchable interstitial space between the feathers that allows animal identity to be born out of difference, and where flourishing, pain, trauma, and demise may literally leave their traces, but modified through social, evolutionary, and intimate practices. In its own peculiar fashion, the chapter on generative human affectivity accordingly focused on the placenta as the exemplary generative organ of the in-between responsible for founding and (re)presenting a "pregnant city," with traces of this pregnant city constantly re-constituting our physiology, pathology, and social-natural relationships. The chapter on human skin for its part focused on the place of the affective, sapient human surface that (re)generates our time, place, and being, and that is—politically and socially—all too easily the victim of distrust and shame, depriving certain skins of life-affirming future-oriented powers.

A third theme of overlap in the accounts of affectivity can be found in the mediation of trauma. In the chapter on plants, this emerged most clearly through, for example, the descriptions of epigenetic changes, traumatic memory, communicative gases, and hybrid, trans-species and trans-generational partnerships. In the chapter on birds, the discussion of the "fault bar allocation hypothesis" clarified that birds have powerful ways to re-signify the meaning of trauma. And in the chapter on generative human affectivity, the placenta and its microchimeric trace emerge as powerful and ambiguous resignifiers of present and future trauma and well-being. Finally, the chapter on human skin argued that the skin's synthetic power points forward toward mediating harm and instituting structures of trust that return a future to otherwise marginalized and traumatized skins.

What has not been discussed so far, and what had to wait until this final, concluding chapter is this: given our current knowledge of these unique, yet intersecting, forms of affectivity in living beings, how might we conceptualize the need for a new form of affectivity, one that allows humans as we currently know them to become transformed and reconstituted into a non-anthropocentric, Latourian "us" with more horizontal, cross-species, affective entanglements? How can we shift our habits and allow ourselves to become more responsive to the needs and sufferings of others, so much needed here and now, at the edge of the anthropocene? Where and how may we find the much-needed opportunity to create and nurture a communal place and time and a new "us," one that cultivates a different epistemic and aesthetic sensitivity and temporality? How can we shift our affective responses and reconstitute an alternative form of affectivity, one that we, preliminarily and ambitiously, might call *e-co-affectivity*?

If it is the case that our global enterprises have failed and have returned us to reconsider the singular ecosphere that is Gaia,[1] then there is an important task lying ahead to think through the web of affective relationships without denying the uniquely human task to position itself differently, to shift its affective responses, and to be reconstituted into a different "us." After Descartes' proclamation of humans as "masters and possessors of nature,"[2] such a transformation is badly needed in light of the ecological havoc left in its wake. Thus, this chapter will explore the possibility for a new affective response, and a new "us," reimagining a different, more participatory entanglement of beings, allowing for ways to suspend the limited and finite horizon of human perspectives. For this reason, the book title *E-Co-Affectivity* resonates particularly strongly in this chapter, in that the focus on participation, solidarity, and place find renewed imagination and articulation in the theme of soil.

The first part of this chapter will conceptualize what co-affectivity or *sym-pathēsis* (as com-passion) means on a more interpersonal, psychological, and physical scale. It discusses two forms of co-affectivity (direct and indirect) in Aristotle's and Haraway's texts, addressing both the use and limitations of their converging approaches. The second part of the chapter has a more ambitious aim, namely to theorize the place, time, and meaning of e-co-affectivity in light of the anthropocene and the consequent need for a new community to be formed. Throughout this chapter, I will draw attention to the meaning of "paying attention" to the suffering of others, and I will index three different kinds of paying attention, one of which addresses the more direct and inter-subjective level of co-affectivity (Haraway's account in *When Species Meet*) and two of which address the macrolevel (Stengers and Stiegler) within which our attention to co-suffering is shaped.

I argue that Aristotle's and Haraway's bifurcation between direct (mimetic) and indirect (non-mimetic) sharing of suffering is crucial to conceptualizing e-co-affectivity, and that there are important elements to their accounts, such as the emphasis on the immanent materiality of sharing suffering, as well as the importance of a nondirect form of co-suffering—witnessing suffering and paying attention—with important ethical, evaluative, and practical consequences. Still, both accounts have shortcomings. Their accounts of direct co-affectivity fall short in that they conceive of direct co-affectivity mostly in the realm of individuated beings interacting with each other in a current time and place; their accounts of indirect co-affectivity are oriented too much toward the realm of human cognitive psychology (pity in Aristotle) and toward specific ethical settings (and this is particularly the case for Haraway's focus in *When Species Meet* on witnessing suffering in nonhuman lab animals).

My account argues that the interface of soil changes the question of access and the conceptual schema of co-affectivity. Since the interface of soil is both the local underpinning for our lives and deaths (and thus direct and physical) and a theme within the global network within which we are connected with all living and nonliving beings (and in that sense indirect) it accesses a broader, different form of affectivity. This different form of e-co-affectivity is focused on ontogenesis versus being; it is one that fosters a form of regenerative noncognitive, material affectivity that births and buries us all; it is one that in its direct touch still leaves open precious pores to contest boundaries between what is and what is not; and finally it opens up to a temporality and a place beyond that of human temporality, thus drawing consolation and hope for a time and place beyond the anthropocene. I will argue that a new affective regime beyond the anthropocene can only be brought about by both (1) direct interaction with the proximate interface of soil, allowing for different kinds of individuations, and (2) indirect interaction with the interface of soil, allowing the theme of soil to move us toward a more percolative, inventive, and regenerative existence within an broader ecological community.

With regard to the discussion of community and the material interface that may make us new, I will use the theories of Stengers (on paying attention) and Haraway (on the chthulucene) to analyze the interface of soil, rather than appealing to Heidegger and the concept of earth. As I indicated in the introduction to this monograph, my argument, while inspired by Heidegger's philosophy (such as his reading of Aristotle and his focus on affectivity), seeks to also sidestep other aspects, such as his focus on individual affectivity and authenticity, to make room for accounts of a broader *eco-community*. Since both Stengers and Haraway appeal to the need to pay attention to suffering and create community, and specifically a posthuman community that fosters connections with what is "odd" and yet akin, their arguments are crucial for this chapter. Second, Stengers's and Haraway's accounts allow us to think through an engagement with the very *materiality* of these interactions, and encourage new forms of material affectivity and habituation with others. As Haraway writes: "We become-with each other or not at all. That kind of material semiotics is always situated, someplace and not noplace, entangled and worldly."[3] Third, rather than romanticizing the "earth" and promoting a return to "art" versus technology in a Heideggerian sense, Stengers and Haraway, along with Stiegler, do not shy away from seeing the benefits of new technology, as long as such technology is part of a transformed epistemic, ethical, and political eco-regime.

Sym-paschō: Direct and Indirect Co-Suffering in Aristotle

> The affection by which I am affected summons *a response*, it draws my attention toward the affecting reality, which, through its affecting, challenges me to react. The particular and individual character of the affecting phenomenon suggests a particular and personal—and thus unique—kind of answer and this suggestion guides my attempt to come up with an *appropriate* response.
>
> —Adriaan T. Peperzak, *Trust* (2013, 40)

Where the overall aim of this chapter is to gain traction on a new notion of e-co-affectivity beyond the era of the anthropocene, the first step here consists in delineating a preliminary grasp of co-affectivity as we find it in the philosophical tradition. Aristotle's writings here prove helpful, even if they are circumscribed within the more limited scope of singular inter-personal or inter-body relationships, beyond which I ultimately seek to center my argument. As I will argue, Aristotle's discussion of (direct and indirect) co-suffering is constructive in proffering a form of co-affectivity that is direct and material, as well as indirect and mediated. While I discern limitations to the specifics of his account of co-suffering, Aristotle's discernment of the two forms of co-affectivity is an essential building-block of my wider claim: that a new affective regime beyond the anthropocene can be effected only by both (1) direct interaction with the proximate interface of soil and (2) indirect interaction with the thematic interface of soil.

To initially think co-affectivity with Aristotle is to find it centered on a distinction between direct (physical and emotional) co-suffering and co-suffering at one step removed. To expand on the first, Aristotle uses the Greek term *sym-paschō* in line with other writers of his time in the context of natural processes. For instance, Aristotle speaks of *sym-paschō* when he argues that it is better for the foot to be split into toes, because if it were unsplit, the entire foot would be affected if one part of it were harmed (*Parts of Animals*, IV.10, 690b4).[4] *Sym-paschō* as used in its physical context connotes literal, simultaneous, unmediated, being-affected together: split toes prevent injury to the foot to be all-pervasive, instead confining harm to partitioned, more localized parts. Thus, the form of co-affectivity that Aristotle here describes is that of physically sharing, that is, participating in, the same suffering. And other works, such as the *Nicomachean Ethics*[5] and the *Rhetoric*,[6] provide important evidence for extending this notion of physical sharing of pain to the realms of sharing human emotions and actions.[7] And this comes particularly clearly into view when we focus on pity (*eleos*) as discussed in the *Rhetoric*, to which we turn next.

The second form of co-suffering is found in the discussion of pity. Pity (*eleos*) is one of the closest kinds of emotion (*pathos*) that connects our own suffering to that of others, but does so at a (mediated) distance. Aristotle defines it in the following way:

> Let pity (*eleos*) be understood as a certain pain (*lupē tis*) at an apparent evil, destructive or painful, which befalls one who

does not deserve (*anaksiou*) it, and which one might expect to suffer (*pathein*) oneself or one of one's own (*tōn hautou*), and moreover when it seems close to hand. (*Rhet.* II.8, 1385b13–16)[8]

For Aristotle, pity is a painful affect[9] that emerges when someone else suffers harm, and specifically when this suffering is undeserved. The latter stipulation ushers in a moral judgment, thus indicating a level of rational mediation in the formation of this affect. What is most productive and enlightening about this definition of pity is the implied personal *vulnerability* to suffering:[10] feeling pity is made possible because one judges oneself, or "one of one's own," vulnerable to similar harms in the future, especially when this suffering seems near.

The personal fragility that Aristotle notes here in his description of pity, however, should not be confused with the direct material sharing of pain that is implied by *sym-paschō*. There are really two different forms of co-affectivity at stake in Aristotle: direct (physical and emotional) co-suffering and co-suffering at one step removed, which entails feeling pain for others as connected to feeling one's own personal fragility.

To illustrate the difference between the two forms of co-affectivity, Aristotle provides a powerful example to distinguish them: the case of King Amasis,[11] who did not weep when his son was led to his death, but did weep when he saw a, presumably distant, friend begging *(Rhet.* II.8, 1386a19–21). According to Aristotle, father and son directly share in the same pain because of their family connection: when the person who suffers is extremely close to us, the suffering of the other is directly related to us and, thus, our own, while the suffering of others at a distance invokes pity.

What exactly can be learned from the distinction between the two forms of co-suffering? Specifically, how might both forms of co-affectivity—that of direct suffering, and that of the articulation of pity as being at one step removed—be productive to push forward the language and experience of co-affectivity needed in light of the anthropocene? And what might be the shortcomings of the discussion of the two forms of co-affectivity that Aristotle discerns?

Sym-paschō Redux: Co-Suffering in Butler and Haraway

> Human beings' learning to share other animals' pain nonmimetically is, in my view, an ethical obligation, a practical problem, and an ontological opening. Sharing pain promises disclosure, promises

becoming. The capacity to respond may yet be recognized and nourished on this earth.

—Haraway, *When Species Meet* (2008, 84)

At one step removed, pity provides an opening to mediate and filter how and that we are affected, involved, and moved by others' suffering. Since it is the case that we, as humans, all suffer and are undone in grief and mourning, Judith Butler has argued that the recognition of suffering and grief in others may allow us to feel a shared humanity, a shared "social vulnerability."[12] In *Precarious Life*, Butler addresses the dynamics of being undone in mourning, and how mourning, along with desire, underlines that rather than being autonomously constituted, we are always also relationally constituted as well as "dispossessed" by our relationships.[13] This has political consequences, in Butler's mind: since there is a differential grievability of different subjects,[14] because precarity is distributed so unequally and unfairly, this "implies the need for a more generalized struggle against precarity"[15] and makes "grief itself into a resource for politics."[16] And, given that our own embodied precarity is part of a network of relations, Butler argues that "we cannot understand bodily vulnerability outside of this conception of its constitutive relations to other humans, living processes, and inorganic conditions and vehicles for living."[17]

It is at this point of connectivity between human and nonhuman sharing of suffering that we may bring in Haraway's work, which articulates the importance of being moved by not only the suffering of human others, but also nonhuman others.[18] In *When Species Meet*, Haraway talks about the important difference between mimetic and nonmimetic sharing of pain in the context of lab animals suffering harm. Haraway differentiates mimetic sharing of suffering—that is, "taking the place of the victim," which is similar to Aristotle's point about direct *sym-paschō* since it equally involves feeling the same, direct pain—from what she calls *true* sharing of suffering: "Sometimes, perhaps, 'taking the place of the victim' is a kind of action ethically required, but I do not think that is sharing."[19] For Haraway, to truly share suffering, we must use a *non-mimetic approach*, which implies carefully and ethically paying attention as a witness. Sharing suffering with those made unequally vulnerable implies an engagement that "has to be material, practical and consequential, the sort of engagement that keeps the inequality from becoming commonsensical or taken as obviously okay."[20]

Thus, Haraway's account of sharing suffering takes note of the need to pay attention to suffering and to take our response seriously, so as to invoke "the mundane grace to eschew separation, self-certainty, and innocence even in our most creditable practices that enforce unequal vulnerability."[21] Accordingly, in her thinking about practices with lab animals and their suffering, she asks us to "do the work of paying attention and making sure that the suffering is minimal, necessary, and consequential."[22]

Haraway's discussion of mimetic and non-mimetic sharing reveals the importance of reflective affective mediation for making sharing suffering true and productive. Over against those thinkers and activists such as Simone Weil who argue that the suffering of others needs to be felt (mostly) directly,[23] Haraway's account pushes us to recognize that non-mimetic sharing of suffering can serve to (1) think through inequalities in suffering,[24] (2) translate sharing suffering into practical and ethical action, ultimately allowing for lessened suffering,[25] and (3) provide impetus for the education and art of paying attention to suffering.[26]

Thus, the important bifurcation that Aristotle already discerned between *direct* physical and emotional sharing of suffering and *indirect* sharing of suffering acquires new prominence with what Haraway calls mimetic and non-mimetic sharing of suffering. The path of non-mimetic sharing of suffering points backward—feeling our responsibility for certain forms of suffering that we ourselves may have caused—and immerses us in the present due to the feeling of pain, and points us forward—toward openness and rethinking new and alternative material, practical and consequential engagement with the suffering of others.

While Haraway, in *When Species Meet*, clearly delineates how such forms of shared suffering should occur in the context of enlightened lab practitioners, the task for us, in this final chapter, is to question what Haraway's call for sharing suffering means for an e-co-affective local-global community to be. In his book *Flight Ways*, Thom van Dooren offers us the technique of telling *narratives*, creating a space for mourning and grief,[27] to carve out the possibility of sharing suffering with species that are on their way to becoming extinct.[28] By telling such stories we may position ourselves in a different affective place and reconnect: "to relearn the world and our place in it."[29] For van Dooren, this also means that, individually and collectively, we are asked "to face up to the dead and to our role in the coming into being of a world of escalating suffering, loss, and extinction."[30]

Van Dooren's emphasis on grief and relearning our place in the world connects us back up with Aristotle's account of pity at one step removed and that of Haraway's non-mimetic suffering: in all cases we are not simply just involved in someone else's suffering, but we reach a mediated affective space where we *reposition* ourselves, take responsibility, and become changed along the way.

Still, there are important shortcomings to the above approach of co-suffering, even if it allows us to feel our own vulnerability and aligns us with the suffering of others through pity or grief. One such shortcoming may be that, as the early Stoics and Adam Smith already noted, co-suffering in the form of compassion is too narrow-minded and "binds us to our own immediate sphere of life,"[31] without seeing others in similar need for attention, and without productive consequences.[32] Along these lines, Hannah Arendt argued that compassion is, politically speaking, irrelevant and problematic, since it forces us into silence and does not invoke "persuasion, negotiation and compromise" needed for law and politics.[33]

For this chapter on e-co-affectivity, where we seek to address the need to participate in and connect with the ways that other kinds of species and beings are affected, not just on the local but the *global* level, this objection of shortsightedness surely resonates. Thus, the focus so far on the individual, psychological, and cognitive aspects of indirect, or non-mimetic, suffering might be insufficient to address the broader, global needs of the wider ecological community in danger. This especially resonates given the thought that e-co-affectivity ideally should speak not only to local, individuated concerns but to the broader need to be affected differently by the totality.

Another important objection, particularly relevant to this chapter, is that the accounts of direct and indirect co-suffering so far formulated are geared at contemporaneous *human* beings, with particular discrete and concrete, finite attributes. Is there a way to envision, beyond the anthropos of the present moment, and even beyond the anthropocene, a form of e-co-affectivity that speaks to a different future, to different possibilities, and possibly to a new "us"? And is there a way to conceive of this new "us" as emerging both out of a direct material *and* indirect interaction with the affectivity and suffering of nonhuman others? Especially since the anthropocene as geological and temporal era seems to exceed our human place and timescale, such a new "us" might need to be envisioned. If so, what might the future geological and temporal era and that new "us" possibly look like? And what material interface might grant us such new opportunities? This is what the second part of this chapter will take on.

E-Co-Affectivity beyond the Anthropocene:
Rethinking the Role of Soil and Soil Pores to
Imagine a New "Us"

> It is up to us to create a manner of responding, for ourselves but also for the innumerable living species that we are dragging into the catastrophe, and, despite this "us" only existing virtually, as summoned by the response to be given.
>
> —Isabelle Stengers, *In Catastrophic Times: Resisting the Coming Barbarism* (2015, 41)

Amid the ongoing and ever-accelerating ecological tragedies of the anthropocene, perhaps more accurately called the capitalocene,[34] Isabelle Stengers zooms in on the human task to shift its affective response. Stengers appeals to us to make us *feel and think* in line with *naming*[35] Gaia's intrusion.[36] In naming that which has been provoked as Gaia (i.e., a "ticklish assemblage of forces")[37] and Gaia's consequent reaction as "intrusion," that is, as being "blind to the damage she causes, in the manner of everything that intrudes,"[38] Stengers does not claim that these names are true, but at least these names have "the power *to make us feel and think* in the mode the name calls for."[39] Instead of hearing one domineering, human voice that answers the question of what is to come,[40] she argues we need to take into account "the voices of many peoples, knowledges and earthy practices."[41]

Gaia's intrusion, for Stengers, steers us to learn to respond and to relearn the art of paying attention.[42] This "creates an obligation to imagine, to check, to envisage consequences that bring into play connections between what we are in the habit of keeping separate. In short, making ourselves pay attention in the sense that attention requires knowing how to resist the temptation to separate what must be taken into account and what may be neglected."[43] Paying attention, for Stengers, implies going beyond habitual ways of making distinctions, and, instead, making room for the interstitial space out of which creativity and new habits (of thinking and feeling) might arise. This is not merely a task for the individual: as her focus on naming already indicates, Stengers is looking for a collective movement: she calls for the "collective reappropriation of the capacity for and art of paying attention."[44] This also implies seeking out other narratives that allow for "new modes of resistance," "which refuse the forgetting of the capacity to think and act together that public order demands."[45]

The new "art" of paying attention needs to go hand in hand with a new "us," that can "'face' Gaia—that is, face the difficult task of participating in an entanglement, the ticklish, touchy character which we are just beginning to understand."[46] The stories that allow us to imagine this new "us" should *decenter* anthropos without seeking substitution:[47] instead, such stories, for Stengers, have "no entity at the centre of the stage. This does not preclude "responsibility," but carries the sense of being able to respond."[48]

For Stengers, one of the topics that can help us "face" Gaia is that of the commons, its expropriation,[49] and the question of what "making common" means.[50] For this investigation, I suggest that thinking through the material and ontogenetic function of *soil* is crucially important to reimagine "us" participating in a new affective entanglement, where entanglement, following Stengers, indicates "entangled coexistence," that is, the emergence of constellations that are not to be grasped as a system of functionality and of parts and whole, but rather as assemblages due to "bricolage," that is, the construction or creation from a diverse range of available things.[51]

Soil and Soil Pores: An Engagement of Soil Science and Plato's *Symposium*

Until the 1870s, soil was mostly conceptualized as an inert layer, the leftover residue of rocks. Only later did soil acquire the status of an active and ontogenetic boundary surface, as "a process in itself, in which a system of layers critical to life on Earth grows out of fine rock particles."[52] Accordingly, researchers have increasingly described soil in terms of both destructive and generative processes, and soil itself has been defined as "the interface between lithosphere, atmosphere, hydrosphere, and biosphere."[53] Ranging from rocks (the lithosphere) and gas (the atmosphere) to liquid (the hydrosphere) and life (the biosphere), soil is an interface on both a macro and micro level. Considered from a macro level, soil is a "reaction layer between rocks and the chemical, physical and biological environment at the atmosphere-lithosphere interface."[54] And from a micro level, we can argue that soil, qua soil, *includes* all these spheres as components of itself (i.e., rocks, air, water, and living organisms); individual soils mix those worlds—of rock, air, water, and living beings[55]—in different proportions.[56] The complexity and productivity[57] of such interactions cannot be understated, and in this regard soil is similar to other intricate environments, such as estuaries.⁵⁸

Perhaps surprisingly, the functioning of soil depends for approximately 50 percent on soil pores:⁵⁹ the mostly invisible interstitial places that form its connective tissue.

> Spaces in soil that are not occupied by soils are called pores. Actually, they are not void; they are filled with either air or water, or both, depending on the soil moisture content and condition of rainfall and irrigation. Roots and soil organisms, both macro- and microflora and fauna, occupy these pores.⁶⁰

This textbook definition establishes the contradictory nature of pores by first defining pores as void of soil, only to subsequently define them in terms of their many functions—absorbing and percolating water and air, providing space to roots and soil organisms—that make soil such a dynamic interface. There is a conceptual hesitancy to make that which is nonsolid (and thus that which is not firm, unstable in shape and with gaps) part of the definition of soil. Still, as Brady and Weil confirm, "the spaces between the particles of solid material are just as important to

Figure 5.1. Soil.

the nature of a soil as are the solids themselves. It is in these pore spaces that air and water circulate, roots grow, and microscopic creatures live."[61]

The conceptual hesitancy to rethink the nature of soil in terms of its interstitial pores parallels the need to provide an ontology of substances and to neglect the material, ontological in-between that makes distinctions between solid versus dynamic (and being vs. nonbeing) fluid and problematic, for instance by linking them through porous boundaries.[62] Along these lines, Merleau-Ponty encourages us to "see as things the intervals between things themselves," allowing us to perceive "another world."[63] And Derrida, in his writings on the conceptual boundaries between animal and human, pleads for "limitrophy": thinking about "what feeds the limit, generates it, raises it, and complicates it."[64]

What would happen if we come to see soil's pores differently, perhaps by following a speculative path rooted in Greek etymology[65] of the term *poros*?[66] And specifically, what results if we trace pores back to Plato's definition of the Greek God Poros in the *Symposium*? In Plato's *Symposium*, Diotima recounts to Socrates the origin of love (Eros), the divine spirit who is born of the male God Poros and the female spirit Penia. Poros is the god of intense pursuit and resourcefulness, and Penia is the embodiment of need and poverty.[67] Resembling his father Poros, Eros

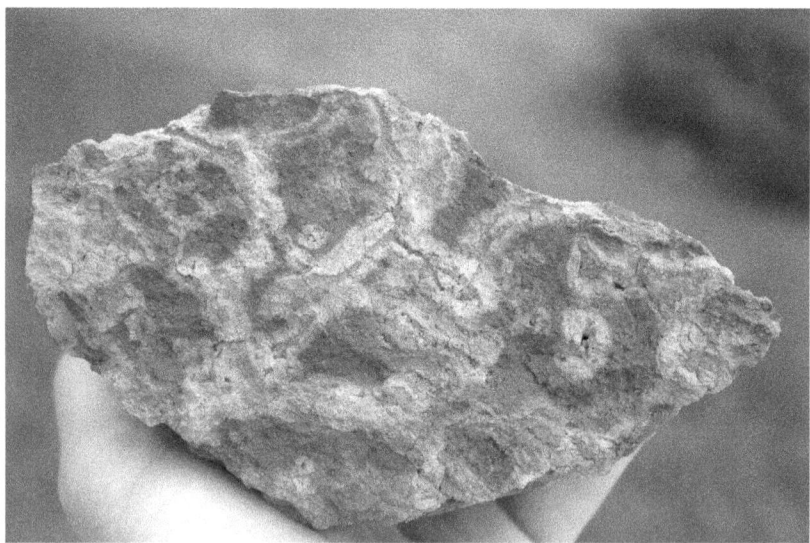

Figure 5.2. Soil pores allow water and gas to move through soil.

is a schemer after the beautiful and the good; he is brave, impetuous and intense, an awesome hunter, always weaving snares, resourceful in his pursuit of intelligence, a lover of wisdom through all his life; a genius with enchantments, potions, and clever pleadings.[68]

If we follow this line of thought, pores are not to be thought of as unsteady, empty, and discontinuous spaces, but instead as places of pursuit and resourcefulness. And certainly when we grasp that pores are embedded within a whole *network* of pores, they emerge as channels and places for connectivity—"weaving snares," as Plato would call it. Moreover, pores—as reflective of Poros' status as parent of love (Eros)—point at a channeling of energy to a new generation, to a new demonic existence that is always in movement.[69] This demonic existence of the in-between (*metaxu*) lets Eros and other *daemons* serve as messengers and hermeneutic mediators between finitude and transcendence. As mediators, they do not just shuttle back and forth, but actually constitute and *connect*, that is, *hold together*, that which is finite and that which transcends it: "Being in the middle of the two, they [spirits, *daemons*] round out the whole and bind fast the all to all."[70]

By birthing Eros, Poros' resourcefulness becomes productive in the lives of finite, material beings through their constant erotic *quests*:

> He [Eros] is by nature neither immortal nor mortal. But now he springs to life when he gets his way; now he dies—all in the very same day. Because he is his father's son, however, he keeps coming back to life, but then the resources he acquires always slip away, and for this reason Love is never completely without resources, nor is he ever rich.[71]

If Poros' nature is to give birth to a fertile, demonic existence immersed in finitude and yet breaking through it, then the soil's pores and what they enable gesture toward a complex combination of finitude, fertility, and generational transcendence. This complex form entails both the limitations of those finite beings involved in it, as well as the creative cultivation of nearly unlimited, yet unthought and unfelt, possibilities enabled through the rupture of finite time.

In sum, focusing on soil as mediating interface for a new "us" is effective in that it offers us a way to imagine a joint, participatory material body that connects—weaves snares—between all of us, yet does so in a way that does not homogenize and overpower. Rather, it empowers invention, resourcefulness, and creativity through that which moves, while being itself non-firm, unstable, and liminal. It may thus allow for the formation of a non-anthropocentric "us," whose name and being is yet to be determined. This would be a Latourian "us" where human agency is not only part of a larger constellation, but mediated and transformed in such a way that we may no longer call such agency by the current name of "human."[72]

Second, soil presents us with an embodiment of an archetypal reaction surface, constantly transforming and reconfiguring itself with incredible resourcefulness. It allows us to see time and place as in-motion, constantly shifting, entailing different temporal and spatial directions. Finally, as an emergent porous body full of opportunities, soil seems to *create* and nurture place and time, rather than the opposite: being the "space" or "place" or "time" in which things are placed. The next section will elaborate on these remarkable dimensions of time and space as they pertain to soil.

Soil, Place, and Temporality and Re-Intervening with Soil

Thinking of soil, and soil pores, on a temporal level holds potential benefit as a prism for shaping a new us. By grasping both the synchronic and diachronic time of soil, soil's temporality lends perspective to our finite human phenomenologies. It has been estimated that "it takes 700 to 1,500 years to generate an inch of soil, or 300 to 600 years for a centimeter of soil."[73] If this is true, then the temporality of soil provides an important contrast to human temporalities, and provides an alternative imagining beyond the minuscule timescale of human, finite time. Moreover, the temporality afforded by soil not only confronts us with its profound and complex past, but also with rich, emergent possibilities yet to come. Rebecca Hill, reading Irigaray's work on the interval, adds important insights here, relevant to understanding the temporal complexity of soil and, specifically, soil pores:

> The interval is a threshold that gestures towards the impossibility of mastering place and time. Why? The past inscribed through and as place remains beyond recuperation in the present, and the futures inscribed as place cannot be anticipated by definition.[74]

Soil pores certainly serve as synchronous limits, holding and limiting content and thereby constituting place and time in the present; pending size and depth of placement, each percolates in its own time. For example, large pores allow for "fast infiltration and percolation of water" and small ones have "strong attractive forces to hold water in the pore."[75] In terms of place, pores are the discrete transit points between the various material "spheres" of soil, thereby suturing the (seemingly) uniform space of soil.

Pores represent and enable diachronic time, a time of slow yet continuous change that we cannot usually readily perceive. For that reason, much like Irigaray's conception of the interval, each pore "is a sensible, porous, and mobile threshold to pasts and to futures that cannot be recuperated or anticipated or said to have being. The interval remains in radical excess of calculation and definition in the inflexible form of a traditional concept."[76] Such radical excess, beyond the concrete now, is also applicable to the place of pores: pores, while constituting definite, concrete spatial limits, also have constant movement and interchange between them, thus influencing beyond their own limits that which passes through them.

That pores hold such a mobile threshold to the past becomes particularly apparent with the development of biopores, which are "macropores created by roots, earthworms, and other organisms."[77] Due to the passing of worms, or the death and decay of plant roots, biopores could be said to contain carved-out traces of the past, constituting the limitations of the present while enabling soil's future; these pores enable the fruition of new life by channeling nutrients and providing a vibrant, dynamic place for plant roots and microorganisms to grow, die, and recycle.

Similar to this conception of the interval, soil pores transcend typically human, short-term reckoning with time. Is there a way to transform our current sense of human temporality to be more responsive to the temporality of the soil? What would such responsiveness look like?

If we take into account the slow, emerging time of soil's origin in combination with its porous, percolating nature, then human practices that engage with such enduring soil temporality and porosity include current popular initiatives such as the shift to "slow food"[78] or even, more generally, "slow living" and "slow movement."[79] Other, similar practices include increased composting of household green waste (another way of using our own waste to "re-invent" soil), the use of green manure, and, in the context of urban construction, keeping current vegetation as "undisturbed" as possible, preserving topsoil for "reapplication," and re-engineering soil after construction, aiming to ensure its quality.[80] Additionally, farming practices[81] that rely on long-term tilling[82] would need to be minimized. Thus, pleas have been made on behalf of "conservation tillage" that decreases soil tillage and keeps the organic residue intact. Many of these suggested changes in farming—less tilling and green manure, for instance—are slowly but surely making their way into mainstream farming, thus indicating that even within the overarching capitalist framework of modern agriculture,[83] such changes can be incorporated, especially when farmers see the immediate financial benefits of these changes, such as through increased monetary yield connected with improved soil fertility and decreased soil erosion.[84]

Still, while the above strategies are promising as we seek to be more responsive to the temporal structures of the soil, they seem to uncritically assume that we need to forsake technology and return to preindustrial techniques such as no tilling. However, don't some current technology-infused strategies, even if limited in scope and technological imagination, show us we *can* engage geological temporality more responsibly without turning back the clock on modern forms of life? These strategies include the use of GPS, Web-based apps, and everyday robotics.[85] For instance, the implementation of satellite navigation may "boost efficiency and cut soil loss by dispersing seed for a cover crop between rows of corn plants well before the corn is harvested."[86] Solar-powered tractors have been developed in conjunction with modern apps that help farmers "keep track of plantings, harvests, and yields."[87] And, if we think along the lines of recent bioengineering technologies that make use of natural microbial consortia to improve soil fertility, or technologies that wean plants off their dependence on fertilizers, we can push this line of argument even further: is there precisely not a distinct need for a form of technics, for a form of prosthesis, that *mediates and re-engineers* our access to geological temporality and changes the agricultural system accordingly?

The progressive development and imagination necessary to push such technologies to an innovative level admittedly takes time, as generations of farmers need to shake up their old habits, usually acquired over decades from previous generations. Often, older generations must die before new habits can truly take hold. As one farmer says: "One of the toughest things about learning to do no-till is having to unlearn all the things that you thought were true."[88] Still, human dependence on soil stands at a critical threshold, with a future looming over us precariously as much as it holds promise. How might we, using the trope of soil, envision a less precarious, more hopeful, future?

Moving Beyond the Anthropocene: Soil and the New "Us"

> What belongs properly to human societies is the question raised by its interstices, at the risk that some social answers to this question may turn against their culture . . .
>
> —Isabelle Stengers, *Thinking with Whitehead* (2011, 328)[89]

In search for the new "us" that, following Stengers, can "face the difficult task of participating in an entanglement,"[90] the material and ontogenetic functions of soil and its pores may offer us ways to imagine ourselves beyond the anthropocene,[91] inspiring hopes for a new future and new indexical "we." Haraway calls for a new epoch, that of the chthulucene, to imagine such a different future. She bases her chosen term for the new epoch, the chthulucene, on the Greek roots *chthōn* and *kainos*, with *chthōn* referring to the Greek term for earth, land, and country.[92] With *chthōn*, Haraway includes "beings of the earth, both ancient and up-to-the-minute . . . replete with tentacles, feelers, digits, cords, whiptails, spider legs, and very unruly hair."[93] *Kainos* refers to time, particularly the sense of what Haraway calls "a thick, ongoing presence."[94]

While there is a close intimacy between my approach and Haraway's, especially given her focus on *chthōn* as related the earth,[95] I suggest, if only playfully, that my argument instead calls for the *soilocene*, to index that I seek an alternative way of being temporalized by the interface of the soil rather than through the figure of individuated animal beings living *in* the earth or beneath its surface, as indicated by *chthōn*.[96]

By suggesting the soilocene rather than the chtulucene, I share Haraway's aim for a future beyond the anthropocene, yet seek to shift her focus on a particular (tentacular) form of life after which we might model ourselves and our future to that of the material and ontogenetic interface of soil. This gestures a shift from figure to interface: rather than thinking from the perspective of individuated critters living in the earth, my focus on soil offers an example of a participatory material body that itself is not one but many in unity, while still bridging divisions between nonliving and living matter: an affective interface that as much as it houses life simultaneously *invents it*. The soilocene thus can effectively express the need to be affected by a *totality*, rather than extending compassion from one being to another—one tentacle at a time. Because of this, it equally satisfies what Haraway seeks, namely the project of "making kin,"[97] albeit in an even more co-affective, communal, material sense.

The soilocene has the additional benefit of emphasizing the importance of *sym-pathēsis* and its ensuing middle voice. While Haraway draws our focus on how the chthulucene will enable *sym-poiēsis*, which, in her words, "enfolds autopoiesis and generatively unfurls and extends it,"[98] my project, while closely connected in affinity to Haraway's, shifts the focus from the subjective act of doing things in community (*sym-poiēsis*) to *being communally and locally affected* (*sym-pathēsis*) and co-emerging together. *Sympathēsis*, in being rooted in *paschein* and thus the root verb for affectivity, has the advantage of emphasizing that any process of emergent generation does not depend solely on already-established individual actors that act in collaboration, but rather on a co-affective process out of which emergent beings unfold and become.

Finally, as a temporal and spatial reaction surface that constantly transforms and reconfigures itself, soil allows us to see time and place in motion, perpetually changing. More particularly, in having multiple layers and thus different senses of place and time (duration), soil yields different temporal and spatial directions and thus different places, pasts and futures.

In short, soil's meaning as interface (and its figurative capacity to link together many entities as well as various temporalities and localities into a new community to be) is promising. Still, the following questions remain: how can we shake up our habits,[99] break through regimes of feeling, and allow ourselves to be co-constructed differently?[100] How can affective and aesthetic cuts, these "revolutions of our senses," as Rancière calls them, happen?[101] And how can we be more aware of this in-between, multilayered, spatiotemporal connective interface? How can we allow for the development of trust,[102] specifically one that indicates one's affirmative engagement in a community that transcends that of humans? On what soil are we standing, or should we be standing? How can we preserve the emphatic middle voice of soil, with its implied destituent power, without losing traction on the meaning and function of human intervention? What emergent possibilities may be created for us once we imagine ourselves created and produced by the material interface of soil, with its mutually implicating spaces?

Stengers's reading of Whitehead, and specifically her analysis of his concept of the interstice, offers an important suggestion for how we may allow this new "us" to emerge. For Whitehead, "life lurks in the interstices of each living cell."[103] And since life, for Whitehead, implies originality and creativity, Stengers analogously argues that only societies that are perceptive to the interstices that bound and ground them can tolerate originality and creativity:

> When a society mobilizes for war, the interstices become imperceptible, and all originality is suspected of treason. Only a society that does not define the environment on which it depends as a threat can tolerate originals.[104]

A culture that embraces its interstices and the imaginations and questions of doubt it holds would "open a human collectivity to an outside whose intrusion suspends habitual social functioning,"[105] and allow such interstices "to propagate themselves," fruitfully leading to "disobedience and desertion."[106]

Following Stengers's ideas, and tracing the import of soil's successful dependence on its vibrant pores, a new "us" may thus appear by allowing interstices to "make themselves felt,"[107] as these are the places where "new possibilities of relevance lurk."[108] Here lies the opportunity to reconstitute ourselves and our perceptions, to bring about new alliances, to break down barriers while constituting a new "us"—all while simultaneously keeping in mind questions of race, class, gender, and species, as much as bios writ large. It is also here where the interstitial cracks may be widened and conceptually intersect with the ambitious vision of Plato's *eros*. Plato's *eros* shows us how the realm of the in-between is immersed in finitude and yet breaks through it: Plato's *eros* shows us that the in-between is fertile with new opportunities that ever emerge as well as disappear. If trust, as Stengers argues, "is one of the many names for love," and if one can "never be indifferent to the trust you inspire,"[109] then Plato's focus on the role of love as dynamically emerging in the in-between may inspire us to put trust in the dynamic, porous interface of soil and to trust the possibilities and new modes of existence arising out of the soil, rather than imposing on them all-too-familiar categories of human sapient meaning that stifle its fertility and block its ever becoming anew.

Along with an aesthetic and epistemic sensitivity to the interstitial boundaries of our culture and nature, our society is in need of aesthetic and epistemic *deceleration and percolation*. A culture can become perceptive to its interstices only once it slows down, relearns patience, and develops endurance. This cannot be a culture that only privileges and lives by chronological standardized time, with its "imperialist regime"[110] that dominates and homogenizes all other forms of time and life. As Jonathan Crary persuasively shows in his book *24/7*, the kind of time we currently encounter is this: 24/7 is "a time without time, a time extracted from any material of identifiable demarcations, a time without sequence or recurrence."[111] This is a homogenized kind of time, dictated by capitalism and its injunctions to constantly perform and to be "on" nonstop: it inscribes into human life "a duration without breaks, defined by a principle of continuous functioning. It is a time that no longer passes."[112] In this world of 24/7, there is no longer any place for deceleration, unplugging, or sleep. The consequence of 24/7, is, according to Crary, "the sweeping abandonment of the pretense that time is coupled to any long-term undertakings, even to fantasies of "progress" or development. An illuminated 24/7 world without shadows is the final capitalist mirage of posthistory, of an exorcism of the otherness that is the motor of historical change."[113]

Thus, Crary diagnoses that the postindustrial capitalist underpinnings of 24/7 deprive us of the opportunity for long-term undertakings, since it offers a world merely identical to itself without offering room for alternate temporalities and discernment of social and ethical valuations.[114] We can only change our form of experiencing time if we rethink our economic and political regimes. Along these same lines, Stiegler argues that we can only resist such a homogenized, and constantly accelerating, form of temporality, and "save time," if there is a "transvaluation of the industrial economy." Only then may we be propelled into a new epoch, provocatively and dialectically called the *Neganthropocene*:

> The Anthropocene is unsustainable: it is a massive and high-speed process of destruction operating on a planetary scale, and its current direction must be reversed. The question and the challenge of the Anthropocene is therefore the "Neganthropocene."[115]

For Stiegler, the Neganthropocene can be brought about only once we employ negentropic forces that, precisely by using alternative forms of technology, transform the speed of current "technological vectors" (merely aimed at increasing entropy) and, literally, allow us "to save time."[116]

Should we pay closer attention to the meaning of "percolation," it becomes clearer what cultivating such a new form of receptivity entails. Percolation is the process of "causing a liquid to permeate through a porous body or medium."[117] The force behind the action, the quality of the medium, the size of its pores, and the contact time all matter. Given this, cultivating an epistemic and aesthetic sensitivity toward percolation implies sensitivity to the *organization* of our affective experience: for instance, awareness of the kind and the size of the forces that drive it toward or away from percolation, its filtering capacity (what it eliminates and keeps and on what basis), and the contact time (speed) it provides to process experiences.

If we link this thought to soil and its temporality, while following soil's enduring diachronic trail, a new "us" would be inclined to create space for a more reflective, percolative, and patient temporal existence, one where possibilities slowly yet steadily emerge out of coincidental assemblages,[118] and where multiple directions and opportunities unfold simply through the gradual passing of time. Making space for this alternative, decelerated, more percolative form of temporality does not preclude urgent action or intervention on the part of current humans: on the contrary, unlearning our own habits and shaping new ones[119] requires the pressing, active work of adapting to a new form of receptivity.

It is here where the various theorists addressing the importance of "paying attention" to suffering come together. Haraway's account of sharing suffering and paying attention in *When Species Meet* alerts us to the inescapable fact of our participatory existence, and levels ethical injunctions at us to care for the nonhuman other and to alleviate and minimize the suffering of others we may have caused. Stengers and Stiegler articulate another way in which paying attention to the suffering of others is important, and do so at the macro level. For Stengers, paying attention to ecological devastation can be mobilized through different epistemologies and languages, and by carefully choosing names and concepts we may gain traction—and alter—our feelings and habitus in light of the catastrophe we face. Stiegler, for his part, also focuses on this macro level, but addresses the need for change to our political-economic systems, which have transformed our affective register and have suspended our creativity and abilities to pay attention to what really matters. According to Stiegler, only through this transformation to our affective regime can we install the Neganthropocene.

The proposed vision for a new "us" might seem improbable if it were not that our predicament calls for this possibility to be realized immediately, especially now, especially here, at the edge of the anthropocene. Similar to recent artistic renditions, including those of Indian artist Tejal Shah that show the possibility to find beauty by embracing the post-apocalypse and dancing on heaps of filthy garbage,[120] the possibility of creating a new "us" will be difficult, but perhaps not impossible. Soil and its pores point the way and provide a living, connective tissue: beyond the concrete and discrete individual, here and now, refusing homogeneous space and standardized chronological time, they direct us toward other places, toward other times, toward solidarity with other beings, toward unexpected assemblages and gatherings,[121] aiming at a future yet unimaginable, but hopefully full of liquidity,[122] deceleration, and percolation.

Epilogue

The autobiographical invocation at the beginning of this chapter has not only affective but also theoretical residue. The soil to which the bodies of our loved ones—and we ourselves—return offers guidance for a philosophical vision of e-co-affectivity. If the poet George Meredith is correct to suggest that soil (or earth, in his words) "knows no desolation. She smells regeneration/in the moist breath of decay,"[123] then my epilogue seeks to address this hopeful figure of the soil: it is precisely soil as proximate and direct interface of our bodies that offers reconfiguration and transformation of life. It is also soil in its direct encounter that gives us life, that feeds us, that creates a place and time, and that keeps us grounded and ungrounded at the same time. Where grief, as exemplified in its etymological rootedness in gravity, pulls us down to the soil,[124] the soil in turn may offer consolation and much more to suggest regeneration and hope.

For Gaston Bachelard, "a material image dynamically experienced, passionately adopted, patiently explored, is an *opening* in every sense of the word, in its real sense and its figurative sense."[125] This is exactly what I think the focus on soil accomplishes: soil is inescapably tangible and material in its reality, yet enigmatic and porous as well. For that reason, it serves not only as an example of a material interface we always already engage with, but also as a powerful metaphor, not only to re-imagine but to change our affects and discourses. Comparable to how certain terms and metaphors such as "immunity" suddenly keep hold of discourses and change our practices, similarly—or so I hope—can the metaphor of soil, following Blumenberg's idea of metaphors, reach down into the substructure of thought and existence,[126] and thus initiate a new way of living, feeling, acting, and thinking.

However, in my view, the levels of direct and indirect interaction with the affectivity of the soil may converge if we look at soil from the broader lens of our political and economic context. If it is the case that, following the ideas of Stiegler, the industrial capture of attention systematically "deforms our attention,"[127] then there is reason to think that we can, once again, *foster* and *reform* attention,[128] and rescue and remake "savoir faire," that is, "knowledge of how to make and do,"[129] if there is a change to current political and economic regimes so as to allow for different ways of (psychic and collective) individuation.

What we need, I argue with Stiegler, is thus a new "politics of individuation,"[130] one that refers to the materiality and community of the soil and intervenes with it creatively and responsibly, fostering attention for long-term goals and dreams that have currently been blocked by the short-term vision and accelerated yet stunted temporality of 24/7 that diminishes and blocks interstitial time and place. As we intervene with the interface of soil, we need not to exclude new forms of technics. On the contrary, following Stiegler, new prosthetics may be key to successful and more responsible interjections.

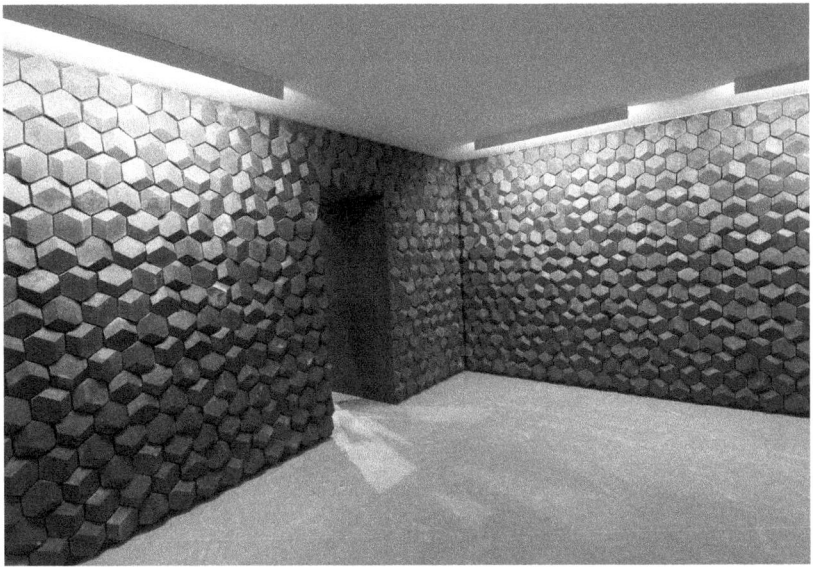

Figure 5.3. *Soil quasi bricks*, 2003. Artwork by Ólafur Elíasson.

Contemporary Danish-Icelandic artist Ólafur Elíasson illustrates the possibility to intervene creatively with soil by making "quasi shapes" out of it, stacked up high like walls. His artwork *Soil quasi bricks* (2003) is made of fired compressed soil tiles and wood.[131]

The quasi brick is "both irregular (at the ends) and regular (the hexagonal section) [which] gives any structure made of quasi brick a chaotic aspect, not seen, for instance, when stacking cubes."[132] Elíasson writes: "The overall shape changes according to how you stack the quasi bricks. So they're quasi shapes, being always open to other ways of building with them. They incorporate time in a way."[133] In stacking the tiles, there is an element of "unpredictable production," which ensures that the artwork is "only constituted in the mesh in which it's entangled and exchanged." It is this element of the nonprescribed and nonpredictable that Elíasson names "quasi."[134] While Elíasson does not address this directly, it is my view that by building these nonprescribed, regular-irregular artworks with soil, Elíasson adds an element of fragility, depth, and unique texture into his artworks, ensuring that temporality is even more visible as a "co-producer of the quasi-project."[135]

Elíasson's artwork illustrates the possibility to engage soil through technics, incorporating soil in his quasi shapes to build walls consisting of both regular patterns as well as open, unpredictable, chaotic ways in which the soil bricks emerge. His artwork shows that careful engineering of the soil[136] can be both responsive to the place and temporality of soil, and evocative of a new e-co-affective regime to come. To counter the "numbing" of existence and what Stiegler calls the affective proletarianization that destroys attention,[137] we would do well to engage the soil more responsibly yet creatively, pausing our lifestyle, and, following the root of the word "attention," encounter a sense of being "stretched" and "waiting."[138] Accordingly, we may reclaim "a sensitivity or responsiveness to both internal and external sensation" and non-metric durations,[139] thus allowing for long-term visions that engage a more sustainable home or *oikos* for all.[140]

Notes

Introduction

1. This is particularly the case for Aristotle's usage of "tode ti" in his *Categories*. See Aristotle, *Categories*, 3b10.

2. In embracing the term "soil" I reject a number of meanings of the term "earth" (*Erde*) as Heidegger formulates them, one of which is that of earth as "the *Heimat* that is both given and yet chosen, the homeland where on has learned to come into one's own." John Sallis, foreword to *The Song of the Earth: Heidegger and the Grounds of the History of Being*, by Michel Haar, trans. Reginald Lilly (Bloomington: Indiana University Press, 1993), xii. Haar distinguishes four meanings of "earth" in Heidegger: (1) the obscure ground of our abode (57); (2) that which is usually called "nature" (59); (3) the "material" of the work (60); and (4) earth as the "terrestrial" (*heimatlicher Grund* [61]).

3. Martin Heidegger, "The Origin of the Work of Art," in *Basic Writings: From "Being and Time" (1927) to "The Task of Thinking" (1964)*, ed. and trans. David Farrell Krell (New York: Harper Collins, 2008), 174. Sheehan speaks lucidly of the relationship between world and earth, addressing the rootedness of our human "possibilities in a specific natural environment." Cf. Thomas Sheehan, "Martin Heidegger," in *Routledge Encyclopedia of Philosophy*, Vol. 4, ed. Edward Craig (London: Routledge, 1998), 318.

4. In his elucidation of the meaning of earth in Heidegger, Haar writes that earth may signal a particular earth, but also signifies for Heidegger "the nonfactual, non-geographic, non-planetary character of the Earth as the *place of rootedness* capable of proffering, given an epoch and a world, a nonhistorical possibility" (Haar, *The Song of the Earth* xvi). And: "Earth which founds art and sustains habitation loses its tangible and purely material or natural obviousness. Communicating with the withdrawal of being, it opens a space which, escaping historical mutations, abides unscathed" (Haar, *The Song of the Earth* 14).

5. In this regard, I find especially the work of Quentin Meillasoux and Ray Brassier useful because Meillasoux and Brassier offer a nuanced view on

the various tiers of materiality as well as the various forms that may emerge out of matter. My interest in Meillasoux's work on new materialism does not mean, however, that I endorse all its tenets: I do not support the anthropocentrism that is also part of Meillasoux's work. Cf. Quentin Meillassoux's *After Finitude: An Essay on the Necessity of Contingency*, trans. Ray Brassier (London: Continuum, 2008).

6. In academic circles, the term "affect" is becoming better known, not only in philosophy proper but also through "affect studies" or "affect theory," a branch of scholarship mostly connected with literary and cultural studies. I will discuss this branch of scholarship, and its connection to my scholarship, more closely in the methodology section of this introduction.

7. *The OED Online*, July 2018, Oxford University Press. s.v. "pathos, n.," accessed November 8, 2018, www.oed.com/view/Entry/138808?redirectedFrom=pathos.

8. The concept of *pathos* emerges across Aristotle's entire oeuvre, in his physics, metaphysics, biology, rhetoric, psychology, and ethics. Within these works, *pathos* shows up with a wide variety of meanings, such as changeable quality, illness, emotion, and excruciating suffering. This spectrum of meanings within Aristotle's works becomes even larger if we also take into consideration related nouns such as *pathēma* and *pathēsis*, and related predicates such as *pathētikos*. It is exactly this wide spectrum of meanings of *pathos* and its related terms that has made it difficult to provide a comprehensive overview. Cf. Hermann Bonitz, *Index Aristotelicus* (Darmstadt: Wissenschaftliche Buchgesellschaft, 1955 [first published 1870]), 555–57.

9. The Oxford English Dictionary (OED) defines *pathos* currently used mostly in two ways: (1) as "a quality which evokes pity, sadness, or tenderness; the power of exciting pity; affecting character or influence," and as (2) "the quality of the transient or emotional, as opposed to the permanent or ideal (contrasted with ethos); emotion, passion. Chiefly with reference to ancient Greek rhetoric and art." *The OED Online*, July 2018, Oxford University Press, s.v. "pathos, n.," accessed November 8, 2018, www.oed.com/view/Entry/138808?redirectedFrom=pathos.

In both cases we see emphasis on *pathos* in terms of fluctuating changes and emotion.

10. Cf. Michael Hardt, "Foreword: What Affects Are Good For," in *The Affective Turn: Theorizing the Social*, ed. Patricia Ticineto Clough with Jean Halley (Durham, NC: Duke University Press, 2007), ix.

11. With thanks to Manuel Vargas for his encouragement and suggestions in formulating this definition.

12. Cf. Adriaan T. Peperzak, *Elements of Ethics* (Palo Alto, CA: Stanford University Press, 2004), 1.

13. James Hart speaks powerfully of a "gracious act of attention" that lies at the origin of our being. Cf. Hart's *The Person and the Common Life: Studies in a Husserlian Social Ethics* (Dordrecht: Kluwer, 1992), 179. With thanks to Peter H. Steeves for drawing my attention to this quote. Also see Irina Aristarkhova,

who argues that the way maternal hospitality is often rendered, namely as merely passive, serves to marginalize the role of the maternal. Instead, Aristarkhova focuses on the maternal activity of offering hospitable space to emphasize the remarkable activity and importance of maternal hospitality for generation: Irina Aristarkhova, *Hospitality of the Matrix: Philosophy, Biomedicine, and Culture* (New York: Columbia University Press, 2012), 46–47.

14. Karen Barad, *Meeting the Universe Halfway: Quantum Physics and the Entanglement of Matter and Meaning* (Durham, NC: Duke University Press, 2007), 393.

15. Michel Henry, *Material Phenomenology*, trans. Scott Davidson (New York: Fordham University Press, 2008), 134.

16. I will offer further definition of my sense of "community" in the methodology section of the Introduction.

17. Cf. François Dagognet, *Faces, Surfaces, Interfaces* (Paris: Librairie Philosophique J. Vrin, 1982), 49.

18. While the term "engineering" has a problematic "hue" due to its association with eugenics in the history of thought, my usage of it seeks to bracket and overcome this baggage by addressing how engineering speaks to the *strategic formation of affective responses* that forms of life and matter create in reaction to what happens to them, not in a totalitarian sense, but anarchically and often in solidarity with others. Speaking of engineering is especially warranted in an ethical and political project such as mine which, ultimately, seeks to (un)ground us in the soil. Given this ungrounding, the process of affective engineering need not imply an engineer or designer, nor imply totalitarianism, since the re-active surfaces I investigate reject the notion of such an autonomous, freestanding, engineer or designer. With special thanks to Amanda Parris for helpful comments on my usage of "engineering." For more on affective engineering, see chapter 5.

19. In Aristotle, the most comprehensive definition of affective change is offered in *Metaphysics* V.21: "*Pathos* means (1) a quality in respect of which a thing can be altered, e.g., white and black, sweet and bitter, heaviness and lightness, and all others of the kind. (2) The actualization of these—the already accomplished alterations. (3) Especially, injurious alterations and movements, and, above all, painful injuries. (4) Misfortunes and painful experiences when on a large scale are called *pathē*. (trans. Ross)." In this definition, note that Aristotle excludes *aisthēsis* from *pathos* proper (see my discussion of this in chapter 2). The range of meanings covered by Aristotle's discussion of *pathos* is wide, echoing the broad scope of meaning of *pathos* in ancient Greek. It extends from the "neutral" potential changes in quality, which beings can experience, to actualized changes, to life-changing experiences of suffering that afflict beings. For further elucidation on the range of meanings of *pathos* in Aristotle's oeuvre and their interconnections, see my article "Passive Dispositions: On the Relationship between *Pathos* and *Hexis* in Aristotle," *Ancient Philosophy* 32, no. 2 (Fall 2012), esp. 355–357.

20. Donna Haraway, *When Species Meet* (Minneapolis: University of Minnesota Press, 2008), 93. As sources for these ideas, Haraway refers to both Isabelle Stengers and Alfred North Whitehead.

21. As Karen Barad has it, from the perspective of new materialism, agency is not undone but has a different focus: it is about "changing the possibilities of change" (Barad, *Meeting the Universe Halfway*, 178).

22. As Braidotti clarifies within the context of posthuman feminism, difference still matters. Rosi Braidotti, *The Posthuman* (Oxford: Polity Press, 2012), 88.

23. Cf. the helpful analysis of the dangers of the turn to materialism in Astrida Neimanis's essay "Thinking with Matter, Rethinking Irigaray: A 'Liquid Ground' for a Planetary Feminism." In this essay, she signals the dangers that materialism may pose for feminism, if this turn is understood to interpret matter as part of "reductive essentialisms" or in terms of "brute and inert matters," which, in turn, may do away with the epistemology and ethics forged so carefully out of feminist concerns with "language, discourse, and representation" (43–44). Instead, Neimanis argues for thinking *with* matter, rather than thinking about it. In her specific case, Neimanis seeks to think with water. Astrida Neimanis, "Thinking with Matter, Rethinking Irigaray: A 'Liquid Ground' for a Planetary Feminism," in *Feminist Philosophies of Life*, eds. Hasana Sharp and Chloe Taylor (Montreal-Kingston: McGill-Queen's University Press, 2016).

24. Here I am very much in line with the thoughts on stratification in the critical ontology of Nicolai Hartmann. As Peterson writes: "Hartmann relates the ontic domains of physical, organic, mental, and socio-cultural reality in terms of the geological metaphor of 'stratification.' Within the framework of these four strata he can consider teleologism to be the error of taking categories from the highest stratum and applying them to lower strata, borrowing principles 'from above' to explain the lower strata, rather than understanding them in terms of their own principles." Keith Peterson, "Stratification, Dependence, and Nonanthropocentrism: Nicolai Hartmann's Critical Ontology," in *Ontologies of Nature: Continental Perspectives and Environmental Reorientations*, eds. Gerard Kuperus and Marjolein Oele (Dordrecht: Springer, 2017), 170. According to Peterson, Hartmann's approach may thus address matter and difference between forms of matters, circumventing both "vulgar materialism" as well as vitalism.

25. In his lecture course *Facing Gaia*, Bruno Latour writes that due to scientific discoveries that measure how certain humanly produced toxins affect the earth, we are coming to realize (think and feel) that "the Earth might be rounded by our own action." Bruno Latour, *Facing Gaia: Six Lectures on the Political Theology of Nature*, Gifford Lectures, February 18–28, 2013, 93–94, www.bruno-latour.fr/sites/default/files/downloads/GIFFORD-ASSEMBLED.pdf.

This turn to a smaller sphere is in radical distinction to previous eras, as Peter Sloterdijk has also observed. Whereas previous ages emphasized universal and imperialist views of the world in "grand narratives," in the current age multi-perspectival foams have taken its place. Cf. Peter Sloterdijk, *Foams: Spheres Volume III: Plural Spherology*, trans. W. Hoban (South Pasadena: Semiotext(e), 2016), 16–25.

26. Aristotle, *Categories* 4, 2a3–4. Cf. my "Attraction and Repulsion: Understanding Aristotle's *Poiein* and *Paschein*," *Graduate Faculty of Philosophy Journal* 33, no. 1 (2012): 85–102.

27. As Stengers writes: "It is up to us to create a manner of responding, for ourselves but also for the innumerable living species that we are dragging into the catastrophe, and, despite this "us" only existing virtually, as summoned by the response to be given." Isabelle Stengers, *In Catastrophic Times: Resisting the Coming Barbarism* (London: Open Humanities Press, 2015), 41.

28. See Heidegger's parsing of the term "phenomenology" in § 7 of the Introduction to *Being and Time*, where he argues that "the expression 'phenomenology' means *legein ta phenomena* (i.e., *apophainesthai ta phenomena*): "to let that which shows itself be seen from itself in the very way in which it shows itself from itself." Martin Heidegger, *Being and Time*, trans. J. Macquarrie and E. Robinson (Malden, MO: Blackwell, 1962), 58. Cf. also Christopher Long, *Aristotle on the Nature of Truth* (Cambridge: Cambridge University Press, 2011), xii.

29. My phenomenological approach has affinity with other phenomenological posthuman thinkers, such as Astrida Neimanis's *Bodies of Water*, which uses a phenomenological approach that incorporates reference to scientific studies. She defends "her use of proxies and syncretic assemblages such as science as ways of getting to 'experience' or 'going back to the things themselves' " (61–62) by referencing Haraway's important proposition that all knowledge is mediated through prosthetics. Astrida Neimanis, *Bodies of Water: Posthuman Feminist Phenomenology* (London: Bloomsbury Academic, 2017). However, my approach is distinct from Neimanis in that it engages phenomena even more radically from the bottom up, and searches for theories and phenomenologists who can best address the phenomena at stake. Moreover, while I am sympathetic to the ethical and feminist register of Neimanis's approach, my attempt is not to insert distinctly *human* valorizations too early into my discourse, so as to truly seek for open and posthuman discourse.

30. Patricia Ticineto Clough, "Introduction," in *The Affective Turn: Theorizing the Social*, eds. Patricia Ticineto Clough with Jean Halley (Durham, NC: Duke University Press, 2007), 9. Ultimately, as Clough articulates it, the "most provocative and enduring contribution of the affective turn" is its pointing to "a dynamism immanent to bodily matter and matter generally—matter's capacity for self-organization in being informational." Patricia Ticineto Clough, "The Affective Turn: Political Economy, Biomedia, and Bodies," in *The Affect Theory Reader*, eds. Melissa Gregg and Gregory J. Seigworth (Durham, NC: Duke University Press, 2010), 207.

31. Clough, "Introduction," 2.

32. Brian Massumi, *Parables for the Virtual: Movement, Affect, Sensation* (Durham, NC: Duke University Press, 2002), 35.

33. This turn from affect to emotion is something that Patricia Clough also recognizes: "Many of the critics and theorists who turned to affect often focused on the circuit from affect to emotion, ending up with subjectively felt states of emotion—a return to the subject as the subject of emotion" (Clough, "The Affective Turn: Political Economy, Biomedia, and Bodies," 207). Clough herself, in this essay, turns to economic-capitalistic forces of production to explore the shift from an understanding of the body-as-organism to what she calls the "biomediated body" (207). While her essay thus addresses a broader grasp of affect, which I endorse, the limiting aspect is her focus on the *human* body.

34. Sara Ahmed's *The Promise of Happiness* interprets affect in terms of feeling and "explores how feelings are attributed to objects, such that some things and not others become happiness and unhappiness causes." Sarah Ahmed, *The Promise of Happiness* (Durham, NC: Duke University Press, 2010), 14.

35. Sara Ahmed, "Happy Objects," in *The Affect Theory Reader*, eds. Melissa Gregg and Gregory J. Seigworth (Durham, NC: Duke University Press, 2010), 29.

36. Clough, "Introduction," 1.

37. Hasana Sharp's *Spinoza and the Politics of Renaturalization* clarifies Spinoza's account of affect, defining it as "those changes in power that belong to finite existence by virtue of being connected necessarily to other beings, immersed in a field of powers and counterpowers that cannot be entirely inventoried, anticipated, or circumscribed by 'human nature'" (25–26). This holds important consequences, as Sharp shows: "As we learn more about our affects, we are better able to gauge our particular 'force of existing,' and whether certain kinds of affections, certain encounters and relationships with others, amplify or diminish our vitality." Hasana Sharp, *Spinoza and the Politics of Renaturalization* (Chicago: University of Chicago Press, 2011), 30.

38. Sharp, *Spinoza and the Politics of Renaturalization*, 34. As Sharp states: "Understanding humanity as vulnerable to the same determinations as beasts, rocks, and vegetables facilitates social harmony and political emancipation. Only when we consider ourselves to be constituted by our constellations of relationships and community of affects can we hope to transform the forces that shape our actions and characters," and may offer "not a better politic of representation and rights, but a posthumanist politics of composition and synergy" (Sharp, *Spinoza and the Politics of Renaturalization*, 15). Sharp pleads for renaturalization, which finds not only inspiration in Spinoza but also in Grosz's embrace of "renaturalism" for redefining feminism, and "seeks local sites of freedom and power without recourse to the figure of an exceptional human faculty, be it reason, moral sensibility, the capacity for autonomy, or even Hegel's desire for recognition." Hasana Sharp and Cynthia Willett, "Ethical Life after Humanism," in *Feminist Philosophies of Life*, eds. Hasana Sharp and Chloe Taylor (Montreal-Kingston: McGill-Queen's

University Press, 2016), 71. Sharp and Willett write: "When we affirm that we are the history of our affective, corporeal, and intellectual involvements, we learn that it is only through transforming a whole network of relations that we can hope to live differently (Sharp and Willett, "Ethical Life after Humanism," 71–72).

39. As Walter Brogan writes: "The fact that Heidegger looked to Aristotle for help in clarifying the many ways of being and knowing that found the possibility of hermeneutic phenomenology complicates the traditional explanation of Heidegger's destruction as a critical movement through the history of philosophy in order to overcome it. In the case of Aristotle at least, Heidegger discovers that the very future of philosophical thinking has already been prepared for but covered over by the scholasticism of the tradition." Walter Brogan, *Heidegger and Aristotle: The Twofoldness of Being* (Albany: State University of New York Press, 2005), 13. An example of Heidegger's reading of Aristotle can be found in his 1924 summer lecture course, *Basic Concepts of Aristotelian Philosophy*. In that course, Heidegger views *De anima* not as a work of psychology or anthropology, but as an ontology of life: it is, as he writes in his 1926 course, "precisely the first-ever phenomenological grasp of life, and it led to the interpretation of motion and made possible the radicalization of ontology." Martin Heidegger, *Basic Concepts of Ancient Philosophy*, trans. R. Rojcewicz (Bloomington: Indiana University Press, 2008), 153; *GA* 22, H. 182.

40. Martin Heidegger, *Basic Concepts of Aristotelian Philosophy*, trans. Robert D. Metcalf and Mark B. Tanzer (Bloomington: Indiana University Press, 2009), 11–12.

41. See also my article "Heidegger's Reading of Aristotle's Concept of *Pathos*," in which I show how Heidegger's reading of Aristotle's concept of *pathos* is extremely rich and innovative as he frees up *pathos* from the narrow confines of psychology and incidental change and places it squarely into the center of the fundamental changes affecting a living being's existence. Marjolein Oele, "Heidegger's Reading of Aristotle's Concept of *Pathos*," *Epoché: A Journal for the History of Philosophy* 16, no. 2 (Spring 2012): 389–406.

42. Bianchi argues that such a strategy "calls us to listen to the Greek assiduously, to attend to the textuality of the text, the philosophical nuance, the rhetorical trope, and especially the resonance of the figures, but also refuses to forget that it is always today that we read or reread Aristotle." Emanuela Bianchi, *The Feminine Symptom: Aleatory Matter in the Aristotelian Cosmos* (New York: Fordham University Press, 2014), 4. Bianchi, in particular, focuses on the question of gender "and in foregrounding that question asks about the legacy of Aristotle's hierarchical system for us" (5). Bianchi writes: "In paying attention to the sexed and gendered symptoms produced in and by the systematicity of these texts, the teleological and hierarchical system may be unsettled from within, or rather, it may be shown to be unsettled in advance, constitutively and incessantly unsettled, and unsettling" (5–6).

43. "community, n." *OED Online*. July 2018. Oxford University Press. www.oed.com/view/Entry/37337?redirectedFrom=community (accessed November 12, 2018).

44. For a constructive account of how collectivity, and the milieu, informs the individual and its ongoing individuations, see Gilbert Simondon, who argues, "The individual is thus no longer either a substance or a simple part of the collectivity. The collective unit provides the resolution of the individual problematic, which means that the basis of the collective reality already forms a part of the individual in the form of the preindividual reality, which remains associated with the individuated reality." Gilbert Simondon, "The Genesis of the Individual," in *Incorporations*, eds. Jonathan Crary and Sanford Kwinter (New York: Zone Books, 1992), 307.

45. John Sallis, *Chorology: On Beginning in Plato's "Timaeus"* (Bloomington: Indiana University Press, 1999), 140.

46. Sallis, *Chorology*, 140.

47. Elizabeth Grosz, *Becoming Undone: Darwinian Reflections on Life, Politics, and Art* (Durham, NC: Duke University Press, 2011).

Chapter 1

1. Stefano Mancuso and Alessandra Viola, *Brilliant Green: The Surprising History and Science of Plant Intelligence* (Washington, DC: Island Press, 2015), 123. As they argue, only 0.3 percent is animal (including human animal) life.

2. Catriona Sandilands, "Phytopolitics: A Critical Foray into Plant Worlds" (lecture at the twentieth annual meeting of the International Association for Environmental Philosophy, Salt Lake City, UT, October 22, 2016). environmentalphilosophy.files.wordpress.com/2017/10/iaep_progream2016.pdf.

3. Francis Hallé, *In Praise of Plants*, trans. David Lee (Portland, OR: Timber Press, 2002),97.

4. The author is also referred to as Pseudo-Aristotle. Pseudo-Aristotle, *De plantis* (Oxford: Clarendon Press), 1908.

5. E.g., in *Enquiry into Plants* III.i.2, Theophrastus discusses the dissemination of willow seeds by floods in Pheneos in Arcadia, and in III.i.3 he discusses the proof that the wind carries the seeds of elm trees. In *Enquiry into Plants* II.ii.7–8, Theophrastus speaks to the effects of soil (*chōra*) differences on the pomegranate, comparing the effect of soil in Egypt with that in Cilicia. He articulates that "the place (*topos*) is more important than cultivation and tendance." Additionally, when he addresses vines, he articulates that the most important aspect for growing and bearing fruit is "suitable soil" (II.v.6). Theophrastus, *Enquiry into Plants Books I–V*, trans. Arthur Hort (London: Putnam's Sons, 1916).

6. The importance and the scale of photosynthetic processes is nearly beyond comprehension. Peter Tompkins and Christopher Bird emphasize that

"without green plants we would neither breathe nor eat," and estimate that "25 million square miles of leaf surface" are engaged with photosynthesis. Peter Tompkins and Christopher Bird, *The Secret Life of Plants: A Fascinating Account of the Physical, Emotional, and Spiritual Relations Between Plants and Man* (New York: Harper Perennial, 1989), viii.

7. As Mancuso and Viola analyze, plants have various systems of communication, namely through "electrical, hydraulic and chemical signals" (*Brilliant Green*, 84).

8. Daniel Chamovitz, *What a Plant Knows: A Field Guide to the Senses* (New York: Scientific American/Farrar, Straus and Giroux, 2012), 44.

9. Chamovitz, *What a Plant Knows*, 43.

10. As Mancuso and Viola write: "even those hundreds of meters away" (Mancuso and Viola, *Brilliant Green*, 56). Those odors allow plants to take measures such as producing phenolic and tannic chemicals to protect them and make themselves "unpalatable to the insects" (Chamovitz, *What a Plant Knows*, 35).

11. Martin J. Hodson and John A. Bryant, *Functional Biology of Plants* (Oxford: Wiley-Blackwell, 2012), 266–67.

12. Hodson and Bryant, *Functional Biology of Plants*, 268.

13. While Hallé writes this in reference to the (presumed) fact that plants do not preserve much from their ancestors as part of their evolutionary lineage (which actually could be contested nowadays based on research of epigenetics), this seems equally if not more applicable to the issue of pain and suffering in plants. See Hallé, *In Praise of Plants*, 288.

14. Chamovitz, *What a Plants Knows*, 139. Chamovitz distinguishes pain from suffering, and writes, "A plant senses when a leaf has been punctured by an insect's jaws; a plant knows when it's been burned in a forest fire. Plants know when they lack water during a drought. But plants do not suffer. They don't have, to our current knowledge, the capacity for an "unpleasant . . . emotional experience." Unlike Chamovitz, I want to grasp affectivity from the plant's perspective, without reference to another form of life with a different materiality, such as that of animals with noci-receptors.

15. Delving into vegetative existence, the adaptable existence of plants may best be grasped as emerging out of a fundamental openness to the power and the role of the accidental and undetermined to "rewrite, resignify, reframe the present." Elizabeth Grosz, "Thinking the New: Of Futures Yet Unthought," in *Becomings: Explorations in Time, Memory, and Futures*, ed. Elizabeth Grosz (Ithaca, NY: Cornell University Press, 1999), 18–19.

16. Hallé, *In Praise of Plants*, 294.

17. The concept of "the active" notably includes an ambiguity, with the distinction between active as in "acting upon another, or upon self qua other," and active as in "in act." Aristotle is sensitive to these ambiguities of the meaning of action and motion. As I have articulated elsewhere in my writings on the meaning of *poiein* and *paschein*, Aristotle clearly understands that motions and processes

can all be "in act" or "in process" but can have various directions and causes: "Aristotle is sensitive to the various directions that motions and activities can take. In other words, there is a difference in meaning at the very root of every motion and activity. This difference is categorized as 'doing' or 'acting' in the most general sense of *poiein* in contrast to that of its antonym, *paschein*, which captures the most general sense of 'being done to,' or 'being acted upon.' What is remarkable is that, although *poiein* and *paschein* are different, they are dependent upon each other as well: as antonyms they cannot be grasped without referring to each other." Marjolein Oele, "Attraction and Repulsion: Understanding Aristotle's *Poiein* and *Paschein*," *Graduate Faculty Philosophy Journal* 33, no. 1 (2012): 87.

18. Charles Scott applies the middle voice to a human- (or Dasein-) centered context in his reading of *Being and Time*. He initially seems to put emphasis on how recognition of the middle voice changes our *thinking*, but he ultimately also includes *living*. Scott writes that "the middle voice creates a need for revised language and thinking" and that it may be necessary "for people to think and live through the question of Being." Charles Scott, "The Middle Voice in *Being and Time*," in *Phaenomenologica: The Collegium Phaenomenologicum, The First Ten Years*, vol 105, eds. John C. Sallis, Giuseppina Moneta, and Jacques Taminiaux (Dordrecht: Kluwer 1988), 165.

19. Rolf Elberfeld, "The Middle Voice of Emptiness: Nishida and Nishitani," in *Japanese and Continental Philosophy: Conversations with the Kyoto School*, eds. B.W. Davis, B. Schroeder and J.M. Wirth (Bloomington: Indiana University Press, 2011), 284.

20. Michael Marder and Luce Irigaray, *Through Vegetal Being: Two Philosophical Perspectives* (New York: Columbia University Press, 2016), 124.

21. Michael Pollan, foreword to *Brilliant Green*, Mancuso and Viola, x, xi.

22. Mancuso and Viola, *Brilliant Green*, 50.

23. Mancuso and Viola, *Brilliant Green*, 3.

24. Mancuso and Viola, *Brilliant Green*, 5, 37, 144. They define intelligence as "the ability to solve problems" (126). Some examples of plant intelligence they provide: "They defend themselves from predators by using complex strategies that not infrequently involve other species, are assisted by trustworthy 'transporters,' in pollination, circumvent obstacles, help one another, can hunt or lure animals, move to reach food, light, oxygen" (129).

25. Rolf Elberfeld makes a persuasive case for why the language of (both classical and modern) Japanese offers a wide field of meanings where the middle voice is still actively operating, simply because in Japanese "the subject can be dropped without further ado, for it does not stand in the center of the sentence" (Elberfeld, "The Middle Voice of Emptiness," 272). As he argues: "it belongs to the ironies of linguistic history that the middle voice up to today remains very

lively in Japanese, but under the influence of European grammar studies since the Meiji period, it is hardly ever still described as the middle voice. It is still in linguistic usage and, above all, it is very vital in one's feeling for the language (Gn. Sprachgefühl) (Elberfeld, "The Middle Voice of Emptiness," 274).

26. Derrida writes about the middle voice: "an operation that cannot be conceived either as passion or as the action of a subject on an object, or on the basis of the categories of agent or patient, neither on the basis of nor moving toward any of these *terms*." Jacques Derrida, *Margins of Philosophy*, trans. A. Bass (Chicago: University of Chicago Press, 1982), 8–9.

27. Benveniste writes: "In the general development of the Indo-European languages, comparatists long ago established that the passive is a modality of the middle, from which it proceeds and with which it keeps close ties even when it has reached the state of a distinct category." Émile Benveniste, *Problems in General Linguistics*, trans. M.E. Meek (Coral Gables: University of Miami Press, 1971), 145.

28. Benveniste, *Problems in General Linguistics*, 147.

29. Benveniste articulates how difficult it is to unlearn our usual thinking in terms of active and passive voice, and to rethink the opposition of voices in terms of active versus middle: "Even the linguist may have the impressions that such a distinction remains incomplete, halting, a little odd, and, in any case, gratuitous, compared to the supposedly understandable and satisfying symmetry between 'active' and 'passive'" (Benveniste, *Problems in General Linguistics*, 150).

30. Linguists have been discerning middle-voiced expressions in English that approximate it ("I am sorry"), or in grammatical forms such as the "get-passive" that come close. Philippe Eberhard, *The Middle Voice in Gadamer's Hermeneutics: A Basic Interpretation with Some Theological Implications* (Tübingen: Mohr Siebeck, 2004), 18–20. We may add to these options ceremonial words of community that echo the middle voice, for instance in saying "congratulations" or "welcome." In these instances, the "I" is not directly invoked but a more participatory, communal process (David Wood, conversation with author, October 2015).

31. Benveniste, *Problems in General Linguistics*, 148.

32. Benveniste, *Problems in General Linguistics*, 149.

33. Eberhard, *The Middle Voice in Gadamer's Hermeneutics*, 15.

34. Eberhard, *The Middle Voice in Gadamer's Hermeneutics*, 16–17.

35. Llewelyn in *The Middle Voice of Ecological Consciousness* points out that for Derrida "the force of deconstruction cannot be likened without qualification to that of the middle voice since the official middle voice of Greek grammar is sometimes tantamount to a reflexive verbs, whereas deconstruction 'does not return to an (individual or collective) *subject* who would take the initiative and apply it to an object, a text, a theme, etc.'" If it is the case that the middle voice in Greek may allow reflexivity, then I am following Scott's lead that the most profound understanding of the middle voice points toward thinking beyond

reflexivity, so in the direction of deconstruction's absent subject. John Llewelyn, *The Middle Voice of Ecological Consciousness: A Chiasmic Reading of Responsibility in the Neighborhood of Levinas, Heidegger and Others* (New York: St. Martin's Press, 1991), 252.

36. Charles Scott, "The Middle Voice of Metaphysics," *Review of Metaphysics* 42, no. 4 (June 1989): 752.

37. Suzanne Kemmer, *The Middle Voice* (Amsterdam: John Benjamins Publishing Company, 1993), 64.

38. Charles Scott, also quoted in Eberhard's *The Middle Voice in Gadamer's Hermeneutics*, 25–26.

39. According to Eberhard, "Scott's account shortchanges the subject," and the volume of the middle voice is so mute, "because it is void . . . Scott stresses the occurrence to such an extent that the relation between the process and the subject falls together with the subject" (Eberhard, *The Middle Voice in Gadamer's Hermeneutics*, 27).

40. For Simondon, the individual occupies only a phase of the whole being, a "phase that therefore carries the implication of a preceding pre-individual state, and that, even after individuation, does not exist in isolation, since individuation does not exhaust in the single act of its appearance all the potentials embedded in the pre-individual state." Gilles Simondon, "The Genesis of the Individual," in *Incorporations*, eds. Jonathan Crary and Sanford Kwinter (New York: Zone Books, 1992), 300.

Simondon also writes that "what individuation makes appear is not the individual alone but the individual-milieu couple." Gilbert Simondon, *L'individuation psychique et collective* (Paris: Aubier, 2007), 12. In this regard, David Scott speaks of how Simondon brings into view the "theater of individuation" (or "drama of individuation"). David Scott, *Gilbert Simondon's "Psychic and Collective Individuation": A Critical Introduction and Guide* (Edinburgh: Edinburgh University Press, 2014), 38, 39. Stiegler addresses this idea of pure ground in terms of a "milieu," and a "potential for individuation"—as a "preindividual fund." Bernard Stiegler, *States of Shock: Stupidity and Knowledge in the 21st Century*, trans. Daniel Ross (Cambridge, UK: Polity, 2015), 52–53.

41. Scott, *Gilbert Simondon's "Psychic and Collective Individuation*," 34.

42. As Mancuso and Viola write: "The purpose of this circulation is readily apparent when you consider that the water absorbed by the roots is lost by the leaves in great quantities through transpiration, and so must be continually restored; meanwhile the sugars produced through photosynthesis . . . must be continuously moved from the site of production (the leaves) to other parts of the organism" (Mancuso and Viola *Brilliant Green*, 85).

43. Ireland defines producers as autotrophs, and consumers as heterotrophs: "producers are autotrophic, meaning they carry out photosynthesis or

chemosynthesis and make food for themselves . . . consumers are heterotrophs. Consumers cannot manufacture organic fuel with solar power but instead must ingest existing organic fuel." Kathleen A. Ireland, *Visualizing Human Biology*, 3rd ed. (Hoboken, NJ: Wiley, 2011), 34–35. The *Oxford English Dictionary* defines "autotrophic" in the following way: "*Biol*. Of an organism: self-nourishing; capable of synthesizing organic compounds from simple inorganic molecules (such as carbon dioxide); not dependent upon organic compounds as a source of energy. Opposed to heterotrophic adj." "autotrophic, adj." *The OED Online*, s.v. "autotrophic," accessed October 12, 2018, 0www.oed.com.ignacio.usfca.edu/view/Entry/250036?redirectedFrom=autotrophic.

44. Another process by way of which plants convert energy is chemosynthesis, an inorganic chemical reaction.

45. As Hallé provocatively writes: "just like the customer at a supermarket, the animal is a consumer and a dispenser of energy" (Hallé, *In Praise of Plants* 289).

46. Hallé, *In Praise of Plants*, 289.

47. Since a plant requires only a simple diet, it has a remarkable ability to find its sources almost everywhere, which contrasts sharply to animals.

48. Hallé, *In Praise of Plants*, 291.

49. Aristotle, *De anima*, trans. Mark Shiffman (Newburyport, MA: Focus Publishing, 2011). (Hereafter cited as *DA*.) For this passage, I used my own translation.

50. Ronald Polansky, *Aristotle's "De anima": A Critical Commentary* (Cambridge, UK: Cambridge University Press, 2007), 216. As Polansky also writes: "*trophē* can, like our term nutrition, be the food that a mortal living being takes or the nutritive process or capacity." Aristotle thus argues that living beings depend on different kinds of food, and also explains this by referring to different nutritive souls (Ron Polansky, email message to author, May 25, 2018).

51. Liddell and Scott distinguish four main meanings for the Greek verb *trephō*: (1) thicken or congeal a liquid; (2) cause to grow or increase, bring up or rear, especially of children bred and brought up in a house; (3) maintain, support; (4) bring up, rear, educate. Henry G. Liddell et al., *A Greek-English Lexicon* (Oxford: Clarendon Press, 1996), 1814.

52. This is similar to many other verbal nouns in Greek, which often have similar flexibility, such as the verbal noun for motion, *kinēsis*: it shares the same root with the active (*to kinoun*) and the middle/passive (*to kinoumenon*).

53. Accordingly, for him this means that the active voice and agent (*to trephon*) of the process of nutrition is centered on "soul in the primary sense"—i.e., that which is concerned with the generation of its offspring (*DA* II.4, 416b23).

54. And the passive voice and patient of the process of feeding (*to trephomenon*) is oriented around its ensouled body (i.e., in terms of plant life, this would be its parts and seeds).

55. With respect to plants, this offers important argumentative counterproof to some of Aristotle's predecessors who deny plants have a soul (Polansky, *Aristotle's "De anima"* 207–8, 211).

56. Chapter 2 of this book is devoted to this account of *aisthēsis*, and in particular to touch.

57. My translation. I am using the term "fully" to speak to the Greek term *enteleicha* and I follow Kosman's suggestion that we should carefully distinguish *energeia* (and translate it as "activity") from *entelecheia* (and translate it as "fulfillment"). Cf. Aryeh Kosman, *The Activity of Being: An Essay on Aristotle's Ontology* (Cambridge, MA: Harvard University Press, 2013), vii–x. See also this book's chapter 2.

58. In this regard, the description here is different from that in *Physics* III.3 where the (passive) process of being taught finds its end in the effect (*pathos*) of acquiring knowledge, as discussed in *Physics* III.3, 212a21–212b22. While we could say that similarly the (passive) process of being nourished finds its end in the effect (*pathos*) of being fed and acquiring nourishment, the difference is that teaching and learning involve qualitative change (at least in the sense of acquiring the *eidos* of knowledge), whereas the focus here is on realization and en-actment without change of the underlying substance. Aristotle, *Aristotle's Physics*, trans. Joe Sachs (New Brunswick, NJ: Rutgers University Press, 1998).

59. This is explored more fully in chapter 2.

60. As Polansky remarks, "the food in the digestive process undergoes alteration and even substantial change as it becomes suitable to feed the plant or animal" (*Aristotle's "De anima"* 215).

61. Polansky examines the sailing analogy (of steersman, hand and rudder) that Aristotle uses to explain the sequence of movers and what is moved. Polansky cites works such as *Generation of Animals* and *On Respiration* to discuss what could serve as "the hand," i.e., as this intermediary moved/mover, citing both fire and pneuma as options (*Aristotle's "De anima"* 220).

62. Cf. Polansky, *Aristotle's "De anima,"* 221. "Assimilation of food is in one way the last step in the process of change, yet in another way, the food has additional work to do in contributing to growth, nourishment, and reproduction."

63. Benveniste, *Problems in General Linguistics*, 149.

64. Aristotle, *Parts of Animals* II.3, 650a21ff., trans. A.L Peck (Cambridge, MA: Harvard University Press, 1937).

65. Giorgio Agamben, "What is a Destituent Power?" *Environment and Planning D: Society and Space* 32, no. 1 (2014): 72.

66. Mancuso and Viola speak of "multiple command centers." See *Brilliant Green*, 3.

67. Cf. Gilles Deleuze, "How Do We Recognize Structuralism?" In *Desert Islands and Other Texts*, ed. David Lapoujade, trans. Michael Taormina (New York: Semiotext[e], 2004), 190.

68. Mancuso and Viola, *Brilliant Green*, 84.

69. Mancuso and Viola write: "the purpose of this circulation is readily apparent when you consider that the water absorbed by the roots is lost by the leaves in great quantities through transpiration, and so must be continually restored; meanwhile the sugars produced through photosynthesis—the plant's main source of energy—must be continuously moved from the site of production (the leaves) to other parts of the organism" (*Brilliant Green* 85).

70. Mancuso and Viola, *Brilliant Green*, 89.

71. Mancuso and Viola, *Brilliant Green*, 89.

72. Mancuso and Viola, *Brilliant Green*, 3.

73. This is with exception of fishes, reptiles and marsupials, as Hallé remarks (*In Praise of Plants*, 97).

74. Hallé, *In Praise of Plants*, 97.

75. Hallé, *In Praise of Plants*, 101. Also see the numerous time-lapse videos that capture the amazing growth and movement of plants. See for instance: "Plants' Stunning Lifecycle Captured in Macro Time-Lapse by Daniel Csobot (VIDEO)," *Huffpost*, July 23, 2013, www.huffingtonpost.com/2013/07/23/plant-time-lapse_n_3582027.html. There may be some exceptions to this, such as tendrils of vines quickly bending, turning, and quivering.

76. Hallé, *In Praise of Plants*, 101.

77. Hallé, *In Praise of Plants*, 97.

78. Hallé, *In Praise of Plants*, 50. He states this and also qualifies it: "In terms of geometry, we can say that animals remain homotopic during their development. In reality, this is only approximate; a baby has a much larger head than an adult relative to its body." Because plants need enough photosynthetic tissue as they develop, their geometrical growth must be open to radical proliferation.

79. Quotation translated by Shiffman; emphasis is mine. Sachs's translation of *De anima* has "all of them that are continually nourished and live for the sake of their ends, so long as they are able to get food." Aristotle, *On the Soul and On Memory and Recollection*, trans. J. Sachs (Santa Fe, NM: Green Lion Press, 2001). Hett has "and they are nourished and continue to live as long as they are able to absorb food." Aristotle, *On the Soul; Parva Naturalia; On Breath*, trans. W.S. Hett (Cambridge, MA: Harvard University Press, 1986).

80. Thus, Aristotle offers a firm response to his (pre-Socratic) predecessors who would have a hard time accounting for the radical oppositional nature of growth in plants without supposing the plant to have a soul. As Polansky writes: "to him [Aristotle] it appears that only soul would prevent the growing thing from being torn asunder as the elements to their separate way." He adds: "soul may employ instrumentally the elemental bodies and their natural directions of motion in arranging the growth of plants and animals, but soul serves as first principle of motion" (*Aristotle's "De anima"* 211).

81. In his interpretation of plant existence in Plato and Aristotle, Nealon argues that they view plants in a "state of constant dissonance, suffering uncontrolled growth without end." As evidence he cites a passage in *DA* II.12, 424b1–3

that speaks to the inability of perception in plants. Jeffrey T. Nealon, *Plant Theory: Biopower and Vegetable Life* (Stanford, CA: Stanford University Press, 2015), 32. However, I take issue with this interpretation, since Aristotle actually argues explicitly *against* unlimited vegetative growth and argues in support of *unified* (*DA* II.4, 416a6–9), *limited* (*peras*), and *ordered* (*logos*) growth (*DA* II.4, 416a16–18) on the principle of *physis* and the soul; this he contrasts with unlimited growth of an element such as fire which does not have such a unifying principle. In addition, the passage in *DA* II.12 that Nealon cites is not meant to demonstrate that there is unlimited growth, rather that plants cannot sense (perceive), since they are affected *together with their matter* by tangible realities as they have no sensuous mean. The absence of a sensuous mean does not imply that plants lack a unifying principle *as such*. See also Theophrastus, who cautions that the growth of plants may *seem* unlimited from the perspective of looking at new shoots; however, when the growth of shoots is understood in light of reproduction (blooming and bearing fruit), plants may seem "more beautiful and more complete" (Theophrastus, *Enquiry into Plants* I.i.2).

82. Joachim specifies how active growing beings themselves are in this process: "the agent of the transformation is not in the food (the food is not of itself transformed into flesh), but in the tissue. The *auksētikon*, immanent in the tissue, converts the food into flesh." Harold H. Joachim, introduction and commentary to *On Coming-to-Be and Passing-Away* = "*De Generatione et Corruptione*," by Aristotle (Oxford: Clarendon Press, 1999), 132. Thus, Joachim stresses the role of (self) transformation—allowing the other, yet adapting and converting the other to suit oneself.

83. Marder, *Plant-Thinking*, 63.

84. If we follow the trope of the locality of plants in terms of earth and soil, then Sloterdijk's words are very promising in that he argues that the earth is a "local area for symbioses of common improbabilities, [is] not a principle, not a foundation. . . . Its way of supporting is that of enabling, not that of securing [*Sicherstellen*]. To this supporting belong the gestures of birth: it delivers, it bears, it generates, it upheaves, it releases." Peter Sloterdijk, *Eurotaoismus: Zur Kritik der politischen Kinetik* (Frankfurt am Main: Suhrkamp, 1989), 326. My translation. See also chapter 5.

85. Polansky, *Aristotle's "De anima,"* 179. He adds helpfully: "therefore the nutritive power is a complete soul, and it seems unlikely that the plant soul is very localized inasmuch as each division of the plant receives a whole soul."

86. As Hallé writes: "the theory of population genetics considers plants and animals as entities at the same level without taking into account that the plant, if it has the structure of a population, can contain several genomes" (Hallé, *In Praise of Plants* 284).

87. Some animals also allow for division, and put the idea of a unified soul in Aristotle even more to the test, since their soul consists of different parts

(perception and nutrition). Polansky argues: "Since the parts of soul all remain together in spite of division of the animal, they seem separate in account rather than separate in place. This is crucial for maintaining that mortal life manifested at different levels presupposes nutritive life and unified soul to account for these levels of life" (*Aristotle's "De anima"* 180).

88. Alfred North Whitehead, "Lecture Two: Expression," in *Modes of Thought* (New York: Macmillan, 1938), 34.

89. The exceptions that Hallé cites include both annual plants such as scarlet pimpernel and wall cress or biennials such as mullein or honesty (Hallé, *In Praise of Plants* 117).

90. Hallé, *In Praise of Plants*, 117.

91. Hallé, *In Praise of Plants*, 110.

92. Hallé, *In Praise of Plants*, 117.

93. Mancuso and Viola, *Brilliant Green*, 3.

94. Michel Luneau, *Paroles d'arbre: Roman* (Paris: Julliard, 1994). Quoted in Hallé, *In Praise of Plants*, 99.

95. Mancuso and Viola, *Brilliant Green*, 145. They define these emergent properties as "properties that single entities develop only by virtue of the unitary functioning of the group; none of the individual components possesses them on their own—just bees or ants, by forming colonies, develop a collective intelligence much greater than that of their individual members" (Mancuso and Viola, *Brilliant Green*, 36).

96. Mancuso and Viola, *Brilliant Green*, 146.

97. Mancuso and Viola, *Brilliant Green*, 141.

98. Agamben, "What is a Destituent Power?" 72.

99. Mancuso and Viola, *Brilliant Green*, 94.

100. Mancuso and Viola, *Brilliant Green*, 94.

101. Marder insightfully circumvents the language of one and many, when he writes that the one plant "is not one—a multiplicity (of growths) that does not merely negate the one, or the One, but reassembles it in a community of growing beings" (Marder and Irigaray, *Through Vegetal Being* 112).

102. Marder and Irigaray, *Through Vegetal Being*, 168.

103. Hallé argues that plants are "indeterminate, undefined, or open," especially when compared to animals (Hallé, *In Praise of Plants* 97).

104. In discussing withering as a *natural* function that is part of the pivotal functions of the soul, Aristotle indicates that withering precludes destruction of life, since this would go counter to Aristotle's idea that the soul is responsible for life (e.g., *DA* II.1, 412a28–29).

105. Joachim, *On Coming-to-Be and Passing-Away*, 131. His complete thought is the following: "it is essential to the soul to animate a corporeal material, i.e. a quantum: and, insofar as the whole tissue is larger or smaller, its 'form' (i.e. its soul or vitality) is expanded or contracted, informing a greater or smaller

quantum." And: "Though what grows is the animated matter as a whole (as a synolon of form and matter), its growth is a uniform expansion of a structural plan—an expansion of the scheme of proportions measuring the matter, not an addition to persisting material constituents."

106. If we examine Aristotle's definition of growth and diminution closely, it becomes clear that both involve change in terms of quantity (*kata to poson*, *DA* II.4, 416b12; cf. *GC* I.4, 319b32).

107. Joachim, *On Coming-to-Be and Passing-Away*, 131. This uniform contraction happens without altering the form of the living being. Polansky: "growth has not only limit in magnitude but also proportion in the parts produced: growth is in all directions with measure so that body parts are suitable organs for the soul" (*Aristotle's "De anima,"* 212). What underlies Aristotle's account of growth is the idea that—as Joachim clarifies—"matter is in constant flux, always flowing in and out, and no material particle endures" (Joachim, *On Coming-to-Be and Passing-Away* 129).

108. In annual plants, "all roots, stems and leaves of the plant die annually. Only the dormant seed bridges the gap between one generation and the next. This is in contrast to perennials, where usually only the top part of the plant dies off, but new parts "regrow from the same root system." Note that a "plant can behave as an annual or a perennial depending on local climatic and geographic growing conditions." Cf. "Annual, Perennial, Biennial?" *Wildflowers in Bloom*, accessed December 30, 2015, aggie-horticulture.tamu.edu/wildseed/growing/annual.html.

109. As Hodson and Bryant explain in their *Functional Biology of Plants*, chilling mostly affects "enzyme systems that are associated with membranes," and chilling-sensitive plants have membranes that solidify at higher temperatures and need to be contrasted with chilling-tolerant plants (Hodson and Bryant, *Functional Biology of Plants* 218). We also need to distinguish between different parts of plants: while some leaves of plants (such as peach trees) can be relatively cold tolerant, its buds may not be.

110. Chamovitz, *What a Plant Knows*, 62.

111. Hallé, *In Praise of Plants*, 97.

112. Cf. Erhun Kula, *Economics of Natural Resources and the Environment* (London: Chapman & Hall, 1993).

113. Such frosts would be particularly harmful for those plants structurally not prepared and set up for it, such as palm trees whose meristems are singular and susceptible to frost.

114. Marder addresses the disruptions of seasonal or daily cycles happening both on a local scale (in hothouses) and global scale (in human-induced climatic changes) in terms of the "disruption of being," and the "unraveling of the measures of vegetal time" (Marder and Irigaray, *Through Vegetal Being* 143).

115. Hallé, *In Praise of Plants*, 123.

116. Hallé, *In Praise of Plants*, 114.

117. Cf. the etymology of the word "endurance" as cited by the OED: "< Old French endure-r to make hard, to endure, = Provençal endurar, Italian indurare < Latin indūrāre, < in (see in- prefix1) + dūrāre to harden, to endure, < dūrus." "endure, v." *The OED Online*, s.v. "endurance," accessed July 17, 2014, en.oxforddictionaries.com/definition/endurance.

118. Hallé, *In Praise of Plants*, 122–23, offers an interesting way of addressing the differences between the nature of death in plants and animals, arguing that plants can "live and die at the same time," which is not the case for animals: they are either "alive or dead."

119. This hardening off is not only in response to cooler temperatures, but also to shortened length of the day. Cf. Chamovitz, *What a Plant Knows*, 126 and cf. assoc.garden.org/courseweb/course1/week4/page20.htm

120. Hallé, *In Praise of Plants*, 122, speaks of "dead points of attachment [that] remain vacant."

121. Hallé states: "In plants, it is as if continual death of used organs has replaced death of the plant itself, the plant having acquired immortality through colonialism" (*In Praise of Plants* 122).

122. Hallé, *In Praise of Plants*, 124.

123. Yulian Wei and Yucheng Dai, "Ecological Function of Wood-Inhabiting Fungi in Forest Ecosystem." *Chinese Journal of Applied Ecology* 15, no. 10 (2004): 1935–38.

124. Interestingly, pioneer plants are often also the ones that offer medicinal value to other kinds of living beings, such as in the case of the dandelions, which have been used to treat urinary problems.

125. Thanks to Christian Douglas for providing these insights on pioneer plants.

126. Chamovitz, *What a Plants Knows*, 129. He writes in reaction to plant research done by Barbara Hohn's laboratory in Basel: "Hohn's astounding study showed that not only do the stressed plants make new combinations of DNA but their offspring also make the new combinations, even though they themselves had never been directly exposed to any stress. The stress in the parents caused a stable heritable change that was passed on to all their offspring: the plants behaved as if they'd been stressed. They remembered that their parents had been through this stress and reacted similarly" (129). The kind of stress these plants underwent included "UV or pathogen stress" (130). As Chamovitz writes: "Hohn's plants, following the UV or pathogen stress, acquired the characteristic of increased genetic variation and passed it on to all of their progeny" (130).

127. Hallé, *In Praise of Plants*, 114.

128. William J. Lewis and D.M.E. Alexander, *Grafting and Budding: A Practical Guide for Fruit and Nut Plants and Ornamentals* (Collingwood, VIC: Landlinks Press, 2008), 2–3.

129. R.J. Garner, *The Grafter's Handbook* (White River Junction: Chelsea Green, 2013), 38.

130. Lewis and Alexander, *Grafting and Budding*, 2–3.

131. Maria Luisa Badenes and David H. Byrne, *Fruit Breeding* (New York: Springer, 2012), 238.

132. In nature, there are also examples of natural grafting, where tree branches or roots of the same species make contact and grow together. Accordingly, such trees may share nutrients such as water and minerals, and form a "larger root mass as an adaptation to promote fire resistance and regeneration." "Wikipedia: Grafting," Wikimedia Foundation, accessed December 30, 2015, 23:38, en.wikipedia.org/wiki/Grafting. This illustrates that plants may *aid* one another directly by allowing resistance to disease to be shared and by reinforcing adaptability to circumstances by joining powers.

133. Mancuso and Viola, *Brilliant Green*, 95.

134. Additionally, "within the nodules the bacteria convert free nitrogen to ammonia, which the host plant utilizes for its development." See: *Encyclopaedia Britannica*, s.v. "nitrogen-fixing bacteria," accessed March 23, 2018, www.britannica.com/science/nitrogen-fixing-bacteria.

135. See Jussi Parikka, *Insect Media: An Archaeology of Animals and Technology* (Minneapolis: University of Minnesota Press, 2010), 129.

136. Benveniste, *Problems in General Linguistics*, 149.

137. Benveniste, *Problems in General Linguistics*, 149.

138. There is much interesting research done on traumatic memory in plants. For instance, research done on flax seedlings shows that a plant can respond to trauma in an interesting way: after removing one of its leaves and cutting its apical bud, flax suppresses growth in the lateral buds closest to its damaged area, while encouraging its lateral bud furthest away to grow, although red light reverses this process, which indicates that the bud closest to the traumatized area still has potential. Even more interesting, plants such as the Spanish needle (*Bidens pilosa*) have ways to memorize the trauma of a wounded leaf, up to a few weeks, as their reaction to another added trauma such as removing the main bud shows. See Chamovitz, *What a Plants Knows*, 122.

139. Christine Dell'Amore, "7 Species Hit Hard by Climate Change— Including One That's Already Extinct," *National Geographic*, April 2, 2014, news.nationalgeographic.com/news/2014/03/140331-global-warming-climate-change-ipcc-animals-science-environment.

140. In a study reporting on the effects of four types of grassland ecosystems, "the researchers found that long-term warming resulted in loss of native species and encroachment of species typical of warmer environments, pushing the plant community toward less productive species." See nau.edu/research/feature-stories/how-climate-change-affects-plants.

Chapter 2

1. Thanks to Christina Garcia Lopez for recommending this passage.

2. Cf. Maurice Merleau-Ponty, *The Visible and the Invisible*, ed. Claude Lefort, trans. Alphonso Lingis (Evanston, IL: Northwestern University Press, 1968), 133–41ff., esp. 141. For a discussion of the meaning of touch in Aristotle as related to chiasmic intertwining in Merleau-Ponty, see Rebecca Steiner Goldner, "Touch and Flesh in Aristotle's *De anima*," *Epoché: A Journal for the History of Philosophy* 15, no. 2 (2011): 439–40.

3. Thus, while I think outlining the conceptual contours of touch is important, certainly in articulating the importance of the untouchable medium, I also think that no account of touch can universally unite animal *aisthēsis* across the different (taxonomical) levels given the difference in materiality of the interfaces that enable touch. Here I am in disagreement with Chrétien, who argues that touch brings with it a triple sense of *universality*: universality as it is found in all its animated subjects, universality in terms of extending and covering the entire body, and "universality on the part of the object," with tangibility constituting sensibility as such. Cf. Jean-Louis Chrétien, *The Call and the Response*, trans. A.A. Davenport (New York: Fordham University Press, 2004), 92–93.

4. For Heidegger, *De anima* is not a work of psychology or anthropology, but an ontology of life: it is, as he writes in his 1926 course, "precisely the first-ever phenomenological grasp of life, and it led to the interpretation of motion and made possible the radicalization of ontology." Martin Heidegger, *Basic Concepts of Ancient Philosophy*, trans. R. Rojcewicz (Bloomington: Indiana University Press, 2008), 153. Aristotle, *De anima*, trans. W.D. Ross (Oxford: Oxford University Press, 1999). (Hereafter cited as *DA*.)

5. Heidegger, *Basic Concepts of Aristotelian Philosophy*, 133. Earlier on, Heidegger writes: "The world, in the character of *hēdu* and *lupēron*, [i.e., of pleasing and unpleasing] is nonobjective; animals do not have the world there as objects. The world is encountered in the mode of the uplifting and the upsetting" (34). And Heidegger writes in *Being and Time*: "And only because the 'senses' [die 'Sinne'] belong ontologically to an entity whose kind of Being is Being-in-the-world with a state-of-mind, can they be 'touched' by anything or 'have a sense for' something in such a way that what touches them show itself in an affect. Under the strongest pressure and resistance, nothing like an affect would come about, and the resistance itself would remain essentially undiscovered, if Being-in-the-world, with its state-of-mind, had not already submitted itself to having entities with-the-world matter to it in a way which its moods have outlined in advance." Martin Heidegger, *Being and Time*, trans. J. Macquarrie and E. Robinson (Malden, MO: Blackwell, 1962), § 29, 176–77.

6. Daniel Heller-Roazen, *The Inner Touch: Archeology of a Sensation* (Brooklyn: Zone Books, 2007), 22.

7. Already Plato's *Theaetetus* brings up the fact that *aisthēsis* has affective components other than pertaining to sight, hearing, smell, etc. so as to include "pleasure and pain, desire and fear," and additional Platonic dialogues bring up connotations such as "seeming" and "believing." It is arguably due to its ambiguous and broad meaning, that *aisthēsis* provides Aristotle with "many possibilities," as Heller-Roazen insightfully adds, to cover the many facets of animal experience (Heller-Roazen, *The Inner Touch* 22–23).

8. Heller-Roazen, *The Inner Touch*, 22.

9. I will be providing my own translation of Aristotle's texts unless otherwise noted.

10. Richard Sorabji, "Aristotle on Demarcating the Five Senses," in *The Senses: Classical and Contemporary Philosophical Perspectives*, ed. F. MacPherson (Oxford: Oxford University Press, 2011), 65.

11. Even if there are "considerable differences in the mechanism involved," such as the medium by way of which an animal perceives (for instance water instead of air as the medium for smell), the *aisthēsis* might still be called similar (for instance "smell") because it pertains to similar objects of each sense ("odor" for instance in the case of smell). Cf. Sorabji, "Aristotle on Demarcating the Five Senses," 66.

12. My translation. As above, I am using the term "fully" to speak to the Greek term *enteleicha* and I follow Kosman's suggestion that we should carefully distinguish *energeia* (and translate it as "activity") from *entelecheia* (and translate it as "fulfillment"). Cf. Aryeh Kosman, *The Activity of Being* (Cambridge, MA: Harvard University Press, 2013), vii–x.

13. He is thereby exploiting the strong linguistic and conceptual link between the verbal sense of being affected (*paschein*) and its noun "affect" (*pathos*) to affirm and contain *pathos* and *paschein* within the boundaries of qualitative change. Notably, in his discussion of *paschein* and *pathos* as part of qualitative change, we could also include the sense of *pathos* as "emotion" or "passion," insofar as Aristotle analyzes *pathos* in the *Nicomachean Ethics* as a way in which we are (temporarily) "moved" and not as a way in which we are "disposed" (*NE* II.5, 1106a3–6). For further exploration of the comparison between *pathos* as emotion and *pathos* as part of qualitative change, see my article "Passive Dispositions: On the Relationship between *Pathos* and *Hexis* in Aristotle," *Ancient Philosophy* 32, no. 2 (Fall 2012): 351–68.

14. Aristotle situates being affected as a process of change, wherein a quality (for instance the quality of coldness) makes place for its contrary (for instance, hotness replacing coldness). This definition of qualitative change as *paschein* is familiar from other passages in Aristotle's oeuvre (such as *On Generation and Corruption* and the *Physics*) and goes so deep and far that Aristotle regularly uses *pathos* as a synonym for the qualities involved in change. Cf. Hermann Bonitz,

Index Aristotelicus (Darmstadt: Wissenschaftliche Buchgesellschaft, 1955 [first published 1870]) 555–57.

15. Aristotle, *On Generation and Corruption*, I.9, II.1–4.

16. Aristotle, *Politics*, trans. C.D.C. Reeve (Indianapolis: Hackett, 1998). Additionally, Aristotle remarks that *aisthēsis* harkens back to the potentialities that arise with birth (*gennēthei*, *DA* II.5, 417b18), further adding evidence to the idea that not only our death, but also our birth is connected to *aisthēsis*. See also Aristotle's *Politics*, where he discusses the issue of the legitimacy of abortion, and aligns birth with *aisthēsis*. He argues that, if abortion is warranted in certain situations, it should only occur "before the onset of sensation and life. For sensation and life distinguish what is pious from what is impious here" (*Politics* VII.16, 1335b25).

17. This idea of categorical contamination could be elaborated more precisely, which I have done elsewhere in a discussion on the correlation between *pathos* and *hexis*. For instance, a sunburn could be an incidental happening (a *paschein* in the "proper" sense, to speak with Aristotle), or be part of other, more permanent changes (for instance, climate change and depletion of ozone) or part of dispositions that make such sunburns more easily or less easily available, such as the color and disposition of one's skin to burn, one's disposition to be careful or careless with regard to exposure to sun, etc. Admittedly, Aristotle on other occasions acknowledges that, in fact, alterations have something to do with dispositions, in that dispositions (*hexeis*) "are some relationship to these [affections] such that they are ordered more or less well." Cf. Ronald Polansky, *Aristotle's "De anima": A Critical Commentary* (Cambridge, UK: Cambridge University Press, 2007), 233; see also *Physics* VII.3. But Aristotle does overall make a serious effort to *separate* one form of change from another, and to distinguish some changes as *expressions* of one's nature from others that are only incidental. Cf. Oele, "Passive Dispositions," 351–68, passim.

18. Christine Battersby, *The Phenomenal Woman: Feminist Metaphysics and the Patterns of Identity* (New York: Routledge, 1998), 58.

19. Battersby, *The Phenomenal Woman*, 58.

20. Elizabeth Grosz, "Thinking the New: Of Futures Yet Unthought," in *Becomings: Explorations in Time, Memory, and Futures*, ed. Elizabeth Grosz (Ithaca, NY: Cornell University Press, 1999), 18–19.

21. We can speak in this regard of the "material secretion of knowledge" associated with *aisthēsis*. We find indications of this idea in Aristotle's *Metaphysics* I.1–2 and *Posterior Analytics* II.19, when Aristotle discusses that learning starts with *aisthēsis* and that *aisthēsis* is fully integrated in the process of learning.

22. Chrétien speaks of the transitive nature of sensibility to address the fact that *aisthēsis* is not inherently reflexive, but finds its origin outside of itself. Chrétien writes: "we always need something other than ourselves in order to

feel, and the organ, to exercise its function of organ, requires the alterity of the object" (*The Call and the Response* 119).

23. Rolf Elberfeld, "The Middle Voice of Emptiness: Nishida and Nishitani," in *Japanese and Continental Philosophy: Conversations with the Kyoto School*, eds. B.W. Davis, B. Schroeder and J.M. Wirth (Bloomington: Indiana University Press, 2011), 271.

24. Erwin W. Straus, *The Primary World of the Senses: A Vindication of Sensory Experience* (New York: Free Press of Glencoe, 1963), 351.

25. In *DA* II.12, 424a17–21, Aristotle offers the example of the signet ring imprinted in wax, writing that just as the ring leaves an imprint on the wax without the iron or gold it is composed of, similarly the sense receives the form of that which it senses without its matter.

26. Elizabeth Grosz, *Chaos, Territory, Art: Deleuze and the Framing of the Earth* (New York: Columbia University Press, 2008), 8. Grosz notes that Deleuze "takes sensation as that which subject and object share, yet is not reducible to either subject or object or their relation."

27. Chrétien, *The Call and the Response*, 120.

28. Chrétien, *The Call and the Response*, 99.

29. Chrétien writes: "for Aristotle, touch is the necessary and sufficient condition for the emergence of an animated body" (Chrétien, *The Call and the Response* 106; cf. 117).

30. Chrétien, *The Call and the Response*, 86.

31. Luce Irigaray, *An Ethics of Sexual Difference*, trans. C. Burke and G.C. Gill (Ithaca, NY: Cornell University Press, 1993), 164. This thought is inspired by her criticism of Merleau-Ponty. Irigaray disputes Merleau-Ponty's ideas to interconnect the sense of the tangible with the visible. Irigaray criticizes Merleau-Ponty for neglecting the sensible medium, and also the *mucous* of the carnal. In his drive to interconnect the sense of the tangible with the visible, he goes, to her mind, too far: "We can agree that there is situating of the visible in the tangible and of the tangible in the visible. But the two maps are incomplete and do not overlap: *the tangible is, and remains, primary in its opening. Its touching on, of, and by means of the other*" (Irigaray, *An Ethics of Sexual Difference*, 162; Irigaray's emphasis).

32. Sorabji, "Aristotle on Demarcating the Five Senses," 75.

33. Chrétien argues that there is a question of a "second" medium in the form of the external, sensory medium based on the passage in *DA* II.11, 423b8–13. He speaks of "a three-dimensional layer of air or water" (Chrétien, *The Call and the Response* 88). However, I think that, in that passage, Aristotle's focus on air and water as surrounding particular objects is to be understood as an analogy for arguing that touch implies mediation as such, without proposing a second form of medium. In other words, for Aristotle, sensible touching is analogous to the seemingly direct touch of two bodies in water or air, insofar as it also seems so direct, but includes us overlooking distance in the form of our flesh: "Still, as we have said before, if we were to perceive all tangible things through a cloth

membrane (*hymenos*) without noticing the separation (*diergei*) caused by it, we should react exactly in the same way (*homoiōs*) as we do now in water and in air; for we seem to touch them directly without the intervention of any medium" (*DA* II.11, 423b8–13).

34. Chrétien, *The Call and the Response*, 89.
35. Chrétien, *The Call and the Response*, 100.
36. Heller-Roazen, *The Inner Touch*, 295.
37. Derrida speaks of "irreducible spacing" in *On Touching*, 221. Earlier, he articulates this as follows: "In thus opening up a gap and making room for the hiatus of noncontact at the heart of contact, this spacing makes for the trial of noncontact as the very condition or experience itself of contact, the selfsame experience itself of the same open forever—and spaced out by the other." Jacques Derrida, *On Touching—Jean-Luc Nancy*, trans. C. Irizarry (Stanford, CA: Stanford University Press, 2005), 179–80.
38. In her analysis of Merleau-Ponty's account of body, Grosz writes that for him body is not just *in* space but inhabits space. Elizabeth Grosz, *Volatile Bodies: Toward a Corporeal Feminism* (Bloomington: Indiana University Press, 1997), 90.
39. The fascination with especially the nightingale and swallow has been long lasting. For instance, see Douglas: "the ancients had a great affection for both nightingale and swallow." Norman Douglas, *Birds and Beasts of the Greek Anthology* (Project Gutenberg Australia, April 2003, last modified March 2009), gutenberg.net.au/ebooks03/0300611h.html.
40. Aristophanes, *The Birds*, trans. W. Arrowsmith (Ann Arbor: University of Michigan Press, 1961), 14.
41. Or, as Abram puts it: "intermediaries between our ground-bound world and that celestial resplendence, that source, the great god of the day-lit world." David Abram, *Becoming Animal: An Earthly Cosmology* (New York: Pantheon Books, 2010), 199.
42. In this regard, Abram speaks with illumination about the winged nature of messengers in different cultures (as angels, as protective spirits, etc.). See also *Becoming Animal*, 198.
43. Catherine Malabou, quoting Sparrow, "Foreword: After the Flesh," in *Plastic Bodies: Rebuilding Sensation after Phenomenology* (London: Open Humanities Press, 2014), 19.
44. Malabou, "Foreword: After the Flesh," 17.
45. Malabou, "Foreword: After the Flesh," 19.
46. Malabou, "Foreword: After the Flesh," 19.
47. Abram, *Becoming Animal*, 190.
48. Abram, *Becoming Animal*, 190.
49. Straus, *The Primary World of the Senses*, 351.
50. Chatterjee details the various mechanisms in place, such as pressure-sensitive sensors and magnetic sensors, that enable processes such as flying and migration: "Like other animals, birds feel with sensitive receptors that are attached

to the nerves. These receptors are scattered all over the body. Birds can sense the speed and direction of the airflow over their wings with the help of feather follicles that act like mechanoreceptors, which are pressure-sensitive sensors. . . . In addition to airflow sensors in the wings, many birds have magnetic sensors, built-in-compasses, probably situated in the eyes that are useful for long-distance migration. Vision and mechanosensing are apparently used at all levels in birds as a sensory response flight control system that is characterized by intricate sensory interconnection and feedback." S. Chatterjee, *The Rise of Birds: 225 Million Years of Evolution* (Baltimore: Johns Hopkins University Press, 2015), 228.

51. Seemingly very different in function and appearance, it is surprising that keratin may unite so many different kinds of material expressions, varying from horns to nails to feathers. Does this indicate that keratin itself is overly plastic qua materiality? (David Madden, personal conversation, October 2015).

52. Tim Birkhead, *Bird Sense: What It's Like to Be a Bird* (New York: Walker and Company, 2012), 84.

53. Birkhead, *Bird Sense*, 84.

54. "filoplume, n." modern Latin filoplūma, badly < Latin filum thread + plūma feather. (The correct Latin form would be *filiplūma.) *The OED Online*, s.v. "filoplume," accessed July 31, 2015, en.oxforddictionaries.com/definition/filoplume.

55. "filoplume, n." *The OED Online* cites Elliot Coues, *Handbook of Field and General Ornitholology: A Manual of the Structure and Classification of Birds* (London: Macmillan, 1890), ii. §3. 128. doi.org/10.5962/bhl.title.57696

56. "filoplume, n." *The OED Online* cites Coues, *Handbook of Field and General Ornitholology*, ii. §3. 128. doi.org/10.5962/bhl.title.57696

57. Thor Hanson, *Feathers: The Evolution of a Natural Miracle* (New York: Basic Books 2011), 278.

58. Hanson writes in this regard that filoplumes "act like telltales on a sail, giving instant data on wind speed and feather position and helping the bird make fine adjustments during flight" (Hanson, *Feathers: The Evolution of a Natural Miracle* 278).

59. Birkhead, *Bird Sense*, 85.

60. Birkhead, *Bird Sense*, 85.

61. See also Gayle Salamon's book *Assuming a Body: Transgender and Rhetorics of Materiality* for an account of the psychical body that is grounded in the phenomenology of Merleau-Ponty and the psychoanalysis of Schilder and Anzieu. Salamon argues that, for Merleau-Ponty, "flesh is neither matter nor mind, but partakes of both these things . . . Merleau-Ponty's description of flesh sounds in several crucial aspects like a description of trangenderism or transsexuality: a region of being in which the subject is not quite unitary and not quite the combination of two different things." Gayle Salamon, *Assuming a Body: Transgender and Rhetorics of Materiality* (New York: Columbia University Press, 2010), 65. In

my discussion of skin in chapter 4, I return to Anzieu's *Skin Ego* given its close connection to that chapter's topic.

62. Cf. Marjorie Grene's commentary on Plessner's ideas on the nonlocalization of the living body in "Positionality in the Philosophy of Helmuth Plessner," *Review of Metaphysics* 20 (1966): 163.

63. Rebecca Steiner Goldner, "Touch and Flesh in Aristotle's *De anima*" (lecture and paper presented at the Annual Meeting of the Ancient Philosophy Society, Michigan State University, East Lansing, MI, April 2010), 5.

64. Chrétien, *The Call and the Response*, 86.

65. Compare to Chrétien, *The Call and the Response*: "the airy or aquatic medium does not give itself to sensation as a distinct object" (89).

66. Chrétien, *The Call and the Response*, 89–90.

67. Bernd Heinrich, *One Man's Owl* (Princeton, NJ: Princeton University Press, 1987), 183.

68. These are Katherine McKeever's words, as reported by Heinrich, *One Man's Owl*, 185.

69. As reported by Heinrich, *One Man's Owl*, 185.

70. Johannes Erritzøe, "Fault Bars—A Review," www.birdresearch.dk/unilang/faultbars/Faultbar5.pdf.

71. Erritzøe, "Fault Bars—A Review."

72. S. David Scott and Casey McFarland, *Bird Feathers: A Guide to North American Species* (Mechanicsburg, PA: Stackpole Books, 2010), 36.

73. Scott and McFarland, *Bird Feathers*, 36.

74. Erritzøe, "Fault Bars—A Review."

75. Erritzøe here cites Russell D. Dawson, Gary R. Bortolotti, and Gillian L. Murza, "Sex-Dependent Frequency and Consequences of Natural Handicaps in American Kestrels," *Journal of Avian Biology* 32 (2001); Erritzøe, "Fault Bars—A Review."

76. Erritzøe here cites Mary E. Murphy, Brian T. Miller, and James R. King, "A Structural Comparison of Fault Bars with Feather Defects Known to Be Nutritionally Induced," *Canadian Journal of Zoology* 67, no. 5 (1989); Erritzøe, "Fault Bars—A Review."

77. The Oxford English Dictionary provides as etymology the following: "Middle English faut(e , < Old French faute (feminine) (also faut masculine) = Provençal falta, Spanish falta, Portuguese falta, Italian falta < popular Latin *fallita, a failing, coming short, < *fallitus, popular Latin past participle of fallĕre: see fail v. Cf. "fault, n." OED Online. July 2018. Oxford University Press. www.oed.com/view/Entry/68601?rskey=FYmxZk&result=1&isAdvanced=false (accessed November 08, 2018).

78. For instance, Møller "has shown that the same barn swallow individual is susceptible and produces fault bars in multiple years" (Johannes Erritzøe, email message to author, October 26, 2015).

79. Erritzøe, "Fault Bars—A Review."

80. Erritzøe, "Fault Bars—A Review,"

81. In personal communication, Erritzøe writes that, after his and Møller's best knowledge, "it is not known if this [traumatic memory in the form of fault bars] can be forwarded to future generations" (Johannes Erritzøe, email message to author, October 26, 2015).

82. Roger Jovani and J. Blas, "Adaptive Allocation of Stress-Induced Deformities on Bird Feathers," *Journal of Evolutionary Biology* 17, no. 2 (2004): 294–301; Cf. Erritzøe, "Fault Bars—A Review."

83. Erritzøe, "Fault Bars—A Review." He continues: "A study of White Storks has shown that the distribution of fault bars was arranged with most of them on the inner wing feathers that have less importance for flight ability . . . As a rule fault bars are found more often in tail- than in wing feathers and in the wings particularly in the inner secondaries and tertials. These feather types are, as already mentioned, of less importance for maneuvering because they have to handle a smaller mechanical load than primaries."

84. Cf. Grosz, "Thinking the New," 18–19.

85. "preen, v.2." OED Online. July 2018. Oxford University Press. www.oed.com/view/Entry/149937?rskey=1QvZum&result=3&isAdvanced=false (accessed November 08, 2018).

86. Birkhead, *Bird Sense*, 82.

87. John M. Marzluff and Tony Angell, *In the Company of Crows and Ravens* (New Haven, CT: Yale University Press, 2005), 166.

88. Eric D. Forsman and Howard Wight, "Allopreening in Owls: What Are Its Functions?" *The Auk* 96, no. 3 (July–September 1979): 528.

89. Marzluff and Angell, *In the Company of Crows and Ravens*, 166.

90. Birkhead, *Bird Sense*, 81.

91. Birkhead, *Bird Sense*, 81.

92. Birkhead, *Bird Sense*, 81.

93. Birkhead, *Bird Sense*, 2012, 80.

94. Chrétien, *The Call and the Response*, 86.

95. Cf. Rebecca Hill, *The Interval: Relation and Becoming in Irigaray, Aristotle, and Bergson* (New York: Fordham University Press, 2012). See my chapter 3 for a more elaborate discussion of the placenta as in-between.

96. Birkhead, *Bird Sense*, 187.

97. Birkhead, *Bird Sense*, 82.

98. Notably, crows additionally get rid of parasites through "anting"—they sit on groups of ants, ruffle their feathers and spread their wings. Thus, we find here possible evidence of interspecies communities relieving and preventing suffering (Heinrich, *One Man's Owl*, 132).

99. www.nwf.org/What-We-Do/Protect-Habitat/Gulf-Restoration/Oil-Spill/Effects-on-Wildlife/Birds.aspx.

100. Birkhead, *Bird Sense*, 83.

101. More references to *synaisthanesthai* may be found in other works by Aristotle: *History of Animals* VIII. 534b18; *EE* XII.1245b22, *EE* XII.1244b25. See also Shane Butler and Alex Purves, eds., *Synaesthesia and the Ancient Senses* (Durham, NC: Acumen, 2013). This editorial volume includes discussion of many classical authors (e.g., Herodotus, Aristophanes, Plato) on *synaesthesia*.

102. Birkhead, *Bird Sense*, 181.

103. John M. Marzluff and Tony Angell, *Gifts of the Crow: How Perception, Emotion and Thought Allow Smart Birds to Behave Like Humans* (New York: Free Press, 2012), 141.

Chapter 3

1. Loke remarks on how the placenta "goes about its duties so unobtrusively, it is easily overlooked and ignored." Y.W. Loke, *Life's Vital Link: The Astonishing Role of the Placenta* (Oxford: Oxford University Press, 2013), 3.

2. In this chapter, I will use the terms "mother," "potential mother," and "woman-becoming-mother" in a predominantly biological way, following the medical scientific literature, referring to how *most* pregnancies gestate, conceive, and give birth, namely, in terms of a female gestational body. This is not to devalue those gestational bodies that are differently gendered (such as those of transgender men) or nongendered. In fact, by emphasizing the *mediatory role of the placenta* and the place it creates for *the pregnant city*, this chapter offers reason to step beyond narrow binary classifications of pregnancy and emphasizes the mixed, complex, material powers of bodies as such. I owe these insights to a helpful discussion with Emily Parker (email message to author, September 2016).

3. Power and Schulkin use the term "extra-fetal organ." Michael L. Power and Jay Schulkin, *The Evolution of the Human Placenta* (Baltimore: Johns Hopkins University Press, 2012), 166.

4. Usha Verma and Nipun Verma, "An Overview of Development, Function, and Diseases of the Placenta," in *The Placenta: Development, Function and Diseases*, ed. Richard Nicholson (Hauppauge: Nova Science Publishers, 2013), 19.

5. Kurt Benirschke and Peter Kaufmann, *Pathology of the Human Placenta* (New York: Springer, 2000), 1–30 passim.

6. Given its permeability of toxins, Mathiesen and Knudsen speak of the placenta as a "xenobiotic-transporting organ." Line Mathiesen and Lisbeth E. Knudsen, "Placental Transport of Environmental Toxicants," in *The Placenta: Development, Function and Diseases*, ed. Richard Nicholson (Hauppauge: Nova Science Publishers, 2013) 187.

7. Along the lines of Hill's interpretation of the interval in Irigaray, the placenta—as place of ontogenetic invention for mother and child—allows us to

think of motherhood not simply as a woman's ultimate essence or function, but rather as a possible function of her body. As Hill writes: "To think the placenta as an interval between woman and fetus is to articulate pregnancy as a function of her body rather than as woman's sole purpose. This prepares for the possibility of thinking woman as place in multiple senses; motherhood must be a component of female corporeal identity rather than a priority of it." Rebecca Hill, *The Interval: Relation and Becoming in Irigaray, Aristotle, and Bergson* (New York: Fordham University Press, 2012), 70.

8. Elizabeth Grosz, "Deleuze, Ruyer and Becoming-Brain: The Music of Life's Temporality," *Parrhesia* 15 (2012): 6.

9. Biologist Hélène Rouch articulates, in conversation with Luce Irigaray: "the difference between the 'self' and other is, so to speak, continuously negotiated. It's as if the mother always knew that the embryo (and thus the placenta) was other, and that she lets the placenta know this, which then produces the factors enabling the maternal organism to accept it as other." Rouch, in conversation with Irigaray, in: Luce Irigaray, *Je, Tu, Nous: Toward a Culture of Difference* (New York: Routledge, 1993), 41.

10. Roberto Esposito, *Bios: Biopolitics and Philosophy*, trans. Timothy Campbell (Minneapolis: University of Minnesota Press, 2008), 108.

11. In the extensive body of scholarship on motherhood, there is ample evidence to suggest that the "pre-pregnant self" and the "motherhood self" or "pregnant self" may encounter a struggle of identity. For instance, Maggie Nelson's *Argonauts* offers a recent example of the description of such a struggle, asking questions whether her pregnancy confronts her with a heteronormative self that she disavows, or whether there may be something "inherently queer about pregnancy itself, insofar as it profoundly alters one's 'normal' state, and occasionally a radical intimacy with—and radical alienation from—one's body" (13). And, expressing her fascination with pregnancy and motherhood, she also admits to separation from the bubble: "I cannot hold my baby at the same time as I write." Maggie Nelson, *The Argonauts* (Minneapolis: Graywolf Press, 2016), 37.

12. Hill, *The Interval*, 70.

13. As Sloterdijk insightfully notes, "the conspiracy of silence against the With has its weak point: in truth, obstetricians know that there are always two units which reach the outside in successful births. . . . Only birth and afterbirth together meet the requirements of a complete delivery." Peter Sloterdijk, *Bubbles: Spheres Volume I: Microspherology*, trans. W. Hoban (Los Angeles: Semiotext(e), 2011), 376.

14. Some of these practices include banking cord blood as a source for stem cells. That these practices can be contested becomes clear in Santoro's writings, who shows that some cases of regulation of cord blood actually led to the development of unregulated transnational markets. Cf. Pablo Santoro, "From (Public?) Waste to (Private?) Value. The Regulation of Private Cord Blood Banking in Spain," *Science*

Studies 22, no. 1 (2009): 3–23 passim. Other processes include drying, cooking, and transforming the placenta into dietary supplements or facial creams to restore health or serve cosmetic benefits. Sloterdijk speaks of the use of the placenta by the cosmetic and pharmaceutical industry, and even reports that placentas have been used as combustive agents in garbage incinerators (Sloterdijk, *Bubbles* 383).

15. Loke, *Life's Vital Link*, 5.
16. Power and Schulkin, *The Evolution of the Human Placenta*, 166.
17. Power and Schulkin, *The Evolution of the Human Placenta*, 166.
18. Power and Schulkin, *The Evolution of the Human Placenta*, 166.
19. Jun-Ming Zhang and Jianxiong An, "Cytokines, Inflammation and Pain," *International Anesthesiology Clinics* 45, no. 2 (Spring 2007): 27. Cf. also Bowen et al., who state that "cytokines are an integral part of a functional regulatory/communication network operating within the placental-maternal unit during normal gestation." J.M. Bowen et al., "Cytokines of the Placenta and Extra-Placental Membranes: Biosynthesis, Secretion and Roles in Establishment of Pregnancy in Women," *Placenta* 23, no. 4 (April 2002): 239–56, at 239.
20. Power and Schulkin, *The Evolution of the Human Placenta*, 166.
21. Power and Schulkin, *The Evolution of the Human Placenta*, 166.
22. Verma and Verma, "An Overview of Development," 7–14.
23. Power and Schulkin note that the placenta "regulates and coordinates metabolism and physiology among the mother, the fetus, and itself" (*The Evolution of the Human Placenta* 163).
24. *Republic* Book III, 416d ff. and the beginning of Book IV discuss the living conditions of the guardians as well as the sacrifice of their happiness.
25. Cf. *Republic* Book II, 374a ff., where Plato discusses the expansion of the *polis* with a professional army to defend it. I will be using the term "guardians" here in an inclusive sense, encompassing the two groups that Plato later distinguishes from each other: the "best of the group" (true guardians) and their helpers (auxiliaries). With regard to the soul, such guardians need to be spirited in order to protect, and thus be "both fearless and unyielding against everything" (375b). But such guardians also need to be "gentle toward their own people" (375b). Thus, Plato concludes that a beautiful and good guardian of the city needs to be "philosophic, spirited, quick, and strong by nature" (376c).
26. Sure enough, insofar as Plato's guardians are also described as having a fundamental role in the selection of partners and their reproduction (*Republic* 457d–471c) we could argue that at least in terms of enabling conditions for life, they have a comparable role in the *genesis* of new life.
27. For a critique of the account of reproductive labor in Plato, for instance in Plato's *Symposium*, see Luce Irigaray, *An Ethics of Sexual Difference*, trans. C. Burke and G.C. Gill (Ithaca, NY: Cornell University Press, 1993). For instance, Irigaray discusses how Plato reappropriates the feminine figure of Diotima, who states that "carnal reproduction is subordinated to the engendering of beautiful and

good things" (31). Page Dubois provides a helpful overview of Plato's problematic reading of feminine labor as well, writing, "Plato uses the tension between the sexes in Greek culture to assert the authority of the male at the scene of philosophy, but also and more importantly, his own desire to appropriate the powers of the female makes that authority a very provisional one and marks the Platonic text as the threshold of a new description of sexual difference. If Plato appropriates the female powers of reproduction to the male philosopher, the philosophical tradition after him stresses the autonomy of that male, his self-sufficiency, his privileged access to the divine and the one, and that tradition describes the female as a defective male, a creature distanced from the absolute presence and union with the divine." Page DuBois, *Sowing the Body: Psychoanalysis and Ancient Representations of Women* (Chicago: University of Chicago Press, 1991), 173.

28. In the *Timaeus*, Plato locates the more masculine and feminine parts of the soul in the following way: "Within the chest, they fastened the mortal kind of soul. And inasmuch as one part thereof is better, and one worse, they built a division within the cavity of the thorax—as if to fence off two separate chambers, for men and for women—by placing the midriff between them as a screen" (69e–70a). In *Sowing the Body*, DuBois writes: "The manly part is closer to the heart, obedient to reason, while the heart must be cooled by the lungs in order that it 'be subservient to the reason (*logoi*) in time of passion.' Women are associated with the heart's blood, which like the womb moves throughout the body and threatens anarchy" (215n7).

29. Sloterdijk, *Bubbles*, 399.

30. Sloterdijk, *Bubbles*, 382.

31. Sloterdijk, *Bubbles*, 358.

32. This in turn forces us to reflect on ourselves as always fundamentally incomplete, with individualism as a naïve, rationalistic dream that forsakes our attachment to others and forgets the sacrifice made through the commitment and ultimate death of another. Sloterdijk speaks in this regard of our modern individualism as reflecting "placental nihilism" (Sloterdijk, *Bubbles* 387).

33. Loke, *Life's Vital Link*, 2.

34. Gail M. Schwab, "Mother's Body, Father's Tongue: Mediation and the Symbolic Order," in *Engaging with Irigaray: Feminist Philosophy and Modern European Thought*, eds. Carolyn Burke, Naomi Schor and Margaret Whitford (New York: Columbia University Press, 1994), 363.

35. Yusuke Marikawa and Vernadeth Alarcón, "Establishment of Trophectoderm and Inner Cell Mass Lineages in the Mouse Embryo," *Molecular Reproduction and Development* 76, no. 11 (2009): 1019, PubMed Central. Based on their study of mice, they write: "The location of blastomeres at this stage, i.e., external or internal of the embryo, in effect defines the commitment towards the TE or ICM lineage, respectively. Some studies implicate the presence of a developmental bias

among blastomeres at 2- or 4-cell stage, although it is unlikely to play a decisive role in the establishment of TE and ICM."

36. Loke, *Life's Vital Link*, 9.

37. Loke addresses the unique nature of the placenta's own program, and speaks (almost hyperbolically) of its goal "to pursue and organize its own program of development totally independent of the baby" (Loke, *Life's Vital Link*, 9).

38. Further evidence for the crucial meaning of the placenta is that in this early stage of differentiation, "over 80 percent of the cells formed are extra embryonic," ultimately composing what will be the placenta (Loke, *Life's Vital Link*, 9).

39. Cf. Loke, *Life's Vital Link*, 9.

40. Loke's focus on the placenta's unique trajectory and autonomy need not be understood as if the placenta's *function* is independent: as Power and Schulkin note, the placenta "regulates and coordinates metabolism and physiology among the mother, the fetus, and itself" (*The Evolution of the Human Placenta* 163). Philosophically, I am interested in questioning until when the remarkable "dominance" of the placenta's existence remains preserved. It seems only "natural" to see this breaking-point at birth, but given the increasing ability of the fetus to digest, "breathe," urinate, etc. (at least in terms of abilities) we might argue that at an earlier age (perhaps around 20–24 weeks) we find an important turning-point in asserting the abilities of the fetus to establish its own boundaries in case of premature birth. Thus, one could argue that the relative dominance of the placenta changes over time and makes place for an increasingly emerging regulatory existence of the fetus.

41. Loke, *Life's Vital Link*, 19.

42. Notably, while the placenta as fully functioning organ is temporary, elements of its structure are all but temporary: see my further account of this enduring trace of the placenta later in this chapter under the heading "Toward a Genuine Sense of Hospitality: Place-Making, Temporality, and Microchimerism."

43. Nicholas Davey, "The Hermeneutics of Seeing," in *Interpreting Visual Culture: Explorations in the Hermeneutics of the Visual*, eds. Ian Heywood and Barry Sandywell (New York: Routledge, 1999), 19.

44. Davey, "The Hermeneutics of Seeing," 19.

45. Hans-Georg Gadamer, *Hermeneutik I: Wahrheit und Methode* (Tübingen: J.C.B. Mohr [P. Siebeck], 1990), 120. English Version: Hans-Georg Gadamer, *Truth and Method*, trans. Joel Weinsheimer and Donald G. Marshall (New York: Continuum, 2003), 114. I slightly modified the translation.

46. Christian Lotz, *The Art of Gerhard Richter: Hermeneutics, Images, Meaning* (New York: Bloomsbury, 2015), 35.

47. Lotz, *The Art of Gerhard Richter*, 36.

48. Power and Schulkin, *The Evolution of the Human Placenta*, 167.

49. Power and Schulkin, *The Evolution of the Human Placenta*, 164.

50. Power and Schulkin, *The Evolution of the Human Placenta*, 164.

51. Gadamer, *Hermeneutik I*, 120; Gadamer, *Truth and Method*, 114.

52. Plato, *Republic* II, 369d, e.

53. Plato especially worries about the happiness of the guardians. Plato prioritizes the happiness of the city as a whole, which is made possible if everyone performs one's work as best as possible. When performing one's work according to one's nature, each group will participate in the kind of happiness that is in accordance with its nature. Plato, *Republic* Book IV, 419a–421c.

54. Loke, *Life's Vital Link*, 6–7. Similarly, Rouch, in her interview with Irigaray, argues that the placenta is the "mediating space between mother and fetus" (Irigaray, *An Ethics of Sexual Difference* 39).

55. This also invokes John Sallis's ideas on the origin as double, for instance in John Sallis, *Double Truth* (Albany: State University of New York Press 1: "to begin will always be (or prove to have been) redoubling."

56. Michael Marder, *Plant-Thinking: A Philosophy of Vegetal Life* (New York: Columbia University Press, 2013), 63.

57. Marder, *Plant-Thinking*, 63.

58. Martin Heidegger, "Bauen Wohnen Denken," in *Vorträge und Aufsätze* Vol. II (Pfullingen: G. Neske, 1954), 28 (German)/ Martin Heidegger, "Building Dwelling Thinking," in *Poetry, Language, Thought*, trans. Albert Hofstadter (New York: Harper and Row, 1971), 154 (English).

59. Robert Mugerauer, "Topos Unbound: From Place to Opening and Back," in *Hermeneutics, Place, and Space*, ed. Bruce Janz (New York: Springer, 2017), 148.

60. Heidegger, "Bauen Wohnen Denken," 26; Heidegger, "Building Dwelling Thinking," 152.

61. Heidegger, "Bauen Wohnen Denken," 28; Heidegger, "Building Dwelling Thinking," 154.

62. Cf. Edward Casey's discussion of the distinction between space and place, in, for instance, Edward Casey, *Getting Back into Place: Toward a Renewed Understanding of the Place-World* (Bloomington: Indiana University Press, 2010). Casey acknowledges his indebtedness on the space-place distinction to Heidegger, but also adds that Heidegger, like Bachelard, did not assess "the role of the human body in the experience of significant places." Casey attempts to "accord to place a position of renewed respect by specifying its power to direct and stabilize us, to memorialize and identify us, to tell us who and what we are in terms of *where we are* (as well as where we are *not*)" (xv).

63. Heidegger, "Bauen Wohnen Denken," 30 / Heidegger, "Building Dwelling Thinking," 156. Heidegger's critique of the abstract notion of space is the following: "the space provided for in this mathematical manner may be called 'space,' the 'one,' space as such. But in this sense 'the' space, 'space,' contains no spaces and no places."

64. Sloterdijk in *Bubbles* speaks about the practice of burial of placentas in cellars or under the staircase so that "the household would profit from its fertile power." He also addresses the "widespread custom to bury it under young fruit trees; one factor in this may have been the morphological connection between the placental issue and the root systems of trees, as a sort of analogy magic" (Sloterdijk, *Bubbles* 378). In addition to burial, other practices such as hanging up and drying, burning, and immersion have been employed. All of these methods show respect to the life-giving power of the placenta and correspond, as Sloterdijk astutely observes, to the four elements (Sloterdijk, *Bubbles* 381).

65. The Māori term *whenua* means both land and placenta: "All life is seen as being born from the womb of Papatūānuku, under the sea. The lands that appear above water are placentas from her womb. They float, forming islands." See: Te Ahukaramū Charles Royal, "Papatūānuku—the Land, Whenua—the Placenta," Te Ara, the *Encyclopedia of New Zealand*, September 24, 2007, www.teara.govt.nz/en/papatuanuku-the-land/page-4.

66. By contrast, in English, place and placenta do not share an etymology: As the OED indicates, the term "placenta" derives from the "post-classical Latin *placenta* (1559 in sense 1), transferred use of classical Latin *placenta* a kind of flat cake < ancient Greek πλακόεντ- , πλακόεις (contracted πλακοῦντ- , πλακοῦς) flat cake, also mallow seed < πλάκ- , πλάξ flat plate (see placo- *comb. form*) + -όεις, suffix generally forming adjectives." The English term "place" derives from "post-classical Latin *platea* . . . < classical Latin *platea* street, in post-classical Latin (also as *placea*, *placia*) also square, public square, marketplace < ancient Greek πλατεῖα street, use as noun (short for πλατεῖα ὁδός) of feminine of πλατύς broad." "placenta, n.," and "place, n." OED Online. July 2018. Oxford University Press. www.oed.com/view/Entry/144884?redirectedFrom=placenta (accessed November 11, 2018); Mugerauer, "Topos Unbound," 148.

67. While Aristotle also refers to artificial objects such as a vessel (*angeion*) to explain place (*Physics* 208b2–23, 210a24), his account of place is primarily rooted in his broader account of nature, motion, and rest, as Helen Lang has argued. Lang writes that "there is no such thing as 'physical space' in Aristotle. Place resembles form and renders place within the cosmos formally determinate, i.e., determinate in respect to direction." Helen Lang, *The Order of Nature in Aristotle's Physics: Place and The Elements* (Cambridge, UK: Cambridge University Press, 1998), 93. Lang's analysis allows us to grasp that place has "formally determinate" qualities, which explain natural motion in Aristotle and allows for accounts such that the elements have an inclination to be in their natural place. See *De Caelo* IV.3, 310b7–12: "And since 'the place' means the boundary of that which encloses it, and the boundaries of all bodies which move upwards and downwards are the extremity and the centre, which in a way constitute the form of the body they enclose, it follows that to move towards its own place is to move towards its like."

68. Hill, *The Interval*, 39.

69. Cf. Lang, *The Order of Nature in Aristotle's Physics*, 35.

70. Heidegger, "Bauen Wohnen Denken," 28–29; Heidegger, "Building Dwelling Thinking," 154; I transliterated Heidegger's use of Greek terms.

71. Jeffrey Malpas, *Heidegger and the Thinking of Place: Explorations in the Topology of Being* (Cambridge, MA: MIT Press, 2012), 8.

72. Lang, *The Order of Nature in Aristotle's Physics*, 93.

73. Lang speaks of the limit here as a "constitutive principle." Cf. Lang, *The Order of Nature in Aristotle's Physics*, 93.

74. Malpas, *Heidegger and the Thinking of Place*, 8.

75. Hill, *The Interval*, 60–61. As Hill points out, "Aristotle takes pains to distinguish *angeion* and *topos*. Place is the motionless limit surrounding a body, while a vessel is a moveable *topos* (209b28–29).

76. Malpas, *Heidegger and the Thinking of Place*, 7.

77. Jeffrey Malpas, "Technology, Spatialisation, and Modernity" (lecture, University of San Francisco, November 9, 2016).

78. Hill, *The Interval*, 45.

79. Irigaray reads Plato's account of *chōra* in the *Timaeus* in terms of a formless receptacle that equals empty space. She rejects the conflation of *chōra* with the feminine or maternal as it places the feminine *outside* any discourse and meaning. Cf. Luce Irigaray, *Speculum of the Other Woman* (Ithaca, NY: Cornell University Press, 1985), 179. Cf. Judith Butler, *Bodies That Matter: On the Discursive Limits of "Sex"* (New York: Routledge, 1993), 40. In his *Chorology*, John Sallis argues that *chōra* is not be confused with (empty) space or place, although—as Sallis notes—Plato's dream suggests that we could easily conflate *topos* with *chōra*. Cf. John Sallis, *Chorology: On Beginning in Plato's "Timaeus"* (Bloomington: Indiana University Press, 1999), 153. Cf. Emanuela Bianchi's *The Feminine Symptom: Aleatory Matter in the Aristotelian Cosmos* (New York: Fordham University Press, 2014), for an account of the receptacle and *chōra*. Bianchi argues that the most notable distinction between the receptacle (*hypodochē*) and *chōra* is that "*hypodochē* envelops within a boundary" and offers "an opening into interiority," while "*chōra* denotes rather an exteriority, an opening, giving room, dimension, depth, and magnitude—spacing—but also, as indicated by the related verb *chōrizō*, separating, dividing, differentiating, and severing" (99).

80. Irigaray, *An Ethics of Sexual Difference*, 36.

81. In this manner, she conceives of an interval that, in Hill's words "cannot be present to thought, because the interval seeps beyond the present to the past and to the future" (Hill, *The Interval* 45).

82. Irigaray, *An Ethics of Sexual Difference*, 41.

83. Irigaray, *An Ethics of Sexual Difference*, 36.

84. Irigaray, *An Ethics of Sexual Difference*, 40. Here she addresses place "as appropriate to and for the other, and towards which he or she may move."

85. Irigaray, "Toward a Mutual Hospitality," 44.
86. Irigaray, "Toward a Mutual Hospitality," 44.
87. Mugerauer, "Topos Unbound," 151; Martin Heidegger, "Art and Space," *Man and World* 6, no. 1 (1973): 5–6.
88. Loke, *Life's Vital Link*, 6.
89. Antoine Malek and Nick A. Bersinger, "Immunology of Human Pregnancy: Transfer of Antibodies and Associated Placental Function" in *The Placenta: Development, Function and Diseases*, ed. Richard Nicholson (Hauppauge: Nova Science Publishers, 2013), 59.
90. This applies to those pregnancies in which the gestational mother is also the biological mother.
91. Verma and Verma, "An Overview of Development, Function, and Diseases of the Placenta," 14.
92. Verma and Verma, "An Overview of Development, Function, and Diseases of the Placenta," 14.
93. Loke, *Life's Vital Link*, 9.
94. The underlying reasoning is, according to Loke, that "the father wants a big placenta to access the maximum amount of food from the mother to feed the baby, whereas the mother restricts this predatory activity in order to conserve her resources for the sake of her own health" (Loke, *Life's Vital Link* 10).
95. As Loke discusses, different kinds of immune systems are operative in our bodies. On the one hand, the archaic, innate system is based on self-recognition (or absence of self) and is designed to work on the organism's internal integrity. On the other hand, the adaptive immune system is based on presence of non-self and works as "defense against external aggressors" (Loke, *Life's Vital Link* 132–33).
96. It "blocks cytotoxic maternal cell effects by secreting various factors" (Verma and Verma, "An Overview of Development, Function, and Diseases of the Placenta," 14).
97. Schwab, "Mother's Body, Father's Tongue," 363.
98. Verma and Verma, "An Overview of Development, Function, and Diseases of the Placenta," 14.
99. Loke, *Life's Vital Link*, 151. In the end, Loke argues, this is evolutionary advantageous, as it allows for expansion of HLA and protection against disease. HLA—human leukocyte (or lymphocyte) antigen—is "a type of molecule found on the surface of most cells in the body. HLAs play an important part in the body's immune response to foreign substances. They make up a person's tissue type, which varies from person to person." For the definition of HLA, see: "HLA," NCI Dictionary of Cancer Terms, n.d., accessed May 29, 2018, www.cancer.gov/publications/dictionaries/cancer-terms/def/hla.
100. Roberto Esposito, *Immunitas: The Protection and Negation of Life*, trans. Zakiya Hanafi (Cambridge, UK: Polity, 2011), 171. Ed Cohen, in *A Body*

Worth Defending: Immunity, Biopolitics, and the Apotheosis of the Modern Body (Durham, NC: Duke University Press, 2010) traces the history of the concept of immunity from law and politics to medicine, and critiques the notion of "defense" associated with biological immunity, since it offers *separation* between (monadic) self and context rather than embeddedness in the context (6). Instead, he aligns himself with immunologist Polly Matzinger, who prefers to speak of biological immunity in terms of integration and living in harmony with one's inner and outer milieu. Given its emphasis on integration, adaptability, and symbiosis rather than defense and hostility, Matzinger's model can thus successfully explain why pregnant bodies do not reject a fetus, and other bodily phenomena that involve changing immune systems, as happens in puberty and aging (Cohen, *A Body Worth Defending* 28–29).

101. Cf. Esposito, *Immunitas*, 171. Regarding pregnancy, he writes that "the force of the immune attack is precisely what keeps alive that which it should normally destroy." The immune response thus becomes "indistinguishable from its opposite, 'community.'"

102. M. Gayed and C. Gordon, "Pregnancy and Rheumatic Diseases," *Rheumatology* 46, no. 11 (2007): 1634–40.

103. For instance, in the case of rheumatoid arthritis, as Buyon argues: "Pregnancy is associated with improvement in the clinical signs and symptoms of rheumatoid arthritis in more than 70% of patients." Conversely, "the course of systemic lupus erythematosus is more variable." Jill P. Buyon, "The Effects of Pregnancy on Autoimmune Diseases," *Journal of Leukocyte Biology* 63, no. 3 (March 1998): 281.

104. Esposito writes: "Indeed, just as the attack of the mother protects the child, the child's attack can also save the mother from her self-injurious tendencies—which explains why autoimmune diseases undergo regression during pregnancy" (Esposito, *Immunitas* 171). Esposito's remark is thought provoking in highlighting the beneficial consequences of pregnancy, but needs some nuance and further complexity, given that some autoimmune diseases actually *develop* or flare up during pregnancy.

105. Insofar as it is theorized that autoimmune diseases are based on mistakenly confusing cells that are "self" for "non-self."

106. Irigaray, "Toward a Mutual Hospitality," 52.

107. This is the view that Gabriel Marcel rejects (Marcel, *Creative Fidelity* 28).

108. Gabriel Marcel, *Creative Fidelity*, trans. Robert Rosthal (New York: Farrar, Straus and Company, 1964), 27. He continues writing that in order to feel at home, "the self does or can seem to itself to impregnate its environment with its own quality, recognizing itself in its surroundings and entering into an intimate relationship with it" (27–28).

109. Marcel, *Creative Fidelity*, 28.

110. Esposito, *Immunitas*, 171.

111. In this regard, I go beyond Aristarkhova's idea that the mother must first be hosted ("at home with herself") before hosting. In my view, placental hospitality goes before and beyond any specific hosting of identities (mother and child). Cf. Irina Aristarkhova, *Hospitality of the Matrix: Philosophy, Biomedicine, and Culture* (New York: Columbia University Press, 2012), 46–47.

112. Esposito, *Bios*, 108.

113. Van Halteren et al. define microchimerism as "a condition where one individual harbors genetically distinct cell populations, and the chimeric population constitutes < 1 % of the total number of cells." Astrid G.S. van Halteren et al., "Meeting Report of the First Symposium on Chimerism," *Chimerism* 4, no. 4 (October–December 2013): 132.

114. J. Lee Nelson, "The Otherness of Self: Microchimerism in Health and Disease," *Trends in Immunology* 33, no. 8 (August 2012): 421, 422.

115. Nelson, "The Otherness of Self," 421.

116. William F.N. Chan: "Our results indicate that fetal DNA and likely cells can cross the human blood-barrier (BBB) and reside in the brain. Changes in BBB permeability occur during pregnancy and may therefore provide a unique opportunity for the establishment of Mc in the brain." William F.N. Chan et al., "Male Microchimerism in the Human Female Brain," *PLoS ONE* 7, no. 9 (2012): 3. doi.org/10.1371/journal.pone.0045592

117. Nelson, "The Otherness of Self," fig. 2, 425. "Male Microchimerism in the Human Female Brain." *PLoS ONE* 7, no. 9 (2012): e45592. doi.org/10.1371/journal.pone.0045592

118. Chan et al., "Male Microchimerism in the Human Female Brain," 3.

119. Nelson, "The Otherness of Self," 424.

120. Robert Martone, "Scientists Discover Children's Cells Living in Mothers' Brains," *Scientific American: Mind*, December 4, 2012, www.scientificamerican.com/article/scientists-discover-childrens-cells-living-in-mothers-brain/.

121. Fetal microchimerism appears to protect against breast cancer, but may promote melanoma, for instance. Cf. Nelson, "The Otherness of Self," 426.

122. Nelson, "The Otherness of Self," 423.

123. Nelson, "The Otherness of Self," box 2, 423.

124. Nelson, "The Otherness of Self," 421; box 2, 423.

125. Cf. Plato, *Republic* Book IV, 419a–421c.

126. Nelson, "The Otherness of Self," 426.

127. This would imply that over time with each pregnancy the maternal body reconstitutes itself through competing with and mixing different residential populations of cells. Moreover, arguably such competition is also already happening in pregnancy itself. For, in the pregnancy-associated illness preeclampsia, the level of fetal microchimerism in maternal blood is far higher than in healthy pregnancies, indicating that there might be healthy forms of competition and levels of increased permeability of fetal cells that may be harmful to both mother and child.

Excessive "leakage" of microchimeric cells has been reported in preeclampsia, with studies reporting on the fact that "women with preeclampsia harbor cellular fetal microchimerism more commonly and at higher concentrations compared with women with uncomplicated pregnancy," Cf. Hilary S. Gammill et al., "Pregnancy, Microchimerism, and the Maternal Grandmother," *PLoS One* 6, no. 8 (2011): e24101. doi.org/10.1371/journal.pone.0024101

128. Van Halteren et al., "Meeting Report of the First Symposium on Chimerism," 133.

129. Van Halteren et al., "Meeting Report of the First Symposium on Chimerism," 133. Moreover, during pregnancy older cell lines—of the pregnant woman's mother (so, cells of the current fetus' maternal grandmother)—may increasingly *re-emerge* in the mother's blood, which researchers have taken as a sign of "healthy maternal adaptation to pregnancy," since the appearance of such cells is diminished in the illness preeclampsia.

130. Nelson, "The Otherness of Self," 426.

131. Nelson, "The Otherness of Self," 424.

132. As Kamper-Jørgensen writes: "Although the biological mechanisms are not precisely known, male microchimerism presence in peripheral blood of women is associated with substantially improved survival in women." Cf. Mads Kamper-Jørgensen et al., "Male Microchimerism and Survival Among Women," *International Journal of Epidemiology* 43, no. 1 (February 2014): 168. doi.org/10.1093/ije/dyt230

133. Nelson, "The Otherness of Self," 426.

134. Further temporal depth may be offered when considering that fetal and maternal cell populations may be in *competition* with each other: in cases of women who have hosted multiple pregnancies *less* maternal microchimerism has been detectable in the woman's blood, suggesting the effects of such competition. Cf. Nelson, "The Otherness of Self," 424.

135. Sure enough, insofar as Plato's guardians are also described as having a fundamental role in the selection of partners and their reproduction (*Republic* 457d–471c) we could argue that at least in terms of enabling conditions for life, they have a comparable role in the *genesis* of new life.

136. This means it provides a *temporary place* and with the progression of a pregnancy much of its boundary-establishing tasks will eventually be taken over by the fetus as such. With thanks to Bob Mugerauer for encouraging me to think through the issues of temporary, portable boundaries, and temporary place (email message to author, November 2015).

137. Hill, *The Interval*, 45.

138. I owe this suggestion to Valerie Broin, whose commentary on my APA paper carefully and insightfully articulated how the placenta also "prepares and allows for the vital and generative "between" to continue after the placenta has done its job . . . its emergence after the birth of the baby signals a new 'after-

birth-between' that extends into the broader world, involving not just the newly developing mother-baby interrelation, but all other relations and involvements that co-constitute and co-develop various identities." Valerie Broin, "Response to Marjolein Oele's 'Placental Mediation: On Mimesis, Immunity and Hospitality,'" Pacific Meeting of the APA, San Francisco, CA, March 30, 2016.

139. As Hill writes: "In Irigarayan terms, the placental relation gestures to the past experience of the mother, her relations with others and with her milieu, to her own prenatal life within her mother's body, and to her future, which is unknowable. The embryo is also virtually human—a boy or a girl—with an incalculable future. For Irigaray, the placental interval unfolds a living rhythm of times that cannot be mastered" (*The Interval* 69).

140. "chimera | chimaera, n.," *The OED Online*, s.v. "chimera," accessed February 24, 2016, www.oed.com/view/Entry/31708?redirectedFrom=chimera#eid.

141. While the placental in-between is not an intersubjective relationship between embryo and mother, it may *become* to be such, according to Hill's interpretation: "Yet, in a virtual sense, the spatiotemporal relation enabled through the placenta is ethical, because the placental relation implies the possible futures of the mother and the fetus that may be born and come to live as a subject" (*The Interval* 70).

142. I would like to thank Stijn De Cauwer and Kim Hendrickx and the anonymous reviewers of *Configurations* for their comments on an earlier version of this chapter published as "Openness and Protection: A Philosophical Analysis of the Placenta's Mediatory Role in Co-Constituting Emergent Intertwined Identities," in *Configurations* 25, no. 3 (July 2017): 347–71. In its earlier formations, this chapter also benefited from the feedback of the participants at the *Immunity and Modernity* conference in Leuven in 2015, organized by Stijn De Cauwer, and from the participants at the *Davies Workshop* at USF in Fall 2015, organized by Gerard Kuperus.

Chapter 4

1. I owe the careful translations of Dagognet's texts to Daniel O'Connell and Anne Mairesse. *La peau découverte* is Dagognet's third and last part of his trilogy devoted to examining living beings. The book title *La peau découverte* is difficult to translate because *découverte* offers a kaleidoscope of meanings, many of which speak to the multiversity of meanings found in the skin. It can mean bare, open, and uncovered; as a noun it can mean "discovery." See *Oxford Dictionaries*, s.v. "découvert," accessed May 11, 2017, 0-premium-oxforddictionaries-com.ignacio.usfca.edu/us/translate/french-english/decouvert.

2. Jablonski defines skin as "the body's interface with the physical, chemical, and biological environment." Nina G. Jablonski, *Living Color: The Biological*

and Social Meaning of Skin Color (Berkeley: University of California Press, 2012), 26.

3. Peter Sloterdijk, *Bubbles: Spheres Volume I: Microspherology*, trans. W. Hoban (South Pasadena: Semiotext(e), 2011), 27. The full quote reads: "an inquiry into our location is more productive than ever, as it examines the place that humans create in order to have somewhere they can appear as those who they are."

4. Sloterdijk's full quote is the following: "Bourgeois-individualist positivism established—against weak resistance from exponents of soul-partnership Romanticism—the radical, imaginary solitary confinement of individuals in the womb, the cot and their own skin throughout society" (Sloterdijk, *Bubbles* 384).

5. Cf. Raylene Phillips, "Uninterrupted Skin-to-Skin Contact Immediately after Birth," *Newborn and Infant Nursing Reviews* 13, no. 2 (2013): 67. Phillips reports that there are both short-term and long-term consequences to early skin-to-skin contact. Not only do "normal, term newborns who are placed skin to skin with their mothers immediately after birth make the transition from fetal to newborn life with greater respiratory, temperature, and glucose stability and significantly less crying," but "being skin to skin with mother protects the newborn from the well-documented negative effects of separation, supports optimal brain development and facilitates attachment, which promotes the infant's self-regulation over time." The author argues for revising hospital protocol to allow for uninterrupted skin-to-skin contact immediately after birth for all deliveries. The hour after birth, according to the author, "is a 'sacred' time that should be honored, cherished and protected whenever possible."

6. According to Aristotle, place is "the first motionless boundary of what surrounds" cf. *Physics* IV.4, 212a21.

7. Martin Heidegger, "Bauen Wohnen Denken," in *Vorträge und Aufsätze Vol. II* (Pfullingen: G. Neske, 1954), 28–29 (German); Martin Heidegger, "Building Dwelling Thinking," in *Poetry, Language, Thought*, trans. Albert Hofstadter (New York: Harper and Row, 1971), 154.

8. Dagognet interestingly sums up the impressive quantitative aspects of the skin's weight and size: "First, the surface of the skin would extend over about 2 square meters; it would weigh 3 kilos for an adult who weighs a total of 70 kilos: In itself, it constitutes the most extended organ as much as the heaviest of the body in its entirety. A square centimeter would contain, grosso modo, 3 blood vessels, 10 hairs, 12 nerves, 15 sebaceous glands, 100 sweat glands, 3 million cells." François Dagognet, *La peau découverte* (Le Plessis-Robinson: Synthélabo 1993), 52. Dagognet's focus on these numbers is not so much to convey the quantitative parameter of the skin but the density, complexity, and most of all the *variety* of its components. Serres equally speaks of the skin in terms of its *variables*. Cf. Michel Serres, *The Five Senses: A Philosophy of Mingled Bodies* (London: Continuum, 2008), 62.

9. Dagognet, *La peau découverte*, 12.
10. Dagognet, *La peau découverte*, 12.
11. Dagognet, *La peau découverte*, 12–13.
12. Taking this thought in a more psychoanalytic direction, Anzieu in *The Skin Ego* suggests that, like the skin, the Ego operates with a containment—envelope—principle. Didier Anzieu, *The Skin Ego*, trans. Chris Turner (New Haven, CT: Yale University Press, 1989), 5.
13. Sloterdijk, *Bubbles*, 90.
14. This quote from Walter Mignolo pertains to the need for decolonial thinking to relate to the meaning of the border between itself and its other, but its main message is very effective for reflections upon the skin. The complete quote reads: "Decolonial thinking means to dwell and think in the border (the slash '/' that divides and unites modernity/coloniality); which means in the exteriority. Exteriority is not the outside, but the outside built from the inside in the process of building itself as inside." Walter Mignolo, "Decolonizing Western Epistemology/ Building Decolonial Epistemologies," in *Decolonizing Epistemologies: Latina/o Theology and Philosophy*, ed. Ada María Isasi-Díaz and Eduardo Mendieta (New York: Fordham University Press, 2012), 26. Thanks to Pedro Lange-Churion for directing me to Mignolo's text.
15. Jeffrey Malpas, "Technology, Spatialisation, and Modernity" (lecture, University of San Francisco, November 9, 2016).
16. Jablonski, *Living Color*, 25–26.
17. Jablonski, *Living Color*, 26.
18. Jablonski, *Living Color*, 26.
19. As Jablonski notes, comparable species such as chimpanzees only produce lots of sweat in their armpits and easily suffer heat exhaustion "because they can't dissipate their excess heat by other means. They compensate for this by being less active in the hottest period of the day" (Jablonski, *Living Color* 26).
20. Vulnerable in the sense of being "exposed to abrasion, plant irritants and UVR damage" (Jablonksi, *Living Color* 27).
21. Jablonski, *Living Color*, 27.
22. Nina G. Jablonski, *Skin: A Natural History* (Berkeley: University of California Press, 2006), 14. Provocatively, we could argue, with Dagognet, that we find ourselves most as ourselves—as sapient affective humans—at the *periphery*. He argues, citing Buffon, that the differences between animals and human animals becomes greater "the further away from the center," culminating in difference at the edge, i.e., the skin. Cf. François Dagognet, *Faces, Surfaces, Interfaces* (Paris: Librairie Philosophique J. Vrin, 1982), 65.
23. Jean-Louis Chrétien, *The Call and the Response*, trans. A.A. Davenport (New York: Fordham University Press, 2004), 86.
24. While Casey admits to the mediating nature of the skin, his analysis of skin still remains caught in a quasi-positivist notion, stating that skin *connects*

to place. This is evident in the following quote: "'Skin' is not just the tissue that covers the body; it is the very medium through which the human person, in and through her living body, relates to her surroundings and most notably to place." Edward Casey, "Skin Deep: Bodies Edging into Place," in *Carnal Hermeneutics*, ed. Brian Treanor and Richard Kearney (New York: Fordham University Press, 2015), 170. Casey tries to clarify the analysis of the skin by speaking of different *axes*: with a first axis running from within the body to without ("inner-to-outer vector"). The second axis "moves from outer to outer": from "the without itself, the very surface of the skin moves outward from itself and links up with the surrounding world in the form of the particular locales that make it into a place-world" (171). Casey speaks of "intentional threads" and "bodily histories" and how they reach out to "whatever 'hooks' that places provide—making them the effective *catchment* areas that draw and capture the outgoing ventures of an enskinned body."

25. In *Bubbles*, Sloterdijk writes, "Thus, an inquiry into our location is more productive than ever, as it examines the place that humans create in order to have somewhere they can appear as those who they are. Here, following a venerable tradition, this place bears the name 'sphere.' The sphere is the interior, disclosed, shared realm inhabited by humans—insofar as they succeed in becoming humans . . . Spheres are immune-systematically effective space creations for ecstatic beings that are operated upon by the outside" (27). He also writes that "We have to speak of space because humans are themselves an effect of the space they create." Peter Sloterdijk, "Talking to Myself about the Poetics of Space." *Harvard Design Magazine no. 30: (Sustainability) + Pleasure, Vol. I: Culture and Architecture* (S/S 2009), www.harvarddesignmagazine.org/issues/30/talking-to-myself-about-the-poetics-of-space. In *Neither Sun nor Death*, Sloterdijk articulates this idea of humans as both involved in created space and being affected by it in the following way. Here he addresses specifically the intimate, dyadic sphere: "Relations of proximity are autogenous vases—a bizarre expression which corresponds to a bizarre reality, because it gives us to understand that, here, the content contains itself. A 'dense' Two is an autogenous container of this type. The connected two *is* first in the interior space that it produces itself, and only afterward in the exterior world-position." Peter Sloterdijk with Hans-Jürgen Heinrichs, *Neither Sun nor Death*, trans. S. Corcoran (Los Angeles: Semiotext(e), 2007), 145.

26. As cited earlier, the active lifestyle of hominids implied important changes in "their digestive system, brain, and skin" (Jablonski, *Living Color* 26).

27. Cf. Claudia Benthien, *Skin: On the Cultural Border Between Self and World*, trans. Thomas Dunlap (New York: Columbia University Press, 2002), 7. Also see the entry for ectoderm in the *Encyclopedia Britannica*: "Ectoderm, the outermost of the three germ layers, or masses of cells, which appears early in the development of an animal embryo. In vertebrates, ectoderm subsequently gives rise to hair, skin, nails or hooves, and the lens of the eye; the epithelia (surface, or

lining, tissues) of sense organs, the nasal cavity, the sinuses, the mouth (including tooth enamel), and the anal canal; and nervous tissue, including the pituitary body and chromaffin tissue (clumps of endocrine cells). In adult cnidarians and ctenophores, the body-covering tissue, or epidermis, is occasionally called ectoderm." Cf. *Encyclopedia Britannica*, s.v. "ectoderm," July 20, 1998, www.britannica.com/science/ectoderm.

28. Moreau and Leclerc explore what underlies this embryological differentiation. In their review, they discuss that the development toward epidermal cells is called an "induced fate," whereas that of the embryological development of neural cells is that of a "default state." In the authors' words: "epidermal fate is an induced fate while neural fate is interpreted as a default state of the ectoderm." The material underpinning for this lies in the role of calcium and calcium dependent signaling pathways, that are either activated (in the case of epidermal fate) or inactive (in the case of development toward neural cell formations). Cf. Marc Moreau and Catherine Leclerc, "The Choice Between Epidermal and Neural Fate: A Matter of Calcium," *The International Journal of Developmental Biology* 48, no. 2–3 (February 2004): 75–78 passim, esp. 75.

29. Anzieu, *The Skin Ego*, 8–9.

30. Benthien, *Skin: On the Cultural Border Between Self and World*, 7, refers for this idea to Anzieu's *The Skin Ego*, 66.

31. Benthien, *Skin: On the Cultural Border between Self and World*, 7.

32. Paul Valéry, "L'Ideé Fixe," in *Oeuvres: Collection Bibliothèque de la Pléiade*, vol. 2 (Villeurbanne: Gallimard, 1960), 215–16.

33. Dagognet, much in line with Valéry, polemically positions himself against Vesalius (so-called "anti-Vésalisme") and his turn to inner organs at the expense of the skin (*La peau découverte* 15).

34. Lisa Guenther's book *Solitary Confinement: Social Death and Its Afterlives* starts off with an impressive account of the devastation brought about by solitary confinement: "There are many ways to destroy a person, but one of the simplest and most devastating is through prolonged solitary confinement. Deprived of meaningful human interaction, otherwise healthy prisoners become unhinged. They see things that do not exist, and they fail to see things that do. Their sense of their own bodies—even the fundamental capacity to feel pain and to distinguish their own pain from that of others—erodes to the point where they are no longer sure if they are being harmed or are harming themselves." Lisa Guenther, *Solitary Confinement: Social Death and Its Afterlives* (Minneapolis: University of Minnesota Press, 2013), xi. Guenther argues the practice of solitary confinement produces "an experiment in living death" (3).

35. Dagognet, *La peau découverte*, 54.

36. Dagognet, *La peau découverte*, 54.

37. Dagognet, *La peau découverte*, 54, 64.

38. Dagognet, *La peau découverte*, 60.

39. Dagognet, *La peau découverte*, 63.
40. Dagognet, *La peau découverte*, 65.
41. Dagognet, *La peau découverte*, 65.
42. Dagognet, *La peau découverte*, 12.
43. Sloterdijk, *Bubbles*, 46.
44. Dagognet, *La peau découverte*, 16.
45. Benthien, *Skin: On the Cultural Border Between Self and World*, 7.
46. Speaking to the conundrum of multiplicity, Aristotle first asks whether touch is single or multiple (*DA* II.11, 422b18ff).
47. For instance, for Aristotle, the sense of sight discriminates colors between the contraries of black and white.
48. I.e., hot-cold, dry-moist, hard-soft, *DA* II.11, 422b27–28.
49. Cf. Aristotle, *DA* II,9, 421a20–26, which addresses how the sensitivity of touch is dependent on the softness of skin and flesh (Ronald Polansky, email message to author, September 23, 2016).
50. According to Aristotle, the other senses are "empty" with regard to that which they perceive (for example, for Aristotle, vision is colorless), while touch brings into play its own embodiment (temperature, hardness, etc.). Cf. Ronald Polansky, *Aristotle's "De anima": A Critical Commentary* (Cambridge, UK: Cambridge University Press, 2007), 332.
51. Polansky, *Aristotle's "De anima,"* 332.
52. Another passage with a similar message: "the sense [of touch] is like a kind of mean (*mesotētos*) of the opposition that is in the sensibles" (*DA* II.11, 424a2–5; Shiffman trans.).
53. Polansky, *Aristotle's "De anima,"* 333.
54. As Chrétien accurately observes: "The mean that we are is the measure of extremes, discerning extremes and differentiating them: the hot is always hotter than us, the cold what is colder than our flesh, and similarly for the hard and the soft (*DA*, II.11, *Meteorology* IV.4, 382a17–21). What is like us is not perceived; we feel only what exceeds us . . . Here as in ethics, the mean is a form of excellence." See Chrétien, *The Call and the Response*, 99–100.
55. Polansky, *Aristotle's "De anima,"* 334.
56. Chrétien, *The Call and the Response*, 100.
57. And even with an appropriate mean, the sense of touch remains at risk. Aristotle articulates how in the case of the other sense organs, an excess of intensity will only destroy that particular organ, but not the animal itself. In the case of touch though, due to its direct involvement through the flesh, "the excess of tangibles, however, such as hot or cold or hard things, does away with an animal" (*DA* III.13, 435b15–16; Shiffman trans.).
58. Serres, *The Five Senses*, 80.
59. This implies that if touch is based on relation and not on purely static quality, then this disrupts a narrow reading of Aristotle where sensation is always simply *adequatio* between the sense and that which it senses.

60. Cf. Catherine Malabou, *What Should We Do with Our Brain?* Trans. Sebastian Rand (New York: Fordham University Press, 2008), 15.

61. Malabou, *What Should We Do*, 15.

62. Cf. Malabou, *What Should We Do*, 15.

63. Malabou, *What Should We Do*, 77.

64. Malabou, *What Should We Do*, 73: "only in making explosives does life give shape to its own freedom."

65. Cf. Malabou, *What Should We Do*, 71.

66. While Malabou speaks of plastic as the ability "to give shape to its own freedom" (73), I reject the notion of freedom and prefer to speak of plasticity's ways of intervening and reordering the aesthetic habitual practices lived on the skin.

67. Serres, *The Five Senses*, 75.

68. Its supposedly fleeting character will precisely be an issue of contestation to be discussed in the following section of this chapter.

69. We need to be careful here, as not all skin blushes when experiencing shame. However, in all cases it does turn warm. In this regard Aristotle's definition of shame in its description of blushing is biased and not cognizant of how various shades of colored skin experience shame.

70. Aristotle's example has limitations in that the sunburn he here addresses in terms of skin coloring red only appeals to certain shades of skin that turn red through sunburn. Still, given the emphasis here on *temporality* his example holds worthwhile insights.

71. I have examined the complex relationship between so-called fleeting qualitative changes (*pathē*) and longer enduring dispositions (*hexeis*) in Aristotle more closely in my article "Passive Dispositions: On the Relationship Between πάθος and ἕξις in Aristotle," *Ancient Philosophy* 32, no. 2 (Fall 2012), 351–68, passim.

72. In *Oneself as Another*, Paul Ricoeur offers a very thoughtful account of temporal synthesis in relationship to the formation of character, addressing the "dialectic of innovation and sedimentation, underlying the acquisition of a habit, and the equally rich dialectic of otherness and internalization, underlying the process of identification." Paul Ricoeur, *Oneself as Another*, trans. Kathleen Blamey (Chicago: University of Chicago Press, 1992), 122.

73. Serres, *The Five Senses*, 75.

74. Ricoeur argues that there is a "twofold sense of "contraction": "abbreviation and affection." Cf. Ricoeur, *Oneself as Another*, 122. The OED notes, among the many meanings of the term "contraction": "shrinking, shortening, narrowing," "the action of contracting, acquiring, or becoming infected with (a disease, habit, etc.) and "the shortening of a muscle from a morbid cause." Cf. *The OED Online*, s.v. "contraction, n.," accessed May 21, 2018, 0-www.oed.com.ignacio.usfca.edu/view/Entry/40343?redirectedFrom=contraction.

75. Gilles Deleuze, *Difference and Repetition*, trans. Paul Patton (London: Athlone Press, 1994), 75.

76. Daniel Smith, review of *Gilles Deleuze's Philosophy of Time: A Critical Introduction and Guide*, by James Williams, *Notre Dame Philosophical Reviews* (September 2013): 205, ndpr.nd.edu/news/42146-gilles-deleuze-s-philosophy-of-time-a-critical-introduction-and-guide. See James Williams's helpful commentary on time and Deleuze: "the contraction of repetitions is a process that gives rise to the living present. Time unfolds thanks to this present, that is, past and future events meet in it, rather than remaining separate entities with no interdependence." James Williams, *Gilles Deleuze's Philosophy of Time: A Critical Introduction and Guide* (Edinburgh: Edinburgh University Press, 2011), 25.

77. The passive synthesis of the present can be contrasted with what Deleuze calls the synthesis of memory, which is the second passive thesis. Several paradoxes help Deleuze to understand how memory grounds the present. For my work on skin, the most relevant paradox is the paradox of coexistence: "if each past is contemporaneous with the present that it was, then *all* off the past coexists with the new present in relation to which it is now past" (Deleuze, *Difference and Repetition* 82).

78. Deleuze, *Difference and Repetition*, 70.

79. Deleuze, *Difference and Repetition*, 76.

80. Daniel Smith, review of *Gilles Deleuze's Philosophy of Time*. See also Williams, *Gilles Deleuze's Philosophy of Time*, 187n10: "Every determinate thing is a combination of singularities, forming a multiplicity that is changing in multiple ways according to the syntheses of time and led by the work of dark precursors and the eternal return of difference, the eternal return of the new" (Williams, *Gilles Deleuze's Philosophy of Time* 187n10).

81. Serres, *The Five Senses*, 61.

82. Aristotle's idea of memory as the "presence now of something earlier absent" acquires depth and complexity once we realize its synthetic and unique nature as *pathos*. Paul Ricoeur, *Memory, History, Forgetting*, trans. Kathleen Blamey and David Pellauer (Chicago: Chicago University Press, 2004), 27.

83. Michel Serres, *The Five Senses*, 75.

84. Benthien writes of aging of the skin that it shows "the marks of all the torrents that originally formed it" (*Skin: On the Cultural Border Between Self and World* 108). She also discusses how skin both betrays and conceals (110) and of wearing the "same outfit" again and again.

85. Ricoeur, *Oneself as Another*, 16.

86. Ricoeur, *Oneself as Another*, 116.

87. Ricoeur argues, more fully, that "self-constancy over time rests on a complex interplay of sameness and ipseity . . . in this equivocal play, the practical and pathetic aspects are more formidable than the conceptual, epistemic ones" (Ricoeur, *Memory, History, Forgetting* 81). Ricoeur also notes that memory need not be seen as personal only but can be part of a collective memory (94). There is also the importance of the fragility of identity and memory as tied to confronting the other (Ricoeur, *Memory, History, Forgetting* 81).

88. Martin Heidegger, *Being and Time*, trans. J. Macquarrie and E. Robinson. Malden, MO: Blackwell, 1962), § 65, 376, H. 328.

89. Heidegger, *Being and Time*, § 68, 386, H. 336.

90. Heidegger, *Being and Time*, § 65, 376, H. 327.

91. Aristotle in *History of Animals* also speaks of how to diagnostically distinguish older animals (in this case quadrupeds) from younger ones through testing the elasticity of the skin and the permanence of wrinkles: "they draw back the skin from the jaw: if it quickly slips back into place (*tachu epaniēi*), the animal is young; if it stays wrinkled up (*errutidōmenon*) for a long time, it is old" (*HA* VI.25, 578a8ff.).

92. Jablonski describes the difference between what are called *dynamic* and *static* wrinkles: "Every time you move one of your limbs or part of your face, your skin moves, developing temporary creases known as dynamic wrinkles. Slowly, over the years, the skin's ability to physically rebound after being creased lessens, and some of the creases—especially on the highly mobile areas of the face—become permanent, or static, wrinkles" (Jablonski, *Skin: A Natural History* 134–35).

93. Dagognet, *La peau découverte*, 52.

94. Dagognet, *La peau découverte*, 52.

95. Immanuel Kant, *Anthropology from a Pragmatic Point of View*, ed. Hans H. Rudnick, trans. Lyle Dowdell (Carbondale: Southern Illinois University Press, 1996), 69. Barbara Cassin juxtaposes Kant's account of nostalgia as returning to eternal youth with Odysseus, whose nostalgia and return home dismisses the eternity and beauty of Calypso and chooses instead the aging Penelope and thereby "chooses the mortal condition and anchors this condition in a place." Barbara Cassin, *Nostalgia: When Are We Ever at Home?* Trans. Pascale-Anne Brault (New York: Fordham University Press, 2016), 12.

96. Cassin, *Nostalgia*, 12.

97. Cassin, *Nostalgia*, 13.

98. Heidegger, *Being and Time*, § 65, 327, H. 328; 387–88, § 68, 387, H. 338.

99. Heidegger, *Being and Time*, § 68, 387, H. 338.

100. Thomas Sheehan, "Martin Heidegger (1889–1976)," in *Routledge Encyclopedia of Philosophy*. Vol. 4, edited by Edward Craig (London: Routledge, 1998).

101. In many Western cultures, wrinkles are to be prevented or corrected since they indicate deterioration. This cultural imperative mostly affects women. Cf. Jablonski, *Skin: A Natural History*, 135.

102. If only temporarily, since Botox treatments generally last only about three to six months. The effects of Botox are due to a temporary relaxation of the facial muscles that underlie and cause wrinkles. Cf. "Botox injections," Mayo Foundation for Medical Education and Research, accessed May 21, 2018, www.mayoclinic.org/tests-procedures/botox/about/pac-20384658.

103. Martin Heidegger, *Fundamental Concepts of Metaphysics: World, Finitude, Solitude*, trans. William McNeill and Nicholas Walker (Bloomington: Indiana University Press, 1995), § 25, 124. Cf. Martin Heidegger, *Die Grundbegriffe der*

Metaphysik: Welt-Endlichkeit-Einsamkeit. Gesamtausgabe Band 29/30 (Frankfurt am Main: Vittorio Klostermann, 1983), § 25, 186. Heidegger writes of the standing still of time: "entirely present to the situation, we bring our time to a stand." And later on, explaining what it means to be entirely present, Heidegger writes: "this entails that we do not turn to whatever, however, or wherever we have been, it entails that we have forgotten it. Entirely present, we have no time either for what we have perhaps planned for tomorrow or for some other time . . . Entirely present for whatever is happening, we are cut off from our having-been and from our future."

    104. Heidegger, *Being and Time*, § 68, 387, H. 338.

    105. Heidegger, *Being and Time*, § 60, 344, H. 298.

    106. Sloterdijk, *Bubbles*, 48. It is worthwhile to cite the entire passage on the death of a sphere here to clarify Sloterdijk's view on death versus Heidegger's: "What Heidegger called being-toward-death means not so much the individual's long march into a final solitude anticipated with panic-stricken resolve; it is rather the circumstance that all individuals will one day leave the space in which they were allied with other in a current, strong relationship. That is why death ultimately concerns the survivors more than the deceased. Human death thus always has two faces: one that leaves behind a rigid body and one that shows sphere residues—those that are sublated into higher spaces and re-animated and those that, as the waste products of things, fallen out of former spaces of animation, are left lying there. In structural terms, what we call the end of the world is the death of a sphere."

    107. Peter Sloterdijk, *Foams: Spheres Volume III: Plural Spherology*, trans. Wieland Hoban (South Pasadena: Semiotext(e) 2016), 48. Sloterdijk discusses aged foam and how it "embodies the ideal of a co-fragile system in which a maximum of interdependence has been reached" (48).

    108. Sloterdijk, *Foams*, 48.

    109. In "Too Late: Racialized Time and the Closure of the Past," Alia Al-Saji, in her reading of Fanon, focuses on the temporality underlying the racialization of the skin. While my temporal focus is on the frozen present, severed from its past and future, and the consequent lack of temporal synthesis, Al-Saji explores the way racialization reconfigures the past, and creates a "closed, anachronistic past" (1) similarly unable to be synthesized. This closed past, she articulates, is "incapable of development on its own terms and cut off from the creativity that gives rise to an open future" (6–7). The "freedom to improvise" is cut off (9). Thus, even though Al-Saji's project analyzes problematic skin practices through a different temporal emphasis than mine, my and Al-Saji's pathways converge in pointing out that racializing practices produce a lack of access to productive, creative temporal synthesis. Alia Al-Saji, "Too Late: Racialized Time and the Closure of the Past," *Insights: Durham University Institute of Advanced Study* 6, no. 5 (2013). I owe thanks to Martina Ferrari for drawing my attention to this article.

    110. I am aware of the limitations of this example as it speaks only to the specifics of the intersection of cultural, biological, and climatological factors

intersecting in regards to people living near the North Pole. However, since the force of the argument lies in the productive *interaction* of these factors and not on the specifics of the situation itself, this example can be extrapolated to different scenarios as well.

111. Jablonski, *Living Color*, 56.

112. Rosamond Rhodes, Nada Gligorov, and Abraham P. Schwab, *The Human Microbiome: Ethical, Legal and Social Concerns* (Oxford: Oxford University Press, 2013), 2.

113. Rhodes, Gligorov, and Schwab, *The Human Microbiome*, 2.

114. Haraway speaks, for instance, of "bodily webbed mortal earthly being and becoming." Cf. Donna Haraway, *When Species Meet* (Minneapolis: University of Minnesota Press, 2008), 71.

115. Alia Al-Saji argues that "the process by which the veiled Muslim woman is 'othered' in western and colonial perception is double—her racialization being inseparably intertwined with gender"—and that "this othering is a form of racism continuous with the racialization that Fanon has described." Alia Al-Saji, "The Racialization of Muslim Veils: A Philosophical Analysis," *Philosophy and Social Criticism* 36, no. 8 (2010): 883–84.

116. Casey lists these depths as "psychical, organic, cognitive, emotional, linguistic." Cf. Casey, "Skin Deep," 170.

117. Aristotle distinguishes two forms of shame: *aidōs* (discussed in the *Nicomachean Ethics*) and *aischynē* (discussed in the *Rhetoric*). Based on *Rhetoric* II.6, it appears that *aidōs* is only prospective, whereas *aischynē* includes both a retrospective, present and prospective outlook. Alessandra Fussi, "Aristotle on Shame," *Ancient Philosophy* 35, no. 1 (2015): 114.

118. Translation by Hippocrates G. Apostle.

119. See my earlier note that we need to be careful in stating that skin blushes when experiencing shame. This is not the case for all shades of skin color, although it is the case that skin warms up. Thus there is bias in Aristotle's description of blushing. We may wonder: is shame felt differently when it is not (directly) visible? However, since this section discusses dispositional shame, this question is not as relevant since the chapter moves away from merely (temporary, incidental, embodied) phenomena of shame to more pernicious, dispositional forms of feeling shame.

120. Modern science adds and complicates this bodily aspect of emotions. For instance, scientific research has shown that the skin's electrical resistance decreases during emotional arousal. See Seçil Uğur's *Wearing Embodied Emotions: A Practice Based Design Research on Wearable Technology* (Dordrecht: Springer, 2013), 8–9.

121. In *Being and Nothingness*, Sartre underlines the importance of both recognition and appearance before the other for feeling shame: in shame "I recognize that I am as the Other sees me," or, as he also puts it: "shame is shame of oneself before the Other." The look of the Other establishes the person feeling shame into "a new type of being." Shame is not just an issue of individuals, but of systems as

well; Sartre refers for instance to "the educational system which consists in making children ashamed of what they are" and how that makes him, as an educator, co-responsible for it. Jean-Paul Sartre, *Being and Nothingness: An Essay in Phenomenological Ontology*, trans. Hazel E. Barns (New York: The Citadel Press, 1966), 198.

122. Günter H. Seidler, *In Others' Eyes: An Analysis of Shame* (Madison, CT: International Universities Press, 2000).

123. The literature here distinguishes shame carefully from embarrassment, since the latter is regarded as far more incidental to the person whereas shame is "weightier and more connected to the self." Cf. Martha Nussbaum, *Hiding from Humanity: Disgust, Shame, and the Law* (Princeton, NJ: Princeton University Press, 2004), 204. Nussbaum here refers to Taylor.

124. Benthien, *Skin: On the Cultural Border Between Self and World*, 100.

125. Benthien, *Skin: On the Cultural Border Between Self and World*, 99.

126. Bernard Williams, *Shame and Necessity* (Berkeley: University of California Press, 1993), 220. Cf. Fussi, "Aristotle on Shame," 128.

127. Max Scheler, "Über Scham und Schamgefühl," in *Schriften aus dem Nachlaß, Band I: Zur Ethik und Erkenntnislehre*, ed. Maria Scheler (Bern: Francke, 1957), 67, 69; Cf. Anthony Steinbock, *Moral Emotions: Reclaiming the Evidence of the Heart* (Evanston, IL: Northwestern University Press, 2014), 69.

128. Anthony Steinbock, *Moral Emotions*, 72, 76, 77.

129. That dermatological diseases may spark loneliness and depression is well known in medicine. It also features in the popular imagination, such as in the 2016 HBO series *The Night Of*, which focuses on a lawyer whose feet are covered in eczema. The eczema is used to explain his isolated, insecure, vulnerable, and eccentric character. *The Night Of*, directed by Steven Zallain, 2016, HBO. With thanks to Erin Brigham for this reference.

130. Fanon describes how he became "the slave not just of the 'idea' that others have of me but of my own appearance." Frantz Fanon, *Black Skin, White Masks* (New York: Grove Press, 1967), 11.

131. Fanon, *Black Skin, White Masks*, 116.

132. As he finds himself othered through the eyes of a white child, Fanon writes about his own experience: "I subjected myself to an objective examination, I discovered my blackness, my ethnic characteristics; and I was battered down by tom-toms, cannibalism, intellectual deficiency, fetishism, racial defects, slave-ships . . . On that day, completely dislocated, unable to be abroad with the other, the white man, who unmercifully imprisoned me, I took myself far off from my own presence, far indeed, and made myself an object. What else could it be for me but an amputation, an excision, a hemorrhage that spattered my whole body with black blood? But I did not want this revision, this thematization. All I wanted was to be a man among other men" (Fanon, *Black Skin, White Masks* 116).

133. I owe these insights to Anne Mairesse. Personal email message to author, May 2016.

134. Cf. Sloterdijk, *Foams*, 53.

135. Valéry, *Oeuvres*, 824.

136. As Edward Casey pointedly notices, the skin is a very vulnerable place, "vulnerable to exploitation by others—to their unwanted incursion in situations of trauma or torture" (Casey, "Skin Deep" 170). I realize that the racialized suffering I discuss in this chapter is admittedly only one form of suffering that the skin directly incurs, and my account is in that regard inadequate to speak to all forms of suffering born in and through the skin.

137. Achille Mbembe, "Necropolitics," *Public Culture* 15, no. 1 (2003), 40, Mbembe's italics. Mbembe's term of the "living dead," while used within the context of racialized politics, shows resemblance to the term that Guenther uses to define solitary confinement, namely as an "experiment in living death" (Guenther, *Solitary Confinement* 3).

138. The political and cultural factors underlying the valorization of skin color are compounded by global capitalism, which offers consumers products that modify such skin colors, either by acquiring a "healthy" tan or to lighten skin color.

139. Adriaan T. Peperzak, *Trust: Who or What Might Support Us?* (New York: Fordham University Press, 2013), 10.

140. Peperzak, *Trust*, 9.

141. Peperzak writes: "To be a *real* (that is, realized and developed) self, I must let others participate in the unfolding of my life. Their trust in me and my trust in them transforms certain elements of their lives, words, convictions, and actions into elements of my existence. We mutually unite and participate in shared existences and this builds mutual trust" (*Trust* 78).

142. Peperzak, *Trust*, 13.

143. Peperzak, *Trust*, 11.

144. This temporal arc of trust emerges clearly when Peperzak writes: "When we have trust in our society, we ask not only whether—on the basis of what it has already shown—it has functioned rather well, but also whether it will continue to do so, and, if it has deficiencies, whether it will be able to correct these" (58).

145. In *History of Animals*, Aristotle writes that, in preparation for fighting each other, wild boars "deliberately thicken their skin as much as they possibly can by rubbing against trees and by repeatedly wallowing in the mud and then letting themselves dry off" (*HA* VI.18, 571b16). His almost casual remark here has significant depth in the sense of recognizing embodied practices of resistance that anticipate danger and decrease vulnerability.

146. Serres speaks of the "experience of mingled bodies," "tangible riots of color and mitigated multiplicities" (Serres, *The Five Senses* 29).

147. Serres, *The Five Senses*, 34.

148. Serres writes: "the most instructive diseases, the diseases of identity, affect the skin and form tattoos that tragically hide the bright colors of birth and experience. They are calls for help and advertise their misery and weakness; we

must learn to read the writing of the enraged gods on the skin of their victims, as on the pages of an open book. The alphabet of pathology is engraved on parchment" (Serres, *The Five Senses* 52). Serres focuses here on medical pathology, it seems, but one could very well read his quote to speak to cultural racial biases that act similar to medical diseases on the skin in distorting identity and well-being.

149. Heidegger, *Being and Time*, § 60, 344, H. 298.

150. Sloterdijk, *Bubbles*, 341.

151. This term is inspired by the title of Logan's book: William Bryant Logan, *Dirt: The Ecstatic Skin of the Earth* (New York: Riverhead Books, 1995). With thanks to Jason Wirth for drawing my attention to this provocative term.

Chapter 5

1. In his lecture course *Facing Gaia*, Bruno Latour writes that due to scientific discoveries that measure how certain humanly produced toxins affect the earth, we are coming to realize (think and feel) that "the Earth might be rounded by our own action." Bruno Latour, *Facing Gaia: Six Lectures on the Political Theology of Nature*, Gifford Lectures, February 18–28, 2013, 93–94, www.bruno-latour.fr/sites/default/files/downloads/GIFFORD-ASSEMBLED.pdf. This turn to a smaller sphere is in radical distinction to previous eras, as Peter Sloterdijk has also observed. Whereas previous ages emphasized universal and imperialist views of the world in "grand narratives," in the current age multi-perspective foams have taken its place. Cf. Peter Sloterdijk, *Foams: Spheres Volume III: Plural Spherology*, trans. W. Hoban (South Pasadena: Semiotext(e), 2016), 16–25 passim.

2. Cf. René Descartes, *Discourse on Method, Optics, Geometry, and Meteorology* (Indianapolis: Hackett, 2001), vi, 62.

3. Donna Haraway, *Staying with the Trouble: Making Kin in the Chthulucene* (Durham, NC: Duke University Press, 2016), 4.

4. Cf. Joachim Ritter and K. Gründer, eds., *Historisches Wörterbuch der Philosophie*, Bd. 7 (Darmstadt: Wissenschaftliche Buchgesellschaft, 1989), 752, which cites the example of infectious yawning as another natural process of *sym-paschein*.

5. For instance, Aristotle uses the Greek prefix *syn* to emphasize the togetherness of friends in pain (*synalgō*, *syllupō*). Thus, in answer to the question whether we can share someone's pain, Aristotle seems to suggest that close friends and family members *can* in fact do this, which may be due to his conception of friends as second selves (*EN* IX.9, 1169b7, 1170b7). Cf. David Konstan, "Pity, Compassion, and Forgiveness: The Moral Terrain," in *The Politics of Compassion*, eds. Michael Ure and Mervyn Frost (New York: Routledge, 2014), 57–58, on friends participating mutually in events.

6. Further evidence for extending this notion of *syn* to the realm of human emotions may be found in the *Rhetoric*. Aristotle argues there that when someone

very close to us suffers something terrible (*deinos*), we actually suffer the same thing. In fact, this kind of suffering "drives out" (*ekkroustikon*) another form of co-affectivity: pity (*Rhet.* II.8, 1386a22).

7. Cf. Marjolein Oele, "Suffering, Pity and Friendship: an Aristotelian Reading of Book 24 of Homer's *Iliad*," *Electronic Antiquity* 14, no. 1 (November 2010), 58.

8. My own translation, modifying and combining Rhys Roberts's translation (1984) and Joe Sachs's translation (2009).

9. The definition of pity in Aristotle is in remarkable contrast to our own tendency to count pity and compassion among the virtues, as well as the Christian account of virtue, which emphasizes transgression of individuality and the need to be compassionate to those who are in need and less well off than we are. Cf. *Rhetorik*, trans. Franz Günter Sieveke, trans., *Rhetorik*, by Aristotle (München: Wilhelm Fink Verlag, 1980), 245. Our modern positive interpretation of pity is mainly argued for in its association with concepts such as sympathy, compassion, or mercy. Modern interpretations of pity are not solely positive, however. Some interpreters argue that pity may deny the autonomous position of the person pitied, and entails a condescending attitude to the person being pitied: Cf. Stephen Leighton, "On Pity and Its Appropriateness," in *Mitleid: Konkretionen eines strittigen Konzepts*, eds. I.U. Dalferth and A. Hunziker (Tübingen: Mohr Siebeck, 2007), 101. Friedrich Nietzsche's famous critique of pity is that pity multiplies suffering and drains strength from those who pity (*Antichrist* §7).

10. Konstan speaks in this regard of "vulnerability to hardship" ("Pity, Compassion, and Forgiveness" 180). Due to the focus on this "personal fragility," commentators such as Konstan have noted an "egotistic dimension" ("Pity, Compassion, and Forgiveness" 180).

11. This example originates with Herodotus' *Histories* III.14.

12. Judith Butler, *Precarious Life: The Powers of Mourning and Violence* (New York: Verso, 2004), 20. To feel and extend suffering to others, and to regard suffering as a central feature for rethinking the basis of humanity, has been a crucial theme in Butler's work of the last fifteen years. Cf. Judith Butler's works *Antigone's Claim: Kinship Between Life and Death* (New York: Columbia University Press, 2000) and *Precarious Life*. Over against Butler's focus on precarity, vulnerability, and death, Bonnie Honig in *Antigone, Interrupted* (Cambridge, UK: Cambridge University Press, 2013) pleads for a reading of Antigone who "not only resists but also quests for sovereignty, who is oriented to life not primarily to death" (191). Honig's reading of Antigone represents an argumentative position *against* the position of "mortalist humanism" that she identifies with Butler, among others. While Honig sees value in addressing the precarity embodied by Antigone's position, and its implications for grasping the human condition accordingly, she wants to emphasize Antigone's *agonistic* nature, and, with that, "the themes of *thumos*, pleasure and eroticism, not just hunger, loss and death" (193). Honig

refuses "to cede lamentation to the humanists who see in shared suffering a new universalism that might (in place of the previous, now discredited, contender, reason) help them to bypass or overcome some of our most intractable conflicts" (194). For Honig, "lamentation (no less than reason!) is itself an essentially contested and politicized practice" (195).

13. Butler, *Precarious Life*, 24.

14. Butler, *Precarious Life*, 32.

15. Judith Butler, *Notes Toward a Performative Theory of Assembly* (Cambridge, MA: Harvard University Press, 2015), 68–69. She continues that the need for a more generalized struggle against precarity "emerges from a felt sense of precarity, lived as slow death, a damaged sense of time, or unmanageable exposure to arbitrary loss, injury, or destitution—this is a felt sense that is at once singular and plural."

16. Butler, *Precarious Life*, 30, cf. 20.

17. Butler, *Notes Toward a Performative Theory of Assembly*, 130.

18. Nussbaum also extends Aristotle's account of pity, arguing that while Aristotle seems to confine feeling pity to those who have "similar possibilities," for our modern sense of compassion, compassion may cross "the species boundary" so that we feel it for humans and nonhuman animals alike." Martha Nussbaum, "Compassion and Terror," in *The Politics of Compassion*, eds. Michael Ure and Mervyn Frost (New York: Routledge, 2014), 194, 199.

19. Donna Haraway, *When Species Meet* (Minneapolis: University of Minnesota Press, 2008), 72.

20. Haraway, *When Species Meet*, 77.

21. Haraway, *When Species Meet*, 75.

22. If not, the enterprise needs to be brought to a halt (Haraway, *When Species Meet* 72).

23. Weil says, "The suffering all over the world obsesses me and overwhelms me to the point of annihilating me. The only way I can release myself from this obsession, is to take on a large share of danger and hardship myself. That alone can save me from being wasted by sterile grief." *An Encounter with Simone Weil*, directed and written by Julia Haslett. 2010, The Netherlands; 2012, USA, 85 min.

24. Nussbaum discerns an "obvious propensity for self-serving narrowness" within the felt nature of pity, given its tendency to be focused on those close to us, within national boundaries (Nussbaum, "Compassion and Terror" 191); Nussbaum's argument thereby intersects with Butler's argument, which similarly pleads for us to imagine grief outside of national boundaries, and contemplating why certain lives are deemed grievable and others not (Butler, *Precarious Life* 32).

25. Konstan speaks of the issue of "translating compassion into practical and ethical action" (Konstan, "Pity, Compassion, and Forgiveness" 187).

26. Nussbaum pleads in this regard for the extension and education of compassion. Children, she argues, should learn to be "tragic spectators . . . through stories and dramas, they should learn to decode the suffering of others, and this

decoding should deliberately lead them into lives both near and far, including the lives of distant humans and the lives of animals" (Nussbaum, "Compassion and Terror" 203–4).

27. "As way into an alternative space—one of acknowledgement of and respect for the dead." Thom van Dooren, *Flight Ways: Life and Loss at the Edge of Extinction* (New York: Columbia University Press, 2014), 126.

28. Van Dooren, in an email correspondence with Haraway, asks, "how might we actually inhabit a shared space of suffering with them ['critters'], and to what end?" As cited in Haraway, *When Species Meet*, 331n5. Cf. also the question that Butler raises given the differential grievability of different subjects. Cf. Judith Butler "Violence, Mourning, Politics," *Studies in Gender and Sexuality* 4, no. 1 (2003): 20.

29. Van Dooren, *Flight Ways*, 141.

30. Van Dooren, *Flight Ways*, 143.

31. Nussbaum discussed in *Upheavals of Thought* the various critics of compassion, ranging from the early Stoics to Adam Smith. She summarizes their critique, arguing compassion "binds u to our own immediate sphere of life, to what has affected us, to what we see before us or can easily imagine. This means . . . that it distorts the world: for it effaces the equal value and dignity of all human lives, their equal need for resources and for aid in time of suffering." Martha Nussbaum, *Upheavals of Thought: The Intelligence of Emotions* (Cambridge: Cambridge University Press, 2001), 360.

32. For these reasons and others, thinkers such as Nussbaum argue the following: "The insights of an appropriate compassion may be embodied in the structure of just institutions so that we will not need to rely on perfectly compassionate citizens" (Nussbaum, *Upheavals of Thought* 403).

33. Hannah Arendt, *On Revolution* (New York: Penguin, 1990), 86–87.

34. The term "capitalocene" was first coined by Jason Moore. See "Anthropocene, Capitalocene, and the Myth of Industrialization," Part I. World-Ecological Imaginations, jasonwmoore.wordpress.com/2013/05/13/anthropocene-or-capitalocene/. Cf. also Donna Haraway, "Anthropocene, Capitalocene, Plantationocene, Chthulucene: Making Kin," *Environmental Humanities* 6 (2015).

35. Seth Denizen also emphasizes the importance of the nominative process for constructing a new ontology, and does so in conjunction with the topic of bringing about, through rhetoric, the thing "hold in the ozone layer," and the thing "soil" that was previously seen identical to rock. Seth Denizen "Three Holes: In the Geological Present," In *Architecture in the Anthropocene: Encounters Among Design, Deep Time, Science and Philosophy*, ed. Etienne Turpin (Ann Arbor: Open Humanities Press, 2013), 7, 10. dx.doi.org/10.3998/ohp.12527215.0001.001

36. Isabelle Stengers, *In Catastrophic Times: Resisting the Coming Barbarism* (London: Open Humanities Press, 2015), 43.

37. Stengers, *In Catastrophic Times*, 46.

38. Stengers, *In Catastrophic Times*, 43. Stengers describes this intrusion as a reaction to Gaia being offended: "And the response that Gaia risks giving might well be without any measure in relation to what we have done, a bit like a shrugging of the shoulder provoked when one is briefly touched by a midge. Gaia is ticklish and that is why she must be named as a being. We are no longer dealing (only) with a wild and threatening nature, nor with a fragile nature to be protected, nor a nature to be mercilessly exploited. The case is new. Gaia, she who intrudes, asks nothing of us, not even a response to the question she imposes" (*In Catastrophic Times* 46).

39. Stengers, *In Catastrophic Times*, 43.

40. Stengers, *In Catastrophic Times*, 50.

41. Stengers, *In Catastrophic Times*, 50.

42. Stengers, *In Catastrophic Times*, 62.

43. Stengers, *In Catastrophic Times*, 62.

44. Stengers, *In Catastrophic Times*, 77.

45. Stengers, *In Catastrophic Times*, 77. Stengers examines one such narrative, that of the expropriation of "commons."

46. Isabelle Stengers, "Matters of Cosmopolitics: On the Provocations of Gaïa: Isabelle Stengers in Conversation with Heather Davis and Etienne Turpin," in *Architecture in the Anthropocene: Encounters Among Design, Deep Time, Science and Philosophy*, ed. Etienne Turpin, 2013, para. 19. dx.doi.org/10.3998/ohp.12527215.0001.001

47. Stengers's proposition is in that regard different from what Puig de la Bellacasa suggests, namely, following Boum and Hartemink, to put "the living earth" in a central position, "from which are derived the limits within which human societies can develop." María Puig de la Bellacasa, "Encountering Bioinfrastructure: Ecological Struggles and the Sciences of Soil," *Social Epistemology* 28, no. 1 (2014): 31.

48. Stengers, "Matters of Cosmopolitics," para. 23.

49. Stengers, *In Catastrophic Times*, 79–89.

50. Stengers, *In Catastrophic Times*, 89.

51. Cf. Isabelle Stengers, *Cosmopolitics* (Minneapolis: University of Minnesota Press, 2010), 34. For instance, in her account of ecology, Stengers argues that ecology is "not a science of functions," but that populations and their formation and functions need to be seen as products of bricolage: "all we can say of which is that it "works more or less," and not of a calculation whose economy and logic would have to be disclosed."

52. Denizen, "Three Holes: In the Geological Present," 12.

53. Nyle C. Brady and Ray R. Weil, *Elements of the Nature and Properties of Soils*, 3rd Edition (Upper Saddle River: Prentice Hall, 2010), 9.

54. Robert Minard Garrels, *A Textbook of Geology* (New York: Harper and Brothers, 1951), 24.

55. Brady and Weil, *Elements of Nature and Properties of Soils*, 11.

56. The relative proportions of these four components greatly influence the behavior and productivity of soils. In a soil, the four components are mixed in complex patterns. Cf. Brady and Weil, *Elements of Nature and Properties of Soils*, 15.

57. Shiva cites a Danish study, which found in a cubic meter of soil the following: "50,000 small earth worms, 50,000 insects and mites, and 12 million roundworms. A gram of the soil contained 30,000 protozoa, 50,0000 algae, 400,000 fungi, and billions of individual bacteria." Vandana Shiva, *Soil Not Oil: Environmental Justice in a Time of Climate Crisis* (London: Zed Books, 2008), 97.

58. Brady and Weil, *Elements of Nature and Properties of Soils*, 9.

59. Brady and Weil describe this well: "although a handful of soil may at first seem to be a solid thing, it should be noted that only about half the soil volume consists of solid material (mineral and organic); the other half consists of pore spaces filled with air or water" (*Elements of Nature and Properties of Soils* 15).

60. Khan Towhid Osman, *Soils: Principles, Properties and Management* (Dordrecht: Springer, 2013), 56–57.

61. Brady and Weil, *Elements of Nature and Properties of Soils*, 15.

62. Jacques Derrida, *The Animal That Therefore I Am*, trans. Marie-Louise Mallet (New York: Fordham University Press, 2008), 29.

63. Maurice Merleau-Ponty, *Phenomenology of Perception* (London: Routledge Classics, 2002), 18.

64. Derrida, *The Animal That Therefore I Am*, 29.

65. One of the standard definitions of pore, as the OED defines it, is "a minute interstice between particles of matter esp. in soil or rock." "pore, n.1." OED Online. July 2018. Oxford University Press. www.oed.com/view/Entry/147956?rskey=HX-SauL&result=1&isAdvanced=false (accessed November 12, 2018). As for its Greek etymology, OED writes: "ancient Greek πόρος passage, channel in the human body." The full etymology as given by OED is the following: Etymology: < Middle French pore opening in the skin (end of 13th cent. in Old French), interstice in porous matter (c1400 or earlier), duct (1478 or earlier as porre), stoma (1765) and its etymon post-classical Latin porus passage, channel in the human body (4th cent.) < ancient Greek πόρος passage, channel in the human body, pore < the same Indo-European base as fare v.1 Compare Old Occitan por (c1350; Occitan pòre), Catalan porus, (now nonstandard) poro, †por (13th cent.), Spanish poro (c1250), Portuguese poro (14th cent.), Italian poro (a1311)."

66. Henry George Liddell and Robert Scott, *A Greek-English Lexicon* (Oxford: Clarendon Press, 1996), 1450–1. Liddell and Scott articulate four main meanings in the ancient Greek: (1) pathway or passage (through the sea, body, etc.); (2) with the genitive: way or means of achieving, accomplishing, or discovering; (3) journey, voyage; and (4) personified as father of Eros, Poros.

67. Plato, *Symposium*, in *Plato on Love*, ed. C.D.C. Reeve, trans. Alexander Nehamas and Paul Woodruff (Indianapolis: Hackett Publishing, 2006), 203d.

68. Plato, *Symposium*, 203d.
69. Plato, *Symposium*, 203e.
70. Plato, *Symposium*, 202e.
71. Plato, *Symposium*, 203e.
72. Stengers argues: "I make a strong distinction between a 'Latourian us' to be composed, who might possibly become able to 'face' Gaïa—that is, face the difficult task of participating in an entanglement, the ticklish, touchy character which we are just beginning to understand—and the 'us' (moderns, Euro-Americans, Western, whatever) for whom the very idea of this task distastefully intrudes, for those whose hairs stick up when they hear the word Gaïa" ("Matters of Cosmopolitics" para. 19).
73. Daniel C. Fouke, "Humans and the Soil," in *Environmental Ethics* 33, no. 2 (Summer 2011): 150.
74. Rebecca Hill, *The Interval: Relation and Becoming in Irigaray, Aristotle, and Bergson* (New York: Fordham University Press, 2012), 66.
75. Osman, *Soils: Principles, Properties and Management*, 57.
76. Hill, *The Interval*, 72.
77. Brady and Weil, *Elements of Nature and Properties of Soils*, 122.
78. Carlo Petrini, *Slow Food Nation: Why Our Food Should Be Good, Clean, and Fair*, trans. Clara Furlan and Jonathan Hunt (New York: Rizzoli Ex Libris, 2013), 11. Petrini describes his visit to one of the faming families involved in the "Quali Project," a project that reintroduces amaranth in a poor, increasingly desert-like area in Mexico. Petrini seeks to illustrate how emphasis on locally grown, sustainable crops may provide farmers stability based on a local economy while also recuperating their own traditional indigenous cuisine.
79. The Slow Movement website addresses both the cultural need for increased connectivity and the need for slowing down. This is discussed in greater detail at www.slowmovement.com.
80. Cf. *Toronto and Region Conservation Authority*, 2018, www.sustainable-technologies.ca/wp/home/healthy-soils.
81. Osman articulates the advantages and disadvantages of farming practices rather conservatively: "Soil management practices such as tillage, irrigation, fertilizer and manure application, liming, and cropping patterns all have positive and negative impacts on soil structure. Over-tilling, over-irrigation, and mono-cropping damage soil structure" (Osman, *Soils: Principles, Properties and Management* 55).
82. Brady and Weil stipulate how short-term tilling has radically different effects, also with regard to porosity, than long-term tilling. "In the short term, stirring the soil often allows it to dry out faster and also mixes in large quantities of air. . . . In the long term, however, tillage may reduce macroporosity" (*Elements of Nature and Properties of Soils* 207).
83. Vandana Shiva casts the current ecological and food crisis in terms of oil vs. soil: "the industrialized, globalized food system is based on oil; biodiverse,

organic, and local food systems are based on living soil. The industrialized system is based on creating waste and pollution; a living agriculture is based on no waste. The industrialized system is based on monocultures; sustainable systems are based on diversity" (*Soil Not Oil* 104).

84. More farmers are abandoning plowing, allowing for more productive soil. Cf. Erica Goode, "Farmers Put Down the Plow for More Productive Soil," *NY Times*, March 9, 2015, www.nytimes.com/2015/03/10/science/farmers-put-down-the-plow-for-more-productive-soil.html.

85. Sites such as FarmHack cater to sharing such inventions to small-scale farmers. Andrew Revkin provides a good overview of such technologies in "On Smaller Farms, Including Organic Farms, Technology and Tradition Meet," *Dot Earth: New York Times Blog*, December 4, 2014, dotearth.blogs.nytimes.com/2014/12/04/on-smaller-farms-including-organic-farms-technology-and-tradition-meet/?_r=1.

86. Revkin, "On Smaller Farms," para. 10.

87. Revkin, "On Smaller Farms," para. 18.

88. Erica Goode, citing McAlister, in "Farmers Put Down the Plow," para. 29.

89. Isabelle Stengers, *Thinking with Whitehead: A Free and Wild Creation of Concepts*, trans. Michael Chase, foreword by Bruno Latour (Cambridge, MA: Harvard University Press, 2011), 328.

90. Stengers, "Matters of Cosmopolitics," para. 19.

91. As Haraway writes in "Anthropocene, Capitalocene, Plantationocene, Chthulucene," we should seek to keep the anthropocene as a geological time as short as possible: "I think our job is to make the Anthropocene as short/thin as possible and to cultivate with each other in every way imaginable epochs to come that can replenish refuge" (160).

92. Liddell and Scott, *Greek-English Lexicon*, 1991.

93. Haraway continues: "Chthonic ones romp in multicritter humus but have no truck with sky-gazing Homo. Chthonic ones are monsters in the best sense; they demonstrate and perform the material meaningfulness of earth processes and critters" (Haraway, *Staying with the Trouble* 2).

94. Haraway, *Staying with the Trouble*, 2.

95. Haraway, *Staying with the Trouble*, 57. Another example of affinity between my approach and Haraway's can be found in Haraway's allusions to compost. As Haraway's focus on compost shows, she is very much in line with a co-emergence and a sense of re-generative "composting" that allows us to move forward: "The unfinished Chthulucene must collect up the trash of the Anthropocene, the exterminism of the Capitalocene, and chipping and shredding and layering like a mad gardener, make a much hotter compost pile for still possible pasts, presents, and futures."

96. If I were to develop this further, beyond the confines of the current argument, I might suggest the term "soliocene," using the Latin root for soil and ground, *solium*. The use of this Latin variation of soil is intended to direct us

away from its current instantiation and alert us to soil's unexplored past, as well as its possibilities yet to come. The OED provides as etymology for soil: "< Anglo-Norman soil, soyl in sense 2b (1292–1305), apparently representing Latin solium (whence also Old French soil, suel: see soil n.2), taken in the sense of Latin solum (French sol) ground. For Scots forms see also sulye n.," "soil, n.1." *OED Online*. July 2018. Oxford University Press. www.oed.com/view/Entry/183967?rskey=7b-wbDF&result=1&isAdvanced=false (accessed November 12, 2018).

97. This requires, according to Haraway, making "oddkin," if we want to stay with the trouble. For, "we require each other in unexpected collaborations and combinations, in hot compost piles. We become-with each other or not at all" (*Staying with the Trouble* 2). Sahlins writes the following about kinship: "This, then, is what I take a 'kinship system' to be: a manifold of intersubjective participations, which is also to say, a network of mutualities of being." Marshall Sahlins, *What Kinship Is—And Is Not* (Chicago: University of Chicago Press, 2013), 20. Deborah Bird Rose, in *Reports from a Wild Country*, speaks of how, for the aboriginal worldview, "kinship includes the natural world" and extends into land. Deborah Bird Rose, *Reports from a Wild Country: Ethics for Decolonisation* (Sydney, NSW: UNSW Press, 2004), 187.

98. Haraway focuses on *sympoiēsis*, "making with," to indicate "worlding with," and being in company: "Sympoiesis enfolds autopoiesis and generatively unfurls and extends it" (*Staying with the Trouble* 58).

99. Stengers, *In Catastrophic Times*, 24.

100. In "The Body We Care For," Vinciane Despret discusses how in certain animal-human interactions we do not just collaborate, but come to co-constitute each other. Both human and animal become "available to the transformation of their identities." Similarly, I want to argue, we should seek to become available to be transformed by the figure of soil. Cf. Vinciane Despret, "The Body We Care For: Figures of Anthropo-Zoo-Genesis," *Body and Society* 10, no. 2–3 (June 2004): 122.

101. Cf. Jacques Rancière, *Dissensus: On Politics and Aesthetics* (London: Bloomsbury, 2015), 151.

102. While Adriaan T. Peperzak words this mostly in an intersubjective, human context, much can be learned from his emphasis on *participation* as crucial to the phenomenon of trust: "Trust creates a kind of participation between you and me, and this changes my life, including my feeling, working, and thinking, at least in some aspect and to a certain extent" (10). The generation of trust takes time, based as it is on past experiences and with an orientation toward the future: "Trust testifies to our dependence; it implies gratitude for the present result of a cooperative past and hope that things will continue to function well." Adriaan T. Peperzak, *Trust: Who or What Might Support Us?* (New York: Fordham University Press, 2013), 80.

103. Alfred N. Whitehead, *Process and Reality* (New York: The Free Press, 1979), 105–6.

104. Stengers, *Thinking with Whitehead*, 327.
105. Stengers, *Thinking with Whitehead*, 328.
106. Stengers, *Thinking with Whitehead*, 332.
107. Stengers, *Thinking with Whitehead*, 437.
108. Stengers, *Thinking with Whitehead*, 484.
109. Isabelle Stengers, "God's Heart and the Stuff of Life" (presentation at the Fourth European Conference on Artificial Life, 1995), as quoted in Despret, "The Body We Care For," 122.
110. Frieling speaks of the "imperialist regime of standardized time." "Rudolf Frieling on *The Refusal of Time*," January 2017. San Francisco Museum of Modern Art, www.sfmoma.org/essay/rudolf-frieling-refusal-time.
111. Jonathan Crary, *24/7: Late Capitalism and the Ends of Sleep* (New York: Verso, 2014), 29.
112. Crary, *24/7*, 8.
113. Crary, *24/7*, 9.
114. Crary, *24/7*, 19, 33.
115. Bernard Stiegler, "Escaping the Anthropocene," trans. Daniel Ross (lecture, Durham University, Durham, North East England, January 2015), www.academia.edu/12692287/Bernard_Stiegler_Escaping_the_Anthropocene_2015_.
116. Stiegler, "Escaping the Anthropocene," 11. By emphasizing negentropic forces, he criticizes the notion of entropic, i.e., static and closed, systems and favors instead dynamic systems aimed at diversification.
117. Cf. OED entry percolation: "the action of causing a liquid to percolate through a porous body or medium; (Pharmacol. and Biochem.) the process of obtaining an extract by passing successive quantities of a solvent through pulverized plant material until all the soluble material has been extracted; an instance of this." *The OED Online*, s.v. "percolation," accessed March, 2017, www.oed.com/view/Entry/140608?redirectedFrom=percolation#eid.
118. For Stengers, slowing down, "is multi-critter thinking, caring for entanglement, learning the art of paying attention" ("Matters of Cosmopolitics" para. 29).
119. Smudgestudio is one of the artist collectives that seeks to connect us to such a deeper notion of time. See the curatorial statement: "We believe that as works made in response to geologic time become more common, human capacities to design, imagine, and live in relation to deep time will expand." Smudgestudio, accessed April 4, 2017, www.smudgestudio.org/smudge/GeoCity.html.
120. Tejal Shah, *Between the Waves*, dOCUMENTA 13, 2012, video, tejalshah.in/project/between-the-waves-collages/. I owe this reference to the insightful presentation by Amanda Boetzkes at the Annual Meeting of IAEP at the Society for Phenomenology and Existential Philosophy, Salt Lake City, UT, October 2016.
121. Thus, whereas Puig de la Bellacasa pleads for "new affective entanglements with invisible workers of the soil," my argument is broader and more future-oriented in that it aims to use the trope of the soil to imagine new affective

entanglements yet to come. Cf. Puig de la Bellacasa, "Encountering Bioinfrastructure," 35.

122. Zygmunt Bauman has associated the liquidity of modern life with our current precarious and uncertain form of living, to be contrasted with what he calls the "solidity" of previous eras. Zygmunt Bauman, *Liquid Modernity* (Cambridge, UK: Polity Press, 2000).

123. George Meredith, "Ode to the Spirit of Earth in Autumn," in *Modern Love*, last modified March 27, 2016, 11:57, eBooks@Adelaide, ebooks.adelaide.edu.au/m/meredith/george/poems-from-the-volume-entitled-modern-love/chapter 17.html.

124. The OED provides the following etymology: "< Old French *grief*, *gref* (masculine), verbal noun < *grever* to grieve v." The Old French grever means "to burden." "grief, n." *OED Online*. July 2018. Oxford University Press. www.oed.com/view/Entry/81389?rskey=oUUHbU&result=1&isAdvanced=false (accessed November 12, 2018).

125. Gaston Bachelard, *Earth and Reveries of Will: An Essay on the Imagination of Matter*, trans. Kenneth Haltman (Dallas: Dallas Institute of Humanities and Culture, 2002), 24.

126. I am thankful to Johannes Türk for bringing this to my attention. Robert Savage, afterword to *Paradigms for a Metaphorology*, by Hans Blumenberg, trans. Robert Savage (Cornell University Press, 2010), 81, EBSCO Publishing, eBook Collection (EBSCO Host).

127. Bernard Stiegler, "Automatic Society, Londres février 2015," *Journal of Visual Art Practice* 15, no. 2–3 (2016): 192.

128. Cf. Stiegler, "Automatic Society," 199.

129. Stiegler, "Automatic Society," 192–93, esp. 192.

130. Stiegler, "Automatic Society," 192–93, 199.

131. The prototype for the brick is based on a study of the I5SSDO, "a 12-faced space-filler built on the rhombic triacatahedron." Ólafur, Elíasson, Anna Engberg-Pedersen, and Philip Ursprung, *Studio Ólafur Elíasson: An Encyclopedia* (Köln: Taschen, 2016), 335.

132. Elíasson, Engberg-Pedersen, and Ursprung, *Studio Ólafur Elíasson*, 335. For images also see: olafureliasson.net/archive/artwork/WEK100991/soil-quasi-bricks, accessed June 3, 2018.

133. Elíasson, Engberg-Pedersen, and Ursprung, *Studio Ólafur Elíasson*, 334.

134. Elíasson, Engberg-Pedersen, and Ursprung, *Studio Ólafur Elíasson*, 333.

135. Elíasson, Engberg-Pedersen, and Ursprung, *Studio Ólafur Elíasson*, 333.

136. While I do see the danger of the concept of "affective engineering" within atmospheres of oppression as outlined by Andreas Philippopoulos-Mihalopoulos in his article "Withdrawing from atmosphere," I think that the kind of "affective engineering" that I plead for avoids such problems. Given the prominence of porosity in soil, and given the imagination it invokes, the affectivity I plead for

eschews totalitarianism and oppression, and invokes coincidental emergences, solidarity, and innovation. Andreas Philippopoulos-Mihalopoulos, "Withdrawing from Atmosphere: An Ontology of Air Partitioning and Affective Engineering," *Environment and Planning D: Society and Space* 34, no. 1 (2015): 151–52.

137. Bernard Stiegler, *Automatic Society: Volume 1: The Future of Work, The Future of Work*, trans. Daniel Ross (Cambridge, UK: Polity Press, 2016), 207.

138. Jonathan Crary, *Suspensions of Perception: Attention, Spectacle, and Modern Culture* (Cambridge, MA: MIT Press, 2001), 10.

139. Crary, *24/7*, 126.

140. I am thankful to the journal *Environmental Philosophy* and its two anonymous reviewers who provided feedback on an earlier version of this chapter published as "E-Co-Affectivity Beyond the Anthropocene: Rethinking the Role of Soil to Imagine a New 'Us,'" *Environmental Philosophy* 16, no. 2 (Fall 2019): 291–317. I also benefited greatly from the feedback of the participants of the workshop "Exemplary Affect: Rethinking the Roots of Modern Sensibility," organized by Johannes Türk and Hall Bjørnstad at Indiana University, Bloomington (April 2018), and from the comments I received from my presentation on soil at the Annual Meeting of IAEP in Memphis in Fall 2017.

Bibliography

Abram, David. *Becoming Animal: An Earthly Cosmology*. New York: Pantheon Books, 2010.
Adkins, Taylor. *Speculative Heresy* (blog). speculativeheresy.wordpress.com/2008/10/06/translation-chapter-1-of-simondons-psychic-and-collective-individuation.
Agamben, Giorgio. "What is a Destituent Power?" *Environment and Planning D: Society and Space* 32, no. 1 (2014): 65–74.
Ahmed, Sara. "Happy Objects." In *The Affect Theory Reader*, edited by Melissa Gregg and Gregory J. Seigworth, 29-51. Durham, NC: Duke University Press, 2010.
———. *The Promise of Happiness*. Durham, NC: Duke University Press, 2010.
Al-Saji, Alia. "The Racialization of Muslim Veils: A Philosophical Analysis." *Philosophy and Social Criticism* 36, no. 8 (2010): 875–902.
———. "Too Late: Racialized Time and the Closure of the Past." *Insights: Durham University Institute of Advanced Study* 6, no. 5 (2013): 1–13.
Anzieu, Didier. *The Skin Ego*. Translated by Chris Turner. New Haven, CT: Yale University Press, 1989.
Arendt, Hannah. *On Revolution*. New York: Penguin, 1990.
Aristarkhova, Irina. *Hospitality of the Matrix: Philosophy, Biomedicine, and Culture* New York: Columbia University Press, 2012.
Aristophanes. *The Birds*. Translated by W. Arrowsmith. Ann Arbor: University of Michigan Press, 1961.
Aristotle. *Aristotle's Metaphysics*. Translated by Joe Sachs. Santa Fe: Green Lion Press, 2002.
———. *Aristotle's "Physics": A Guided Study*. Translated by Joe Sachs. New Brunswick, NJ: Rutgers University Press, 1998.
———. *Categories and de Interpretatione*. Translated by J. L. Ackrill. Oxford: Clarendon Press, 1993.
———. *De anima*. Translated by W. D. Ross. Oxford: Oxford University Press, 1999.
———. *De anima, Books II and III*. Translated by D. W. Hamlyn. Oxford: Clarendon Press, 2002.

———. *De anima*. Translated by Mark Shiffman. Newburyport, MA: Focus Publishing, 2011.

———. *On the Soul. Parva Naturalia. On Breath*. Translated by W. S. Hett. Cambridge, MA: Harvard University Press, 1986.

———. *On the Soul and On Memory and Recollection*. Translated by Joe Sachs. Santa Fe: Green Lion Press, 2001.

———. *De Caelo*. In: *The Works of Aristotle: Vol. 2*. Oxford: Clarendon Press, 1970.

———. *History of Animals: Books IV–VI*. Translated by A. L. Peck. Cambridge, MA: Harvard University Press, 1970.

———. *History of Animals. Books VII–X*. Translated by D. M. Balme. Cambridge, MA: Harvard University Press, 1991.

———. *The Nicomachean Ethics*. Edited by D.A. Rees with commentary by H. H. Joachim. Oxford: Clarendon Press, 1970.

———. *Nicomachean Ethics*. Translated by Hippocrates G. Apostle. Grinnell: Peripatetic Press, 1984.

———. *Nicomachean Ethics*. Translated, glossary, and introduction by Joe Sachs. Newburyport, MA: Focus Publishing, 2002.

———. *On Coming-to-Be and Passing-Away = "De Generatione et Corruptione."* A revised text with introduction and commentary by Harold H. Joachim. Oxford: Clarendon Press, 1999. First published 1926.

———. *On the Parts of Animals*. Translated with a commentary by J.G. Lennox. Oxford: Clarendon Press, 2001.

———. *Parts of Animals*. Translated by A. L Peck. Cambridge, MA: Harvard University Press, 1937.

———. *Physics*. Edited by W. D. Ross. Oxford: Oxford University Press, 1998.

———. *Physics, Books III and IV*. Translated by E. Hussey. Oxford: Clarendon Press, 1983.

———. *Politics*. Translated with an introduction by C.D.C. Reeve. Indianapolis: Hackett, 1998.

———. *Posterior Analytics*. Translated by Jonathan Barnes. Oxford: Clarendon Press, 2002.

———. *Aristotle: Rhetoric and Plato: Gorgias*. Translated by Joe Sachs. Newburyport, MA: Focus, 2009.

———. *The Rhetoric and the Poetics of Aristotle*. Translated by W. Rhys Roberts. New York: McGraw-Hill, 1954.

———. *The Rhetoric and the Poetics of Aristotle*. Translated by W. Rhys Roberts and Ingram Bywater. New York: The Modern Library, 1984.

———. *Rhetorik*. Translated by Franz Günter Sieveke. München: Wilhelm Fink Verlag, 1980.

Bachelard, Gaston. *Earth and Reveries of Will: An Essay on the Imagination of Matter*. Translated by Kenneth Haltman. Dallas: Dallas Institute of Humanities and Culture, 2002.

Badenes, Maria Luisa, and David H. Byrne. *Fruit Breeding*. New York: Springer, 2012.
Barad, Karen. *Meeting the Universe Halfway: Quantum Physics and the Entanglement of Matter and Meaning*. Durham, NC: Duke University Press, 2007.
Battersby, Christine. *The Phenomenal Woman: Feminist Metaphysics and the Patterns of Identity*. New York: Routledge, 1998.
Bauman, Zygmunt. *Liquid Modernity*. Cambridge, UK: Polity Press, 2000.
Benirschke, Kurt, and Peter Kaufmann. *Pathology of the Human Placenta*. New York: Springer, 2000.
Bentham, Jeremy. *An Introduction to the Principles of Morals and Legislation*. Kitchener: Batoche Books, 1999.
Benthien, Claudia. *Skin: On the Cultural Border Between Self and the World*. Translated by Thomas Dunlap. New York: Columbia University Press, 2002.
Benveniste, Émile. *Problems in General Linguistics*. Translated by M. E. Meek. Coral Gables, FL: University of Miami Press, 1971.
Bianchi, Emanuela. *The Feminine Symptom: Aleatory Matter in the Aristotelian Cosmos*. New York: Fordham University Press, 2014.
Bird Rose, Deborah. *Reports from a Wild Country: Ethics for Decolonisation*. Sydney, NSW: UNSW Press, 2004.
Birkhead, Tim. *Bird Sense: What It's Like to Be a Bird*. New York: Walker and Company, 2012.
Blumenberg, Hans. *Paradigms for a Metaphorology*. Translated by Robert Savage. Cornell University Press, 2010. EBSCO Publishing, eBook Collection (EBSCO Host).
Bonitz, Hermann. *Index Aristotelicus*. Darmstadt: Wissenschaftliche Buchgesellschaft, 1955. First published 1870.
Bowen, J. M., L. Chamley, M. D. Mitchell, and J. A. Keelan. "Cytokines of the Placenta and Extra-Placental Membranes: Biosynthesis, Secretion and Roles in Establishment of Pregnancy in Women." *Placenta* 23 no. 4 (April 2002): 239–56.
Braidotti, Rosi. *The Posthuman*. Oxford: Polity Press, 2012.
Brady, Nyle C., and Ray R. Weil. *Elements of the Nature and Properties of Soils*. 3rd Edition. Upper Saddle River: Prentice Hall, 2010.
Brogan, Walter. *Heidegger and Aristotle: The Twofoldness of Being*. Albany: State University of New York Press, 2005.
Butler, Judith. *Antigone's Claim: Kinship Between Life and Death*. New York: Columbia University Press, 2000.
———. *Bodies That Matter: On the Discursive Limits of "Sex."* New York: Routledge, 1993.
———. *Notes Toward a Performative Theory of Assembly*. Cambridge, MA: Harvard University Press, 2015.
———. *Precarious Life: The Powers of Mourning and Violence*. New York: Verso, 2006.

———. "Violence, Mourning, Politics." *Studies in Gender and Sexuality* 4, no. 1 (2003): 9–37.

Butler, Shane, and Alex Purves, eds. *Synaesthesia and the Ancient Senses*. Durham, NC: Acumen, 2013.

Buyon, Jill P. "The Effects of Pregnancy on Autoimmune Diseases." *Journal of Leukocyte Biology* 63, no. 3 (March 1998): 281–87.

Casey, Edward. *Getting Back into Place: Toward a Renewed Understanding of the Place-World*. Bloomington: Indiana University Press, 2010.

———. "Skin Deep: Bodies Edging into Place." In *Carnal Hermeneutics*, edited by Brian Treanor and Richard Kearney, 159–72. New York: Fordham University Press, 2015.

Cassin, Barbara. *Nostalgia: When Are We Ever at Home?* Translated by Pascale-Anne Brault. New York: Fordham University Press, 2016.

Chamovitz, Daniel. *What a Plant Knows: A Field Guide to the Senses*. New York: Scientific American/Farrar, Straus and Giroux, 2012.

Chan, William F. N., Cécile Gurnot, Thomas J. Montine, Joshua A. Sonnen, Katherine A. Guthrie, J. Lee Nelson. "Male Microchimerism in the Human Female Brain." *PLoS ONE* 7, no. 9 (2012): e45592. doi.org/10.1371/journal.pone.0045592

Chatterjee, S. *The Rise of Birds: 225 Million Years of Evolution*. Baltimore: Johns Hopkins University Press, 2015.

Chrétien, Jean-Louis. *The Call and the Response*. Translated by A. A. Davenport. New York: Fordham University Press, 2004.

———. *L'Appel et La Réponse*. Paris: Les Éditions de Minuit, 1992.

Clough, Patricia Ticineto. "Introduction." In *The Affective Turn: Theorizing the Social*, edited by Patricia Ticineto Clough with Jean Halley. Durham, NC: Duke University Press, 2007.

———. "The Affective Turn: Political Economy, Biomedia, and Bodies." In *The Affect Theory Reader*, edited by Melissa Gregg and Gregory J. Seigworth, 206–22. Durham, NC: Duke University Press, 2010.

Cohen, Ed. *A Body Worth Defending: Immunity, Biopolitics, and the Apotheosis of the Modern Body*. Durham, NC: Duke University Press, 2010.

Coues, Elliot. *Handbook of Field and General Ornithology: A Manual of the Structure and Classification of Birds*. London: Macmillan, 1890. doi.org/10.5962/bhl.title.57696

Crary, Jonathan. *24/7: Late Capitalism and the Ends of Sleep*. New York: Verso, 2014.

———. *Suspensions of Perception: Attention, Spectacle, and Modern Culture*. Cambridge, MA: MIT Press, 2001.

Csobot, Daniel, dir. "Plants' Stunning Lifecycle Captured in Macro Time-Lapse." *Huffpost*, July 23, 2013. www.huffingtonpost.com/2013/07/23/plant-time-lapse_n_3582027.html.

Dagognet, François. *Faces, Surfaces, Interfaces*. Paris: Librairie Philosophique J. Vrin, 1982.

---. *La peau découverte*. Le Plessis-Robinson: Synthélabo, 1993.
Davey, Nicholas. "The Hermeneutics of Seeing." In *Interpreting Visual Culture: Explorations in the Hermeneutics of the Visual*, edited by Ian Heywood and Barry Sandywell, 3–29. New York: Routledge, 1999.
Dawson, Russell D., Gary R. Bortolotti, and Gillian L. Murza. "Sex-Dependent Frequency and Consequences of Natural Handicaps in American Kestrels." *Journal of Avian Biology* 32 (2001): 351–57.
Deleuze, Gilles. *Difference and Repetition*. Translated by Paul Patton. London: Athlone Press, 1994.
---. "How Do We Recognize Structuralism?" In *Desert Islands and Other Texts*. Edited by David Lapoujade. Translated by Michael Taormina. New York: Semiotext(e), 2004.
Dell'Amore, Christine. "7 Species Hit Hard by Climate Change—Including One That's Already Extinct." *National Geographic*. April 2, 2014. news.nationalgeographic.com/news/2014/03/140331-global-warming-climate-change-ipcc-animals-science-environment.
Denizen, Seth. "Three Holes: In the Geological Present." In *Architecture in the Anthropocene: Encounters Among Design, Deep Time, Science and Philosophy*. Edited by Etienne Turpin. Ann Arbor, MI: Open Humanities Press, 2013. dx.doi.org/10.3998/ohp.12527215.0001.001
Derrida, Jacques. *Margins of Philosophy*. Translated by A. Bass. Chicago: University of Chicago Press, 1982.
---. *On Touching—Jean-Luc Nancy*. Translated by C. Irizarry. Stanford, CA: Stanford University Press, 2005.
---. *The Animal That Therefore I Am*. Translated by Marie-Louise Mallet. New York: Fordham University Press, 2008.
Descartes, René. *Discourse on Method, Optics, Geometry, and Meteorology*. Indianapolis: Hackett, 2001.
Despret, Vinciane. "The Body We Care For: Figures of Anthropo-Zoo-Genesis." *Body and Society* 10, no. 2–3 (June 2004): 111–34.
Douglas, Norman. *Birds and Beasts of the Greek Anthology*. Project Gutenberg Australia. April 2003, last modified March 2009. gutenberg.net.au/ebooks03/0300611h.html.
DuBois, Page. *Sowing the Body: Psychoanalysis and Ancient Representations of Women*. Chicago: University of Chicago Press, 1991.
Eberhard, Philippe. *The Middle Voice in Gadamer's Hermeneutics: A Basic Interpretation with Some Theological Implications*. Tübingen: Mohr Siebeck, 2004.
Elberfeld, Rolf. "The Middle Voice of Emptiness: Nishida and Nishitani." In *Japanese and Continental Philosophy: Conversations with the Kyoto School*. Edited by B. W. Davis, Brian Schroeder, and J. M. Wirth, 269–85. Bloomington: Indiana University Press, 2011.

Elíasson, Ólafur, Anna Engberg-Pedersen, and Philip Ursprung. *Studio Ólafur Elíasson: An Encyclopedia*. Köln: Taschen, 2016.
Erhun, Kula. *Economics of Natural Resources and the Environment*. London: Chapman and Hall, 1993.
Erritzøe, Johannes. "Fault Bars—A Review." www.birdresearch.dk/unilang/fault-bars/Faultbar5.pdf.
Esposito, Roberto. *Bios: Biopolitics and Philosophy*. Translated by Timothy Campbell. Minneapolis: University of Minnesota Press, 2008.
———. *Immunitas: The Protection and Negation of Life*. Translated by Zakiya Hanafi. Cambridge, UK: Polity, 2011.
Fanon, Frantz. *Black Skin, White Masks*. New York: Grove Press, 1967.
Forsman, Eric D., and Howard Wight. "Allopreening in Owls: What Are Its Functions?" *The Auk* 96, no. 3 (July–September 1979): 525–31.
Fouke, Daniel C. "Humans and the Soil." *Environmental Ethics* 33, no. 2 (Summer 2011): 147–61.
Frieling, Rudolf. "Rudolf Frieling on *The Refusal of Time*." January 2017. San Francisco Museum of Modern Art. www.sfmoma.org/essay/rudolf-frieling-refusal-time.
Fussi, Alessandra. "Aristotle on Shame." *Ancient Philosophy* 35, no. 1 (2015): 113–35.
Gadamer, Hans-Georg. *Hermeneutik I: Wahrheit und Methode*. Tübingen: J.C.B. Mohr (P. Siebeck), 1990.
———. *Truth and Method*. Translation revised by Joel Weinsheimer and Donald G. Marshall. New York: Continuum, 2003.
Gammill, Hilary S., Kristina M. Adams Waldorf, Tessa M. Aydelotte, Joëlle Lucas, Wendy M. Leisenring, Nathalie C. Lambert, and J. Lee Nelson. "Pregnancy, Microchimerism, and the Maternal Grandmother." *PLoS One* 6, no. 8 (2011): e24101. doi.org/10.1371/journal.pone.0024101
Garner, R. J. *The Grafter's Handbook*. White River Junction, VT: Chelsea Green, 2013.
Gayed, M., and C. Gordon. "Pregnancy and Rheumatic Diseases." *Rheumatology* 46, no. 11 (2007): 1634–40.
Goode, Erica. "Farmers Put Down the Plow for More Productive Soil." *New York Times*. March 9, 2015. www.nytimes.com/2015/03/10/science/farmers-put-down-the-plow-for-more-productive-soil.html.
Gregg, Melissa, and Gregory J. Seigworth, eds. *The Affect Theory Reader*. Durham, NC: Duke University Press, 2010.
Grene, Marjorie. "Positionality in the Philosophy of Helmuth Plessner." *Review of Metaphysics* 20 (1966): 250–77.
Grosz, Elizabeth. *Becoming Undone: Darwinian Reflections on Life, Politics, and Art*. Durham, NC: Duke University Press, 2011.

———. *Chaos, Territory, Art: Deleuze and the Framing of the Earth.* New York: Columbia University Press, 2008.
———. "Deleuze, Ruyer and Becoming-Brain: The Music of Life's Temporality." *Parrhesia* 15 (2012): 1–13.
———. "Thinking the New: Of Futures Yet Unthought." In *Becomings: Explorations in Time, Memory, and Futures*, edited by Elizabeth Grosz, 15–28. Ithaca, NY: Cornell University Press, 1999.
———. *Volatile Bodies: Toward a Corporeal Feminism.* Bloomington: Indiana University Press, 1997.
Guenther, Lisa. *Solitary Confinement: Social Death and Its Afterlives.* Minneapolis: University of Minnesota Press, 2013.
Haar, Michel. *The Song of the Earth: Heidegger and the Grounds of the History of Being.* Translated by Reginald Lilly and with a foreword by John Sallis. Bloomington: Indiana University Press, 1993.
Hallé, Francis. *In Praise of Plants.* Translated and with a foreword by David Lee. Portland, OR: Timber Press, 2002.
Hanson, Thor. *Feathers: The Evolution of a Natural Miracle.* New York: Basic Books, 2011.
Haraway, Donna. "Anthropocene, Capitalocene, Plantationocene, Chthulucene: Making Kin." *Environmental Humanities* 6 (2015): 159–65.
———. *Simians, Cyborgs and Women: The Reinvention of Nature.* New York: Routledge, 1990.
———. *Staying with the Trouble: Making Kin in the Chthulucene.* Durham, NC: Duke University Press, 2016.
———. *When Species Meet.* Minneapolis: University of Minnesota Press, 2008.
Hardt, Michael. "Foreword: What Affects Are Good For." In *The Affective Turn: Theorizing the Social.* Edited by Patricia Ticineto Clough with Jean Halley. Durham, NC: Duke University Press, 2007.
Hart, James. *The Person and the Common Life: Studies in a Husserlian Social Ethics.* Dordrecht: Kluwer, 1992.
Haslet, Julia, writer and director. *An Encounter with Simone Weil.* Documentary, 2010, The Netherlands; 2012, USA, 85 min.
Heidegger, Martin. "Art and Space." *Man and World* 6, no. 1 (1973): 3–8.
———. *Basic Concepts of Ancient Philosophy.* Translated by R. Rojcewicz. Bloomington: Indiana University Press, 2008.
———. *Basic Concepts of Aristotelian Philosophy.* Translated by Robert D. Metcalf and Mark B. Tanzer. Bloomington: Indiana University Press, 2009.
———. *Grundbegriffe der aristotelischen Philosophie.* Frankfurt am Main: V. Klostermann, 2002.
———. *Being and Time.* Translated by J. Macquarrie and E. Robinson. Malden, UK: Blackwell, 1962.

———. "Building Dwelling Thinking." In *Poetry, Language, Thought*. Translated by Albert Hofstadter. New York: Harper and Row, 1971.
———. "Bauen Wohnen Denken." In *Vorträge und Aufsätze* Vol. II, pp. 19–36. Pfullingen: G. Neske, 1954.
———. *Fundamental Concepts of Metaphysics*: World, Finitude, Solitude. Translated by William McNeill and Nicholas Walker. Bloomington: Indiana University Press, 1995.
———. *Die Grundbegriffe der Metaphysik: Welt-Endlichkeit-Einsamkeit. Gesamtausgabe Band 29/30*. Frankfurt am Main: Vittorio Klostermann, 1983.
———. "The Origin of the Work of Art." In *Basic Writings: from "Being and Time" (1927) to "The Task of Thinking" (1964)*. Translated and edited by David Farrell Krell. New York: Harper Perennial Modern Thought, 2008.
Heinrich, Bernd. *One Man's Owl*. Princeton, NJ: Princeton University Press, 1987.
Heller-Roazen, Daniel. *The Inner Touch: Archeology of a Sensation*. Brooklyn, NY: Zone Books, 2007.
Henry, Michel. *Material Phenomenology*. Translated by Scott Davidson. New York: Fordham University Press, 2008.
Herodotus. *Herodotus: The Histories: The Complete Translation, Backgrounds, Commentaries*. Edited by Walter Blanco and Jennifer T. Roberts. Translated by Walter Blanco. New York: W.W. Norton and Company, 2013.
Hill, Rebecca. *The Interval: Relation and Becoming in Irigaray, Aristotle, and Bergson*. New York: Fordham University Press, 2012.
Hodson, Martin J., and John A. Bryant. *Functional Biology of Plants*. Oxford: Wiley-Blackwell, 2012.
Hogan, Linda. *Dwellings: A Spiritual History of the Living World*. New York: Norton, 1995.
Honig, Bonnie. *Antigone, Interrupted*. Cambridge, UK: Cambridge University Press, 2013.
Ireland, Kathleen A. *Visualizing Human Biology*. Hoboken, NJ: Wiley, 2011.
Irigaray, Luce. *An Ethics of Sexual Difference*. Translated by C. Burke and G.C. Gill. Ithaca, NY: Cornell University Press, 1993.
———. *In the Beginning, She Was*. London: Bloomsbury, 2013.
———. *Je, Tu, Nous: Pour une culture de la différence*. Paris: Grasset, 1990.
———. *Je, Tu, Nous: Toward a Culture of Difference*. New York: Routledge, 1993.
———. *Speculum of the Other Woman*. Ithaca, NY: Cornell University Press, 1985.
———. "Toward a Mutual Hospitality." In *Conditions of Hospitality: Ethics, Politics, and Aesthetics on the Threshold of the Possible*, edited by Thomas Claviez, 42–54. New York: Fordham University Press, 2013.
Jablonski, Nina G. *Living Color: The Biological and Social Meaning of Skin Color*. Berkeley: University of California Press, 2012.
———. *Skin: A Natural History*. Berkeley: University of California Press, 2006.
Jovani, Roger, and J. Blas. "Adaptive Allocation of Stress-Induced Deformities on Bird Feathers." *Journal of Evolutionary Biology* 17, no. 2 (2004): 294–301.

Kamper-Jørgensen, Mads, Henrik Hjalgrim, Anne-Marie Nybo Andersen, Vijayakrishna K. Gadi, and Anne Tjønneland. "Male Microchimerism and Survival Among Women." *International Journal of Epidemiology* 43, no. 1 (February 2014): 168–73. doi.org/10.1093/ije/dyt230

Kant, Immanuel. *Anthropology from a Pragmatic Point of View*. Edited by Hans H. Rudnick. Translated by Lyle Dowdell. Carbondale: Southern Illinois University Press, 1996.

Keats, John. "Ode to a Nightingale." Malvern East, VIC: Electio Editions, 2005.

Kemmer, Suzanne. *The Middle Voice*. Amsterdam: John Benjamins Publishing Company, 1993.

Konstan, David. "Pity, Compassion, and Forgiveness: The Moral Terrain." In *The Politics of Compassion*. Edited by Michael Ure and Mervyn Frost, 179–88. New York: Routledge, 2014.

Kosman, Aryeh. *The Activity of Being*. Cambridge, MA: Harvard University Press, 2013.

Lang, Helen. *The Order of Nature in Aristotle's Physics: Place and The Elements* Cambridge, UK: Cambridge University Press, 1998.

Latour, Bruno. *Facing Gaia: Six Lectures on the Political Theology of Nature*. Gifford Lectures. February 18–28, 2013. www.bruno-latour.fr/sites/default/files/downloads/GIFFORD-ASSEMBLED.pdf

Leighton, Stephen. "On Pity and Its Appropriateness." In *Mitleid: Konkretionen eines strittigen Konzepts*. Edited by I.U. Dalferth and A. Hunziker, 99–118. Tübingen: Mohr Siebeck, 2007.

Lewis, William J., and D.M.E. Alexander. *Grafting and Budding: A Practical Guide for Fruit and Nut Plants and Ornamentals*. Collingwood, VIC: Landlinks Press, 2008.

Liddell, Henry G., Robert Scott, Henry S. Jones, and Roderick McKenzie. *A Greek-English Lexicon*. Oxford: Clarendon Press, 1996.

Llewelyn, John. *The Middle Voice of Ecological Consciousness: A Chiasmic Reading of Responsibility in the Neighborhood of Levinas, Heidegger and Others*. New York: St. Martin's Press, 1991.

Logan, William Bryant. *Dirt: The Ecstatic Skin of the Earth*. New York: Riverhead Books, 1995.

Loke, Y. W. *Life's Vital Link: The Astonishing Role of the Placenta*. Oxford: Oxford University Press, 2013.

Long, Christopher. *Aristotle on the Nature of Truth*. Cambridge, UK: Cambridge University Press, 2011.

Lotz, Christian. *The Art of Gerhard Richter: Hermeneutics, Images, Meaning*. New York: Bloomsbury, 2015.

Luneau, Michel. *Paroles d'arbre: Roman*. Paris: Julliard, 1994.

Malabou, Catherine. "Foreword: After the Flesh." In *Plastic Bodies: Rebuilding Sensation after Phenomenology*, by Tom Sparrow. London: Open Humanities Press, 2014.

---. *What Should We Do with Our Brain?* Translated by Sebastian Rand. New York: Fordham University Press, 2008.

Malek, Antoine, and Nick A. Bersinger. "Immunology of Human Pregnancy: Transfer of Antibodies and Associated Placental Function." *The Placenta: Development, Function and Diseases*, ed. Richard Nicholson, 59–79. Hauppauge: Nova Science Publishers, 2013.

Malpas, Jeffrey. *Heidegger and the Thinking of Place: Explorations in the Topology of Being.* Cambridge, MA: MIT Press, 2012.

---. "Technology, Spatialisation, and Modernity." Lecture at the University of San Francisco. San Francisco, CA. November 9, 2016.

Mancuso, Stefano, and Alessandra Viola. *Brilliant Green: The Surprising History and Science of Plant Intelligence.* Translated by Joan Benham. Washington, DC: Island Press, 2015.

Marcel, Gabriel. *Creative Fidelity.* Translated by Robert Rosthal. New York: Farrar, Straus and Company, 1964.

Marder, Michael. *Plant-Thinking: A Philosophy of Vegetal Life.* New York: Columbia University Press, 2013.

Marder, Michael, and Luce Irigaray. *Through Vegetal Being: Two Philosophical Perspectives.* New York: Columbia University Press, 2016.

Marikawa, Yusuke, and Vernadeth Alarcón. "Establishment of Trophectoderm and Inner Cell Mass Lineages in the Mouse Embryo." *Molecular Reproduction and Development* 76, no. 11 (2009): 1019–32. PubMed Central.

Martone, Robert. "Scientists Discover Children's Cells Living in Mothers' Brains." *Scientific American: Mind.* December 4, 2012. www.scientificamerican.com/article/scientists-discover-childrens-cells-living-in-mothers-brain.

Marzluff, John M., and Tony Angell. *Gifts of the Crow: How Perception, Emotion and Thought Allow Smart Birds to Behave Like Humans.* New York: Free Press, 2012.

---. *In the Company of Crows and Ravens.* New Haven, CT: Yale University Press, 2005.

Massumi, Brian. *Parables for the Virtual.* Durham, NC: Duke University Press, 2002.

Mathiesen, Line, and Lisbeth E. Knudsen. "Placental Transport of Environmental Toxicants." In *The Placenta: Development, Function and Diseases*, edited by Richard Nicholson, 187–216. Hauppauge: Nova Science Publishers, 2013.

Mbembe, Achille. "Necropolitics." *Public Culture* 15, no. 1 (2003): 11–40.

Meillassoux, Quentin. *After Finitude: An Essay on the Necessity of Contingency.* Translated by Ray Brassier. London: Continuum, 2008.

Meredith, George. "Ode to the Spirit of Earth in Autumn." In *Modern Love.* Last modified March 27, 2016, 11:57. eBooks@Adelaide. ebooks.adelaide.edu.au/m/meredith/george/poems-from-the-volume-entitled-modern-love/chapter17.html.

Merleau-Ponty, Maurice. *Phenomenology of Perception*. London: Routledge Classics, 2002.

———. *The Visible and the Invisible*. Edited by Claude Lefort. Translated by Alphonso Lingis. Evanston, IL: Northwestern University Press, 1968.

Mignolo, Walter. "Decolonizing Western Epistemology/Building Decolonial Epistemologies." In *Decolonizing Epistemologies: Latina/o Theology and Philosophy*, edited by Ada María Isasi-Díaz and Eduardo Mendieta, 19–43. New York: Fordham University Press, 2012.

Minard Garrels, Robert. *A Textbook of Geology*. New York: Harper and Brothers, 1951.

Møller, A. P., Johannes Erritzøe, and J. Nielsen. "Frequency of Fault Bars in Feathers of Birds and Susceptibility to Predation." *Biological Journal of the Linnean Society* 97, no. 2 (May 2009): 334–45.

———. "Viability Cost of Male Tail Ornaments in a Swallow." *Nature* 339 (1989): 132–35.

Moore, Jason W. "Anthropocene, Capitalocene, and the Myth of Industrialization, Part I." In *World-Ecological Imaginations*. May 13, 2013. jasonwmoore.wordpress.com/2013/05/13/anthropocene-or-capitalocene/.

Moreau, Marc, and Catherine Leclerc. "The Choice Between Epidermal and Neural Fate: A Matter of Calcium." *The International Journal of Developmental Biology* 48, no. 2–3 (February 2004): 75–84.

Mugerauer, Robert. "Topos Unbound: From Place to Opening and Back." In *Hermeneutics, Place, and Space*, edited by Bruce Janz, 143–56. New York: Springer, 2017.

Murphy, Mary E., Brian T. Miller, and James R. King. "A Structural Comparison of Fault Bars with Feather Defects Known to Be Nutritionally Induced." *Canadian Journal of Zoology* 67, no. 5 (1989): 1311–1317.

Nealon, Jeffrey T. *Plant Theory: Biopower and Vegetable Life*. Stanford, CA: Stanford University Press, 2015.

Neimanis, Astrida. *Bodies of Water: Posthuman Feminist Phenomenology*. London: Bloomsbury Academic, 2017.

———. "Thinking with Matter, Rethinking Irigaray: A 'Liquid Ground' for a Planetary Feminism." In *Feminist Philosophies of Life*, edited by Hasana Sharp and Chloe Taylor, 42–65. Montreal-Kingston: McGill-Queen's University Press, 2016.

Nelson, J. Lee. "The Otherness of Self: Microchimerism in Health and Disease." *Trends in Immunology* 33, no. 8 (August 2012): 421–27.

Nelson, Maggie. *The Argonauts*. Minneapolis: Graywolf Press, 2016.

Nietzsche, Friedrich. *The Anti-Christ, Ecce Homo, Twilight of the Idols, and Other Writings*. Edited by Aaron Ridley and Judith Norman. Cambridge, UK: Cambridge University Press, 2010.

Nussbaum, Martha. "Compassion and Terror." In *The Politics of Compassion*, edited by Michael Ure and Mervyn Frost, 189–207. New York: Routledge, 2014.
———. *Hiding from Humanity: Disgust, Shame, and the Law*. Princeton, NJ: Princeton University Press, 2004.
———. *Upheavals of Thought: The Intelligence of Emotions*. Cambridge, UK: Cambridge University Press, 2001.
Oele, Marjolein. "Attraction and Repulsion: Understanding Aristotle's *Poiein* and *Paschein*." *Graduate Faculty Philosophy Journal* 33, no. 1 (2012): 85–102.
———. "Heidegger's Reading of Aristotle's Concept of *Pathos*." *Epoché: A Journal for the History of Philosophy* 16, no. 2 (Spring 2012): 389–406.
———. "Passive Dispositions: On the Relationship Between πάθος and ἕξις in Aristotle." *Ancient Philosophy* 32, no. 2 (Fall 2012): 351–68.
———. "Suffering, Pity and Friendship: an Aristotelian Reading of Book 24 of Homer's *Iliad*." *Electronic Antiquity* 14, no. 1 (November 2010): 51–65.
Osman, Khan Towhid. *Soils: Principles, Properties and Management*. Dordrecht: Springer, 2013.
Parikka, Jussi. *Insect Media: An Archaeology of Animals and Technology*. Minneapolis: University of Minnesota Press, 2010.
Peperzak, Adriaan T. *Elements of Ethics*. Palo Alto, CA: Stanford University Press, 2004.
———. *Trust: Who or What Might Support Us?* New York: Fordham University Press, 2013.
Peterson, Keith. "Stratification, Dependence, and Nonanthropocentrism: Nicolai Hartmann's Critical Ontology." In *Ontologies of Nature: Continental Perspectives and Environmental Reorientations*, edited by Gerard Kuperus and Marjolein Oele, 159–80. Dordrecht: Springer, 2017.
Petrini, Carlo. *Slow Food Nation: Why Our Food Should Be Good, Clean, and Fair*. Translated by Clara Furlan and Jonathan Hunt. New York: Rizzoli Ex Libris, 2013.
Philippopoulos-Mihalopoulos, Andreas. "Withdrawing from Atmosphere: An Ontology of Air Partitioning and Affective Engineering." *Environment and Planning D: Society and Space* 34, no. 1 (2015): 150–67.
Phillips, Raylene. "Uninterrupted Skin-to-Skin Contact Immediately After Birth." *Newborn and Infant Nursing Reviews* 13, no. 2 (2013): 67–72.
Plato. *Republic*. Translated by J. Sachs. Newburyport, MA: Focus Publishing, 2006.
———. *Symposium*. In *Plato on Love*. Edited by C.D.C. Reeve. Translated by Alexander Nehamas and Paul Woodruff. Indianapolis: Hackett Publishing, 2006.
Plessner, Helmuth. *Die Stufen des Organischen und der Mensch*. Berlin: De Gruyter, 1965.
Polansky, Ronald. *Aristotle's "De anima": A Critical Commentary*. Cambridge, UK: Cambridge University Press, 2007.

Pollan, Michael. Foreword to *Brilliant Green: The Surprising History and Science of Plant Intelligence*, by Stefano Manusco and Alessandra Viola. Translated by Joan Benham. Washington, DC: Island Press, 2015.
Power, Michael L., and Jay Schulkin. *The Evolution of the Human Placenta*. Baltimore: Johns Hopkins University Press, 2012.
Pseudo-Aristotle. *De plantis*. In Aristotle, *Works*. Translated and edited by W.D. Ross. Oxford: Clarendon Press, 1908.
Puig de la Bellacasa, María. "Encountering Bioinfrastructure: Ecological Struggles and the Sciences of Soil." *Social Epistemology* 28 no. 1 (2014): 26–40.
Rancière, Jacques. *Dissensus: On Politics and Aesthetics*. London: Bloomsbury, 2015.
Revkin, Andrew. "On Smaller Farms, Including Organic Farms, Technology and Tradition Meet." *Dot Earth: New York Times Blog*. December 4, 2014. dotearth.blogs.nytimes.com/2014/12/04/on-smaller-farms-including-organic-farms-technology-and-tradition-meet/?_r=1.
Rhodes, Rosamond, Nada Gligorov, and Abraham P. Schwab. *The Human Microbiome: Ethical, Legal and Social Concerns*. Oxford: Oxford University Press, 2013.
Ricoeur, Paul. *Memory, History, Forgetting*. Translated by Kathleen Blamey and David Pellauer. Chicago: Chicago University Press, 2004.
———. *Oneself as Another*. Translated by Kathleen Blamey. Chicago: University of Chicago Press, 1992.
Ritter, Joachim, and K. Gründer, eds. *Historisches Wörterbuch der Philosophie*, Bd. 7. Darmstadt: Wissenschaftliche Buchgesellschaft, 1989.
Royal, Te Ahukaramū Charles. "Papatūānuku—the Land, Whenua—the Placenta." Te Arab, *Encyclopedia of New Zealand*. September 24, 2007. www.teara.govt.nz/en/papatuanuku-the-land/page-4.
Sahlins, Marshall. *What Kinship Is—And Is Not*. Chicago: The University of Chicago Press, 2013.
Salamon, Gayle. *Assuming a Body: Transgender and Rhetorics of Materiality*. New York: Columbia University Press, 2010.
Sallis, John. *Chorology: On Beginning in Plato's "Timaeus."* Bloomington: Indiana University Press, 1999.
———. *Double Truth*. Albany: State University of New York Press, 1995.
Sandilands, Catriona. "Phytopolitics: A Critical Foray into Plant Worlds." Lecture at the Twentieth Annual Meeting of the International Association for Environmental Philosophy. Salt Lake City, UT. October 22, 2016. environmentalphilosophy.files.wordpress.com/2017/10/iaep_progream2016.pdf.
Santoro, Pablo. "From (Public?) Waste to (Private?) Value. The Regulation of Private Cord Blood Banking in Spain." *Science Studies* 22, no. 1 (2009): 3–23.

Sartre, Jean-Paul. *Being and Nothingness: An Essay in Phenomenological Ontology*. Translated by Hazel E. Barns. New York: The Citadel Press, 1966.
Scheler, Max. "Über Scham und Schamgefühl." In *Schriften aus dem Nachlaß, Band I: Zur Ethik und Erkenntnislehre*, edited by Maria Scheler, 63–154. Bern: Francke, 1957.
Schwab, Gail M. "Mother's Body, Father's Tongue: Mediation and the Symbolic Order." In *Engaging with Irigaray: Feminist Philosophy and Modern European Thought*, edited by Carolyn Burke, Naomi Schor, and Margaret Whitford, 351–78. New York: Columbia University Press, 1994.
Scott, Charles. "The Middle Voice in *Being and Time*." In *Phaenomenologica: The Collegium Phaenomenologicum, The First Ten Years*. Vol. 105. Edited by John C. Sallis, Giuseppina Moneta and Jacques Taminiaux, 159–73. Dordrecht: Kluwer, 1988.
———. "The Middle Voice of Metaphysics." *Review of Metaphysics* 42, no. 4 (June 1989): 743–64.
Scott, David. *Gilbert Simondon's "Psychic and Collective Individuation": A Critical Introduction and Guide*. Edinburgh: Edinburgh University Press, 2014.
Scott, David S., and Casey McFarland. *Bird Feathers: A Guide to North American Species*. Mechanicsburg, PA: Stackpole Books, 2010.
Seidler, Günter H. *In Others' Eyes: An Analysis of Shame*. Madison, CT: International Universities Press, 2000.
Serres, Michel. *The Five Senses: A Philosophy of Mingled Bodies*. Translated by Margaret Sankey and Peter Cowley. London: Continuum, 2008.
Shah, Tejal. *Between the Waves*, dOCUMENTA 13, 2012, video. tejalshah.in/project/between-the-waves-collages.
Sharp, Hasana. *Spinoza and the Politics of Renaturalization*. Chicago: The University of Chicago Press, 2011.
Sharp, Hasana, and Cynthia Willett. "Ethical Life after Humanism." In *Feminist Philosophies of Life*. Edited by Hasana Sharp and Chloe Taylor, 67–84. Montreal-Kingston: McGill-Queen's University Press, 2016.
Sheehan, Thomas. "Martin Heidegger (1889–1976)." In *Routledge Encyclopedia of Philosophy*. Vol. 4. Edited by Edward Craig, 307–23. London: Routledge, 1998.
Shiva, Vandana. *Soil Not Oil: Environmental Justice in a Time of Climate Crisis*. London: Zed Books, 2008.
Simondon, Gilbert. *L'individuation psychique et collective*. Paris: Aubier, 2007.
Simondon, Gilbert. "The Genesis of the Individual." In *Incorporations*, edited by Jonathan Crary and Sanford Kwinter, 297–319. New York: Zone Books, 1992.
Sloterdijk, Peter. *Bubbles: Spheres Volume I: Microspherology*. Translated by W. Hoban. South Pasadena, CA: Semiotext(e), 2011.
———. *Eurotaoismus: Zur Kritik der politischen Kinetik*. Frankfurt am Main: Suhrkamp, 1989.
———. *Foams: Spheres Volume III: Plural Spherology*. Translated by W. Hoban. South Pasadena, CA: Semiotext(e), 2016.

———. "Talking to Myself about the Poetics of Space." *Harvard Design Magazine* no. 30: (Sustainability) + Pleasure, Vol. I: Culture and Architecture (S/S 2009) www.harvarddesignmagazine.org/issues/30/talking-to-myself-about-the-poetics-of-space.
Sloterdijk, Peter, with Hans-Jürgen Heinrichs. *Neither Sun nor Death*. Translated by S. Corcoran. Los Angeles: Semiotext(e), 2007.
Smith, Daniel. Review of *Gilles Deleuze's Philosophy of Time: A Critical Introduction and Guide*, by James Williams. *Notre Dame Philosophical Reviews* (September 2013): 205. ndpr.nd.edu/news/42146-gilles-deleuze-s-philosophy-of-time-a-critical-introduction-and-guide.
Sorabji, Richard. "Aristotle on Demarcating the Five Senses." In *The Senses: Classical and Contemporary Philosophical Perspectives*. Edited by F. MacPherson, 64–82. Oxford: Oxford University Press, 2011.
Steinbock, Anthony. *Moral Emotions: Reclaiming the Evidence of the Heart*. Evanston, IL: Northwestern University Press, 2014.
Steiner Goldner, Rebecca. "Touch and Flesh in Aristotle's *De anima*." *Epoché: A Journal for the History of Philosophy* 15, no. 2 (2011): 435–46.
———. "Touch and Flesh in Aristotle's *De anima*." Paper presented at the Annual Meeting of the Ancient Philosophy Society at Michigan State University, East Lansing, Michigan, April 2010.
Stengers, Isabelle. *Cosmopolitics I*. Translated by Robert Bononno. Minneapolis: University of Minnesota Press, 2010.
———. *In Catastrophic Times: Resisting the Common Barbarism*. London: Open Humanities Press, 2015.
———. "Matters of Cosmopolitics: On the Provocations of Gaïa: Isabelle Stengers in conversation with Heather Davis and Etienne Turpin." In *Architecture in the Anthropocene: Encounters Among Design, Deep Time, Science and Philosophy*, edited by Etienne Turpin, 2013. dx.doi.org/10.3998/ohp.12527215.0001.001
———. *Thinking with Whitehead: A Free and Wild Creation of Concepts*. Translated by Michael Chase with a foreword by Bruno Latour. Cambridge, MA: Harvard University Press, 2011.
Stiegler, Bernard. "Automatic Society, Londres février 2015. *Journal of Visual Art Practice* 15, no 2–3 (2016): 192–203.
———. *Automatic Society, Volume 1: The Future of Work*. Translated by Daniel Ross. Cambridge, UK: Polity Press, 2016.
———. "Escaping the Anthropocene." Translated by Daniel Ross. Lecture at Durham University. Durham, North East England. January 2015. www.academia.edu/12692287/Bernard_Stiegler_Escaping_the_Anthropocene_2015_.
———. *States of Shock: Stupidity and Knowledge in the 21st Century*. Translated by Daniel Ross. Cambridge, UK: Polity, 2015.
Straus, Erwin W. *The Primary World of the Senses: A Vindication of Sensory Experience*. New York: Free Press of Glencoe, 1963.

Theophrastus. *Enquiry into Plants Books I–V.* Translated by Arthur Hort. London: G.P. Putnam's Sons, 1916.

Tompkins, Peter, and Christopher Bird. *The Secret Life of Plants; A Fascinating Account of the Physical, Emotional, and Spiritual Relations between Plants and Man.* New York: Harper Perennial, 1989.

Uğur, Seçil. *Wearing Embodied Emotions: A Practice Based Design Research on Wearable Technology.* Dordrecht: Springer, 2013.

Valéry, Paul. "Dialogue with a Tree." In *The Collected Works of Paul Valéry: Dialogues.* Vol. 4. Translated by W. M. Stewart. Princeton, NJ: Princeton University Press, 1971.

———. "L'Ideé Fixe." In *Oeuvres: Collection Bibliothèque de la Pléiade.* Vol. 2. Villeurbanne: Gallimard, 1960.

van Dooren, Thom. *Flight Ways: Life and Loss at the Edge of Extinction.* New York: Columbia University Press, 2014.

van Halteren, Astrid G. S., Peter Sedlmayr, Thomas Kroneis, William J. Burlingham, and J. Lee Nelson. "Meeting Report of the First Symposium on Chimerism." *Chimerism* 4, no. 4 (October–December 2013): 132–35.

Verma, Usha, and Nipun Verma. "An Overview of Development, Function, and Diseases of the Placenta." In *The Placenta: Development, Function and Diseases*, edited by R. Nicholson, 1–30. Hauppauge: Nova Science Publishers, 2013.

Wei, Yulian, and Yucheng Dai. "Ecological Function of Wood-Inhabiting Fungi in Forest Ecosystem." *Chinese Journal of Applied Ecology* 15, no. 10 (2004): 1935–1938.

Whitehead, Alfred North. "Lecture Two: Expression." In *Modes of Thought.* New York: Macmillan, 1938.

———. *Process and Reality.* Corrected edition by D.R. Griffin and D.W. Sherburne. New York: The Free Press, 1979.

Williams, Bernard. *Shame and Necessity.* Berkeley: University of California Press, 1993.

Williams, James. *Gilles Deleuze's Philosophy of Time: A Critical Introduction and Guide.* Edinburgh: Edinburgh University Press, 2011.

Zhang, Jun-Ming, and Jianxiong An. "Cytokines, Inflammation and Pain." *International Anesthesiology Clinics* 45, no. 2 (Spring 2007): 27–37.

Index

Page numbers in *italics* refer to figures.

Abram, David, 63, 189nn41–42
active voice. *See* passive-active bifurcation
affect theory, 11–12, 166n6
affective turn, 7, 11–12
affectivity: concept of, 4–5; concrete tangible interfaces and, 1–3, 7–9, 10, 139–41; locality of, 10, 140. *See also* place; methodology and, 11–15; *pathos* and, 4–5; research questions on, 9–10; science and, 3–4, 14–15; significance of, 5–8. *See also* co-affectivity (*sym-pathēsis*); e-co-affectivity
affirmative deconstruction, 13
Agamben, Giorgio, 21
agency, 22
Ahmed, Sara, 170n34
aisthēsis (sensation): Aristotle on, 27–30, 51–60, 62, 76–77, 167n19; community and, 75–76; as middle-voiced phenomenon, 56; Plato on, 186n7. *See also* bird feathers; human skin; touch
aisthetic synthesis, 116–19
Alarcón, Vernadeth, 196–97n35
alloiōsis (qualitative change), 53–54, 76–77

allopreening, 72–74, *73*, 77
Al-Saji, Alia, 214n109, 215n115
anarchy: placenta and, 104; plants and, 32, 37, 49
Ancient Greek: middle voice in, 21, 22. *See also specific terms*
anthropocene, 10, 149–50
Anzieu, Didier, 114, 207n12
Arendt, Hannah, 148
Argonauts (Nelson), 194n11
Aristarkhova, Irina, 166–67n13
Aristophanes, 61–62
Aristotle: on affections (*pathē*), 120–21; on affectivity, 7, 11, 12–13; on *aisthēsis*, 27–30, 51–60, 62, 76–77, 167n19; on co-affectivity, 142, 143–45; on community (*koinōnia*), 14, 75–76; contemporary questions and, 13; on friendship (*philia*), 75–76; Heidegger and, 12–13, 51–52; on memory, 212n82; on motion, 9–10; on nutrition, 24, 25–30, 31; on *pathos*, 3–4, 167n19; on pity (*eleos*), 144–45, 147–48; on place, 14, 81, 93–95, 96–97, 110; on plants, 31, 33, 35, 36, 37–38; on *poiein* (to act) and *paschein* (to be affected, to be acted upon),

247

Aristotle *(continued)*
  9–10, 25–27, 173–74n17; on shame
  (*aidōs*), 130; on skin, 213n91,
  217n145; on "some this" (*tode ti*),
  2; on touch (*haphē*), 53–56, 59–60,
  65, 74, 116–18, 119, 121
Assuming a Body (Salamon),
  190–91n59
atmosphere, 150
Augenblick (moment of vision),
  124–25
autoimmune diseases, 100, 102
autotrophy (self-feeding), 24–25, 32

Bachelard, Gaston, 162, 198n62
Barad, Karen, 6–7, 168n21
*Basic Concepts of Aristotelian
  Philosophy* (Heidegger), 13, 51–52,
  171n39
Battersby, Christine, 54–55
Bäumel, Sonja, *128*
Becoming Animal (Abram), 63
Becoming Undone (Grosz), 15
Being and Nothingness (Sartre),
  215–16n121
Being and Time (Heidegger), 169n28,
  185n5
Benthien, Claudia, 114, 131
Benveniste, Émile, 20, 21–22, 24
Bergson, Henri, 15
Bianchi, Emanuela, 13, 200n79
biosphere, 150
Bird, Christopher, 172–73n6
bird feathers: allopreening and,
  72–74, *73*, 77; community and, 74,
  75–76; interstitial spaces between,
  64–67, 74, 77; molting and, 67–68;
  plasticity and, 61–63; trauma and,
  68–72, *69*, 74–75, 141; types of, 64,
  65; untouchable *hiatus* and, 60–61,
  66, 74
Bird Sense (Birkhead), 76

Birds (Aristophanes), 61–62
Birkhead, Tim, 73, 75, 76
Black Skin, White Masks (Fanon), 131
Blumenberg, Hans, 162–63
Bodies of Water (Neimanis), 169n29
A Body Worth Defending (Cohen),
  201–202n100
Botox treatments, 125, 126
Bowen, J. M., 195n19
Braidotti, Rosi, 168n22
brain, 113–16
Brassier, Ray, 165–66n5
Brogan, Walter, 171n39
Broin, Valerie, 104, 204–205n138
Bryant, John A., 182n109
Bubbles (Sloterdijk), 86–87, 208n25
Building Dwelling Thinking
  (Heidegger), 93
burial, 139
Butler, Judith, 6, 7, 146
Buyon, Jill P., 202n103

capitalocene. *See* anthropocene
Casey, Edward, 113, 198n62, 217n136
Cassin, Barbara, 124, 213n95
categorical contamination, 9, 13,
  51–55, 76–77, 120–21
Categories (Aristotle), 9–10, 120–21
Chamovitz, Daniel, 173n14, 183n126
Chan, William F. N., 203n116
Chatterjee, Sankar, 189–90n50
chimera, 105. *See also* microchimerism
chōra, 96, 172n5
Chrétien, Jean-Louis: on *aisthēsis*, 58,
  187–88n22; on extremes, 210n54;
  on touch, 60, 66, 74, 112–13,
  185n3
chthulucene, 143, 157
climate change, 38–39
Clough, Patricia Ticineto, 11–12
co-affectivity (*sym-pathēsis*): Aristotle
  on, 142, 143–45; Butler and, 146;

van Dooren and, 147–48; Haraway and, 142, 146–48; soil and, 142–43, 158
Cohen, Ed, 201–202n100
community: *aisthēsis* and, 75–76; Aristotle on, 14, 75–76; birds and, 74, 75–76; co-affectivity and, 143; concept of, 13–14; e-co-affectivity and, 5, 6–7; human skin and, 132–36; plants and, 37, 40–45, *44*, 46; pregnant city and, 82, 84, 85–86, 91, 102–104. See also *polis* (city-state)
compassion: concept of, 148; as co-suffering, 145–48, 161; plants and, 126–27; soil and, 11, 137, 158. See also co-affectivity (*sym-pathēsis*)
Continental Thought, 3–4, 6, 11
contour feathers, 64, 68–72, *69*
Crary, Jonathan, 160

Dagognet, François, 11, 111, 115, 116, 124, 125–26
Darstellung (to present something to someone), 88–91, 104
Darwin, Charles, 15
Dasein, 6, 123–25, 136
dative, 134
De anima (Aristotle): on *aisthēsis*, 52–54, 56–58; Chrétien and, 74; Heidegger on, 171n39; on touch (*haphē*), 116–18, 119
De plantis (Pseudo-Aristotle), 18–19
death: human skin and, 123–24, 126, 133; plants and, 39–42
Deleuze, Gilles, 12, 14–15, 121
Derrida, Jacques, 21, 152, 175n35, 189n37
Descartes, René, 141
Dirt (Logan), 218n151
disease. See illness and disease
Dooren, Thom van, 147–48

Douglas, Norman, 189n39
down feathers, 64
Dubois, Page, 196n27

earth (*Erde*), 2–3, 143
Eberhard, Philippe, 20, 22–23, 24, 176n39
e-co-affectivity: anthropocene and, 10, 149–50; community and, 5, 6–7; concept of, 4–5, 141–43; politics of, 9; soil and, 9, 162–64. See also affectivity; co-affectivity (*sym-pathēsis*)
eco-community, 143
Elberfeld, Rolf, 56, 174–75n25
Elíasson, Ólafur, *163*, 164
emotion. See feeling and emotion
Enquiry into Plants (Theophrastus), 19
epigenetic research, 42–43, 44–45
eros, 159
Eros (Greek God), 152–53
Erritzøe, Johannes, 68–69, 71
Esposito, Roberto, 100
ethics of responsivity, 6–7
evolution theory, 15
"Expanded Self" (Bäumel), *128*

Facing Gaia (Latour), 168n25
Fanon, Frantz, 131
fault bars, 68–72, *69*, 74–75
feeling and emotion: affectivity and, 7; Aristotle on, 144–45; co-suffering and, 145–48, 161; human skin and, 127, 129–32, 136–37; *pathos* and, 4–5; placenta and, 82. See also affective turn
fetal microchimerism, 102–104
filoplumes (thread-feathers), 64–67
finitude: birds and, 76; human skin and, 123–26, 135–36; placenta and, 103–104; plants and, 39–42, *41*
flexibility, 54

Flight Ways (van Dooren), 147–48
fluidity, 54–55, 57, 62–63
Foucault, Michel, 133
friendship (*philia*), 75–76
Fundamental Concepts of Metaphysics (Heidegger), 125

Gadamer, Hans-Georg, 21, 89–91
Gammill, Hilary S., 204n127
Garner, R. J., 43
genitive, 134
Gewissen (conscience), 126
grafting, 43
Grosz, Elizabeth, 14–15, 55, 80–81, 189n38
Guenther, Lisa, 209n34

Haar, Michel, 165n2, 165n4
Habermas, Jürgen, 13
Hallé, Francis: on animals, 177n45, 179n78, 183n118; on death, 183n118; on plants, 20, 40, 173n13, 180n86, 181n103, 183n118
Halteren, Astrid G. S. van, 203n113
Hanson, Thor, 190n58
Haraway, Donna: on categorical deconstruction, 8; on chthulucene, 143, 157; co-affectivity and, 142, 146–48; on microbiome, 128–29; on paying attention, 161; soil and, 11
Hart, James, 166n13
Hartmann, Nicolai, 168n24
Heidegger, Martin: on affectivity, 6, 7; Aristotle and, 12–13, 51–52; Casey and, 198n62; on earth, 2–3, 143; on finitude, 123–26, 135–36; on middle voice, 21; on phenomenology, 169n28; on place, 81, 93, 94, 95, 96, 110
Heller-Roazen, Daniel, 60, 186n7
Henry, Michel, 6–7
heterotrophy, 25

hexis (disposition), 53–54
Hill, Rebecca, 82, 154, 193–94n7
History of Animals (Aristotle), 213n91, 217n145
Hodson, Martin J., 182n109
Hohn, Barbara, 183n126
hospitality, 99–104
human skin: aisthetic synthesis and, 116–19; Botox treatments and, 125, 126; brain and, 113–16; as concrete tangible interface, 2, 7, 136–37; emotional, cultural, and political atmosphere of, 127–36; etymology of skin and, 131; evolution, place and meaning of, 110–13; human *pathos* and, 107–10; place and, 110–13, 117–18; Serres on, 11, 117–18, 121, 206n8, 217n146; temporality and, 119–27, 135–36; trauma and, 141
hydrosphere, 150

illness and disease: human skin and, 131, 133; *pathos* and, 4–5; placenta and, 100, 102–104; plants and, 20, 40, 43–44, 46, 50
Immunitas (Esposito), 100
immunology, 98–100
interface: affectivity and, 1–3, 7–9, 10, 139–41; human skin as, 2, 7, 136–37; placenta as, 2; soil as, 1–3, 8, 9, 153–54, 157–62. *See also specific interfaces*
interstice, 159
interval: Irigaray on, 96–97, 154–55, 193–94n7; placenta as, 82, 98, 193–94n7; soil pores as, 154–55
Ireland, Kathleen A., 176–77n43
Irigaray, Luce: on affectivity, 7; on *chōra*, 96; Hill and, 154, 193–94n7; on interval, 96–97, 154–55, 193–94n7; on middle voice, 21; on

place, 96–98; Plato and, 195–96n27; scientific discoveries and, 14–15; on touch, 59

Jablonski, Nina G., 112, 127, 205–206n2, 213n92
Joachim, Harold H., 180n82, 181–82n105

Kamper-Jørgensen, Mads, 204n132
Kant, Immanuel, 124
Keats, John, 62
Knudsen, Lisbeth E., 193n6
Kosman, Aryeh, 186n12

Lang, Helen, 199n67
Latour, Bruno, 168n25
Leclerc, Catherine, 209n28
Levinas, Emmanuel, 6, 126
Liddell, Henry G., 177n51
limitrophy, 152
lithosphere, 150
Living Color (Jablonski), 112
Llewelyn, John, 175–76n35
Logan, William Bryant, 218n151
Loke, Y. W., 84, 92, 99, 193n1, 201n94&95
loss and mourning: birds and, 76; co-suffering and, 146–48; plants and, 18, 35. *See also* death
Lotz, Christian, 89
Luneau, Michel, 36

Malabou, Catherine, 62–63, 118–19, 133–34, 135
Malpas, Jeffrey, 95–96, 111–12
Mancuso, Stefano: on 'command centers' in plants, 20–21, 32, 36; on emergent properties of plants, 178n66; on photosynthesis, 176n42, 179n69; on plant communication, 173n7, 173n10

Marcel, Gabriel, 101
Marder, Michael, 33–34, 92, 181n101, 182n114
Marikawa, Yusuke, 196–97n35
Marzluff, John M., 73
Massumi, Brian, 12
maternal hospitality, 99–104
Mathiesen, Line, 193n6
Matzinger, Polly, 202n100
Mbembe, Achille, 133
McKeever, Katherine, 67–68
medicine, 3
Meillasoux, Quentin, 165–66n5
memory and memories, 119, 122
Meredith, George, 162
Merleau-Ponty, Maurice, 11, 62, 152, 188n31, 190–91n59
Metaphysics (Aristotle), 167n19, 187n21
methodology, 11–15
microbiome, 128–29, 132
microchimerism, 101–105
middle voice: *aisthēsis* and, 56; as alternative ontology of motion, 10; concept of, 21–24; plant affectivity and, 20–21, 23–25, 45–47, 50; plant growth and, 32–39, *34*; plant nutrition and, 24–25, 30–32; temporal and spatial zones of indeterminacy and, 140; as voice of openness and resilience in plants, 39–45
The Middle Voice of Ecological Consciousness (Llewelyn), 175–76n35
Mignolo, Walter, 207n14
mimesis, 84, 86–91
Møller, A. P., 191n78, 192n81
molting, 67–68
Moreau, Marc, 209n28
mother: definition of, 193n2. *See also* placenta

motion, 9–10
mourning. *See* loss and mourning
Mugerauer, Robert, 93
multigenerational microchimerism, 102, 103–104

Nealon, Jeffrey T., 179–80n81
necropower and necropolitics, 133
Neganthropocene, 160
Neimanis, Astrida, 168n23, 169n28
Neither Sun nor Death (Sloterdijk), 208n25
Nelson, Maggie, 194n11
new materialism, 3–4
Nicomachean Ethics (Aristotle), 75–76, 144, 186n13
Nicotiana attenuata, 19
The Night Of (HBO series), 216n129
nitrogen-fixing bacteria, 43–44, *44*
nutrition: Aristotle on, 25–30, 31; plants and, 24–25, 30–32

"Ode to a Nightingale" (Keats), 62
On Generation and Corruption (Aristotle), 186n14
On Touching (Derrida), 189n37
ontogenesis: affectivity and, 7–8, 11; birds and, 54–55; human skin and, 111, 126–27; placenta and, 84, 89–91; plants and, 18, 24; soil and, 142

Parables for the Virtual (Massumi), 12
partnership, 63
Parts of Animals (Aristotle), 31
paschein (to be affected, to be acted upon): *aisthēsis* and, 52–54; Aristotle on, 9–10, 25–27, 56, 173–74n17; co-affectivity and, 158; *pathos* and, 4–5. See also *aisthēsis* (sensation)
passive-active bifurcation, 9–10, 20–22, 49–51. *See also* middle voice
pathē (affections), 120–21

pathos: affectivity and, 4–5; Aristotle on, 3–4, 167n19; definitions of, 166n9; etymology of, 4; skin and, 133. *See also* affectivity
La peau découverte (Dagognet), 111, 115, 116, 124, 125–26
Peperzak, Adriaan, 134
percolation, 159–60, 161
Peterson, Keith, 168n24
phenomenology, 2–3, 169n28, 169n29. *See also* Heidegger, Martin
Phillips, Raylene, 206n5
photosynthesis, 25
Phylloxera, 43
Physics (Aristotle), 58, 95, 178n58, 186n14
physis (nature), 27, 53–54, 57–58, 81, 91–98
pioneer plants, 42
pity (*eleos*), 144–45, 147–48
place: Aristotle on, 14, 81, 93–95, 96–97, 110; Heidegger on, 81, 93, 94, 95, 96, 110; human skin and, 110–13, 117–18; interstitial spaces between bird feathers and, 64–67, 74, 77; Irigaray on, 96–98; Malpas on, 95–96, 111–12; nutrition and, 29–30; placenta and, 91–98; Plato on, 14
placenta: as boundary, 91–98; in clinical hospital setting, 82–84, *83*; as concrete tangible interface, 2; *Darstellung* and, 88–91, 104; etymology of, 199n66; finitude and, 103–104; hospitality and, 99–104; immunology and, 98–100; inner logic of, 79–82; Loke on, 92, 99, 193n1, 201n94&95; microchimerism and, 101–105; *mimesis* and, 84, 86–91; placement, origin, and function of, 84–85, 197n40; Plato's *polis* and, 85–86, 88, 91, 103–104; Sloterdijk on, 87, 194n13, 195n14,

199n64; temporality and, 103–104
plants: adaptive and responsive strategies of, 19–20; Aristotle on, 31, 33, 35, 36, 37–38; community and, 37, 40–45, *44*, 46; concept of middle voice and, 20–21, 23–25, 45–47, 50; finitude and, 39–42, *41*; growth and middle voice in, 32–39, *34*; middle voice as voice of openness and resilience in, 39–45; nutrition and middle voice in, 24–25, 30–32; paradoxes and contradictions of, 17–19; trauma and, 140–41
plasticity, 61–63, 68, 118–19, 133–34
Plato: on *aisthēsis*, 186n7; on *chōra*, 96; contemporary questions and, 13; on *eros*, 159; on place, 14; on *polis*, 14, 82, 85–86, 88, 91, 103–104; soil and, 152–53
Plessner, Helmuth, 66
poiein (to act), 9–10, 25–27, 173–74n17. See also passive-active bifurcation
Polansky, Ronald: on nutrition and growth, 177n50, 178n60–61, 179n80, 180n85, 181n87, 182n107; on touch, 117
polis (city-state): placenta and, 85–86, 88, 91, 103–104; Plato on, 14, 82, 85–86, 88, 91, 103–104; skin and, 127
Politics (Aristotle), 187n17
Poros (Greek God), 152–53
Posterior Analytics (Aristotle), 187n21
Power, Michael L., 193n3, 197n40
Precarious Life (Butler), 146
preeclampsia, 204n127
pregnancy. See placenta
pregnant city, 82, 84, 85–86, 91, 102–104

The Primary World of the Senses (Straus), 57
The Promise of Happiness (Ahmed), 170n34
Pseudo-Aristotle, 18–19

reflexivity, 23
Republic (Plato), 14, 85–86, 88, 91, 103–104
research questions, 9–10
resilience, 39–40
Rhetoric (Aristotle), 144–45
Rhodes, Rosamond, 128
Ricoeur, Paul, 122–23
Rouch, Hélène, 194n9, 198n54

Salamon, Gayle, 190–91n59
Sallis, John, 14, 198n55, 200n79
Sanskrit, 21, 22
Santoro, Pablo, 194–95n14
Sartre, Jean-Paul, 215–16n121
Scheler, Max, 131
Schulkin, Jay, 193n3, 197n40
science, 3–4, 14–15
Scott, Charles, 23–24, 174n18, 177n51
self-feeding (autotrophy), 24–25, 32
Serres, Michel: on medical pathology, 217n146; on mingled bodies, 217–18n148; on skin, 11, 117–18, 121, 206n8, 217n146
shame (*aidōs*), 130–31
Sharp, Hasana, 12
Sheehan, Thomas, 165n3
Simondon, Gilbert, 24, 172n44
skin. See human skin
Sloterdijk, Peter: on affectivity, 7; on Dasein, 136; on death, 126; on earth and soil, 180n84; on foams, 132, 168–69n25; on place, 208n25; on placenta, 86–87, 194n13, 195n14, 199n64; on skin, 111
slow movement, 155
Smith, Adam, 148

soil: burial and, 1–2, 139; co-affectivity and, 142–43, 158; as concrete tangible interface, 1–3, 8, 9; vs. earth, 2–3; e-co-affectivity and, 9, 162–64; as mediating interface for new "us," 153–54, 157–62; nature of, 150–52, *151–52*; Plato's *Symposium* and, 152–53; as skin of the earth, 137; Sloterdijk on, 180n84; temporality and, 154–57, 160–61; Theophrastus on, 172n5

soil pores, 151–55, *152*, 159, 162

Soil quasi bricks (Elíasson), *163*, 164

soilocene, 157–58

Solitary Confinement (Guenther), 209n34

Sorabji, Richard, 59

Sparrow, Tom, 62–63

spider plants, 35

Spinoza, Baruch, 12

Spinoza and the Politics of Renaturalization (Sharp), 12

Stengers, Isabelle: on interstice, 159; on paying attention, 143, 149–50, 161; soil and, 11; on "us," 157, 169n27

Stiegler, Bernard, 11, 160, 161, 163, 164

Stoics, 148

Straus, Erwin, 57, 63

sym-pathēsis. *See* co-affectivity (*sym-pathēsis*)

sym-poiēsis, 158

Symposium (Plato), 152–53

synaisthanesthai (sensing-together), 75–76

temporality: birds and, 67, 76; human skin and, 119–27, 135–36; nutrition and, 28–29; placenta and, 103–104; soil and, 154–57, 160–61; as synchronic and diachronic, 40–45, 154–55, 161

Theaetetus (Plato), 186n7

Theophrastus, 19

Timaeus (Plato), 196n28

Tompkins, Peter, 172–73n6

topos, 81

touch: allopreening and, 72–74; Aristotle on, 53–56, 59–60, 65, 74, 116–18, 119, 121; Chrétien on, 60, 66, 74, 185n3; Derrida on, 189n37; Irigaray on, 59. *See also aisthēsis* (sensation); bird feathers; human skin

trauma: bird feathers and, 68–72, *69*, 74–75, 141; human skin and, 141; plants and, 45, 140–41

trust, 134–35

Truth and Method (Gadamer), 89–91

24/7 (Crary), 160

Valéry, Paul, 114–15, 132

Verma, Nipun, 201n96

Verma, Usha, 201n96

Viola, Alessandra: on 'command centers' in plants, 20–21, 36; on emergent properties of plants, 178n66; on photosynthesis, 176n42, 179n69; on plant communication, 173n7, 173n10

water hyacinth (*Eichhornia crassipes*), 39

Weil, Simone, 147

When Species Meet (Haraway), 142, 146–48, 161

Whitehead, Alfred North, 35, 159

Willett, Cynthia, 170–71n38

Williams, James, 131, 212n76

www.ingramcontent.com/pod-product-compliance
Ingram Content Group UK Ltd.
Pitfield, Milton Keynes, MK11 3LW, UK
UKHW041917140426
5217IPUK00013B/188